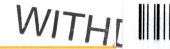
WITHD

D1758083

Intraocular Inflammation and Uveitis

Section 9

2012–2013

(Last major revision 2011–2012)

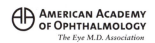

AMERICAN ACADEMY
OF OPHTHALMOLOGY
The Eye M.D. Association

LEO

LIFELONG
EDUCATION FOR THE
OPHTHALMOLOGIST®

The Basic and Clinical Science Course (BCSC) is one component of the Lifelong Education for the Ophthalmologist (LEO) framework, which assists members in planning their continuing medical education. LEO includes an array of clinical education products that members may select to form individualized, self-directed learning plans for updating their clinical knowledge. Active members or fellows who use LEO components may accumulate sufficient CME credits to earn the LEO Award. Contact the Academy's Clinical Education Division for further information on LEO.

The American Academy of Ophthalmology is accredited by the Accreditation Council for Continuing Medical Education to provide continuing medical education for physicians.

The American Academy of Ophthalmology designates this enduring material for a maximum of 10 *AMA PRA Category 1 Credits*™. Physicians should claim only the credit commensurate with the extent of their participation in the activity.

The BCSC is designed to increase the physician's ophthalmic knowledge through study and review. Users of this activity are encouraged to read the text and then answer the study questions provided at the back of the book.

To claim *AMA PRA Category 1 Credits*™ upon completion of this activity, learners must demonstrate appropriate knowledge and participation in the activity by taking the post-test for Section 9 and achieving a score of 80% or higher. For further details, please see the instructions for requesting CME credit at the back of the book.

The Academy provides this material for educational purposes only. It is not intended to represent the only or best method or procedure in every case, nor to replace a physician's own judgment or give specific advice for case management. Including all indications, contraindications, side effects, and alternative agents for each drug or treatment is beyond the scope of this material. All information and recommendations should be verified, prior to use, with current information included in the manufacturers' package inserts or other independent sources, and considered in light of the patient's condition and history. Reference to certain drugs, instruments, and other products in this course is made for illustrative purposes only and is not intended to constitute an endorsement of such. Some material may include information on applications that are not considered community standard, that reflect indications not included in approved FDA labeling, or that are approved for use only in restricted research settings. **The FDA has stated that it is the responsibility of the physician to determine the FDA status of each drug or device he or she wishes to use, and to use them with appropriate, informed patient consent in compliance with applicable law.** The Academy specifically disclaims any and all liability for injury or other damages of any kind, from negligence or otherwise, for any and all claims that may arise from the use of any recommendations or other information contained herein.

Cover image courtesy of E. Mitchel Opremcak, MD.

Basic and Clinical Science Course

Gregory L. Skuta, MD, Oklahoma City, Oklahoma, *Senior Secretary for Clinical Education*

Louis B. Cantor, MD, Indianapolis, Indiana, *Secretary for Ophthalmic Knowledge*

Jayne S. Weiss, MD, New Orleans, Louisiana, *BCSC Course Chair*

Section 9

Faculty Responsible for This Edition

Ramana S. Moorthy, MD, *Chair,* Indianapolis, Indiana
P. Kumar Rao, MD, St Louis, Missouri
Russell W. Read, MD, PhD, Birmingham, Alabama
Russell N. Van Gelder, MD, PhD, Seattle, Washington
Albert T. Vitale, MD, Salt Lake City, Utah
Bahram Bodaghi, MD, PhD, *Consultant,* Paris, France
Carrie M. Parrish, MD, Nashville, Tennessee
  Practicing Ophthalmologists Advisory Committee for Education

The Academy wishes to acknowledge Mary Lou Jackson, MD, *Vision Rehabilitation Committee,* for her review of this edition.

The Academy wishes to acknowledge the American Uveitis Society for recommending faculty members to the BCSC Section 9 committee.

Financial Disclosures

Academy staff members who contributed to the development of this product state that they have no significant financial interest or other relationship with the manufacturer of any commercial product discussed in this course or with the manufacturer of any competing commercial product.

The authors state the following financial relationships:

Dr Bodaghi: Allergan, consultant; Bausch & Lomb Surgical, consultant; Lux Biosciences, grant recipient; Novartis Pharmaceuticals, grant recipient

Dr Rao: National Eye Institute, grant recipient; Genentech, grant recipient

Dr Read: Alcon Laboratories, consultant; EyeSight Foundation of Alabama, grant recipient; GlaxoSmithKline, consultant; International Retinal Research Foundation, grant recipient; Research to Prevent Blindness, grant recipient; Lux Biosciences, consultant

Dr Van Gelder: Alcon Laboratories, consultant, grant recipient; Novartis Pharmaceuticals, consultant; Photoswitch Therapeutics, grant recipient

Dr Vitale: Bausch & Lomb Surgical, consultant; Acient, consultant

The other authors state that they have no significant financial interest or other relationship with the manufacturer of any commercial product discussed in the chapters that they contributed to this course or with the manufacturer of any competing commercial product.

Recent Past Faculty

Janet Davis, MD
C. Stephen Foster, MD
Careen Yen Lowder, MD, PhD
Nalini S. Bora, PhD

In addition, the Academy gratefully acknowledges the contributions of numerous past faculty and advisory committee members who have played an important role in the development of previous editions of the Basic and Clinical Science Course.

American Academy of Ophthalmology Staff

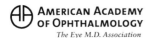

AMERICAN ACADEMY
OF OPHTHALMOLOGY
The Eye M.D. Association

655 Beach Street
Box 7424
San Francisco, CA 94120-7424

Contents

General Introduction

The Basic and Clinical Science Course (BCSC) is designed to meet the needs of residents and practitioners for a comprehensive yet concise curriculum of the field of ophthalmology. The BCSC has developed from its original brief outline format, which relied heavily on outside readings, to a more convenient and educationally useful self-contained text. The Academy updates and revises the course annually, with the goals of integrating the basic science and clinical practice of ophthalmology and of keeping ophthalmologists current with new developments in the various subspecialties.

The BCSC incorporates the effort and expertise of more than 80 ophthalmologists, organized into 13 Section faculties, working with Academy editorial staff. In addition, the course continues to benefit from many lasting contributions made by the faculties of previous editions. Members of the Academy's Practicing Ophthalmologists Advisory Committee for Education serve on each faculty and, as a group, review every volume before and after major revisions.

Organization of the Course

The Basic and Clinical Science Course comprises 13 volumes, incorporating fundamental ophthalmic knowledge, subspecialty areas, and special topics:

1 Update on General Medicine
2 Fundamentals and Principles of Ophthalmology
3 Clinical Optics
4 Ophthalmic Pathology and Intraocular Tumors
5 Neuro-Ophthalmology
6 Pediatric Ophthalmology and Strabismus
7 Orbit, Eyelids, and Lacrimal System
8 External Disease and Cornea
9 Intraocular Inflammation and Uveitis
10 Glaucoma
11 Lens and Cataract
12 Retina and Vitreous
13 Refractive Surgery

In addition, a comprehensive Master Index allows the reader to easily locate subjects throughout the entire series.

References

Readers who wish to explore specific topics in greater detail may consult the references cited within each chapter and listed in the Basic Texts section at the back of the book.

These references are intended to be selective rather than exhaustive, chosen by the BCSC faculty as being important, current, and readily available to residents and practitioners.

Related Academy educational materials are also listed in the appropriate sections. They include books, online and audiovisual materials, self-assessment programs, clinical modules, and interactive programs.

Study Questions and CME Credit

Each volume of the BCSC is designed as an independent study activity for ophthalmology residents and practitioners. The learning objectives for this volume are given on page 1. The text, illustrations, and references provide the information necessary to achieve the objectives; the study questions allow readers to test their understanding of the material and their mastery of the objectives. Physicians who wish to claim CME credit for this educational activity may do so by following the instructions given at the end of the book.

Conclusion

The Basic and Clinical Science Course has expanded greatly over the years, with the addition of much new text and numerous illustrations. Recent editions have sought to place a greater emphasis on clinical applicability while maintaining a solid foundation in basic science. As with any educational program, it reflects the experience of its authors. As its faculties change and as medicine progresses, new viewpoints are always emerging on controversial subjects and techniques. Not all alternate approaches can be included in this series; as with any educational endeavor, the learner should seek additional sources, including such carefully balanced opinions as the Academy's Preferred Practice Patterns.

The BCSC faculty and staff are continuously striving to improve the educational usefulness of the course; you, the reader, can contribute to this ongoing process. If you have any suggestions or questions about the series, please do not hesitate to contact the faculty or the editors.

The authors, editors, and reviewers hope that your study of the BCSC will be of lasting value and that each Section will serve as a practical resource for quality patient care.

Objectives

Upon completion of BCSC Section 9, *Intraocular Inflammation and Uveitis,* the reader should be able to

- outline the immunologic and infectious mechanisms involved in the occurrence and complications of uveitis and related inflammatory conditions, including acquired immunodeficiency syndrome (AIDS)

- identify general and specific pathophysiologic processes that affect the structure and function of the uvea, lens, intraocular cavities, retina, and other tissues in acute and chronic intraocular inflammation

- differentiate and identify infectious and noninfectious uveitic entities

- choose appropriate examination techniques and relevant ancillary studies based on whether an infectious or noninfectious cause is suspected

- develop appropriate differential diagnoses for ocular inflammatory disorders

- describe the principles of medical and surgical management of infectious and noninfectious uveitis and related intraocular inflammation, including indications for and complications of immunosuppressive agents

- describe the structural complications of uveitis and their treatments

- describe criteria that can be applied to differentiate the masquerade syndromes from true uveitis

Introduction

This section of the BCSC is divided into 2 parts. Part II, Intraocular Inflammation and Uveitis, will come as no surprise to the reader opening a volume of the same name. Part II introduces the clinical approach to uveitis and devotes a chapter each to infectious and noninfectious forms of uveitis and to endophthalmitis. The chapter on noninfectious uveitis is organized anatomically. Because infectious uveitic conditions can involve any part of the uveal tract, the chapter on infectious uveitis is organized by causative agents. Part II then discusses the masquerade syndromes, both nonneoplastic and neoplastic. The following chapter discusses the complications of all forms of uveitis, and the final chapter of Part II covers ocular involvement in AIDS, offering the most complete summary of this topic in the BCSC series.

The reader may, however, not expect to find Part I of the book, Ocular Immunology, going into such great depth. Why are so many pages given to this topic? What relevance does it have to Part II? Progress in basic immunology, as well as in the regional immunology of the eye, has translated into major advances in recent years. Our understanding of the mechanisms by which uveitis and other intraocular diseases develop has helped clinicians to identify and establish uveitic entities and to develop specific treatments directed at altered immune processes. These clinically relevant advances include the discovery of unique immune responses in the intraocular cavities and subretinal space; the delineation of the association between HLA and various uveitic entities; and the detection of infectious agents by immunologic methods, such as Western blot and enzyme-linked immunosorbant assay (ELISA), and genetic methods, such as polymerase chain reaction (PCR). Lymphocytic studies for cell surface markers and in vitro studies based on antibodies have helped in clearly separating those uveitic entities that are mediated by immune mechanisms, in particular those resulting from organ-specific antibodies, from those caused by altered lymphocyte functions. The latter mechanism appears to be prevalent in posterior uveitis, and altered cell-mediated immunity can be directed to retinal proteins or other ocular antigens in these intraocular inflammations. These immunologic discoveries continue to shape new immunomodulatory therapies, including powerful cytokine-inhibiting biologic agents.

The section on immunology describes basic aspects of the human immune response, including responses specific to the ocular structures; the effector mechanisms of immunity, including antibody-mediated and lymphocyte-generated mechanisms; and the various pro- and anti-inflammatory cytokines and other effector molecules, including reactive oxygen species and nitric oxide products. Clinical examples are interspersed throughout the immunology text, discussing the clinical relevance of the issues covered in diagnosis and management of uveitis. A clear understanding of the immune mechanisms will enhance an appreciation of the clinical features and principles behind the management of uveitis triggered by either an infectious agent or another insult.

PART I

Ocular Immunology

Introduction to Ocular Immunology and Immune-Mediated Eye Disease

Immune-mediated eye diseases are a leading cause of visual disability and blindness worldwide. Understanding the pathogenesis, diagnosis, and treatment of this class of diseases requires familiarity with basic concepts of immunology, as well as an understanding of the unique aspects of immune function in the eye. The next 4 chapters provide a basic overview of ocular immunology in the healthy and diseased eye. This introduction is not a substitute for a full immunology course; the reader unfamiliar with modern immunology is directed to one of several excellent texts covering this material.

Abbas AK, Lichtman AH. *Basic Immunology: Functions and Disorders of the Immune System.* 3rd ed. Philadelphia, PA: WB Saunders; 2010.

Abbas AK, Lichtman AH, Pillai S. *Cellular and Molecular Immunology.* New York, NY: Elsevier Health Sciences; 2009.

Murphy K, Travers P, Walport M. *Janeway's Immunobiology.* 7th ed. London: Taylor & Francis; 2007.

CHAPTER **1**

Basic Concepts in Immunology: Effector Cells and the Innate Immune Response

Definitions

An immune response is a sequence of cellular and molecular events designed to rid the host of an offending pathogenic organism, toxic substance, cellular debris, or neoplastic cell. There are 2 broad categories of immune responses, *adaptive* and *innate*. Adaptive (or *acquired*) responses are directed against unique antigens with an immunologic response specific for that antigen and will be discussed in detail in Chapter 2.

In contrast, innate immune responses, or *natural immunity*, require no prior contact with or "education" about the stimulus against which they are directed. In the present chapter we will introduce the critical cells of the immune system, and discuss their function in innate immunity.

Components of the Immune System

Leukocytes

White blood cells, or *leukocytes*, are nucleated cells that can be distinguished from one another by the shape of their nuclei and the presence or absence of granules. They are further defined by uptake of various histologic stains.

Neutrophils

Neutrophils are the most abundant granulocytes in the blood. These polymorphonuclear leukocytes feature cytoplasmic granules and lysosomes. Neutrophils are efficient phagocytes that readily clear tissues and degrade ingested material. They act as important effector cells through the release of granule products and cytokines.

Neutrophils dominate the infiltrate in experimental models and clinical examples of active bacterial infections of the conjunctiva, sclera (scleritis), cornea (keratitis), and vitreous (endophthalmitis). Neutrophils are also dominant in many types of active viral infections of the cornea (herpes simplex virus keratitis) and retina (herpes simplex virus retinitis). Neutrophils also constitute the principal cell type in ocular inflammation induced by lipopolysaccharides (see below) and after direct injection of most cytokines into various ocular tissues.

Eosinophils

Eosinophils, a second type of polymorphonuclear leukocyte, also contain abundant cytoplasmic granules and lysosomes. However, the biochemical nature of the granules in eosinophils consists of more basic protein (thus acidic dyes, such as eosin, will bind to these proteins), and eosinophils differ from neutrophils in the way they respond to certain triggering stimuli. Eosinophils have receptors for, and become activated by, many mediators; interleukin-5 (IL-5) is especially important. Eosinophil granule products, such as major basic protein or ribonucleases, are efficient at destroying parasites. Not surprisingly, these cells accumulate at sites of parasitic infection. Eosinophils are also numerous in skin infiltrates during the late-phase allergic response, in atopic lesions, and in lung infiltrates during asthma.

Eosinophils are abundant in the conjunctiva and tears in many forms of atopic conjunctivitis, especially vernal and allergic conjunctivitis. However, eosinophils are not considered major effectors for intraocular inflammation, with the notable exception of helminthic infections of the eye, especially uveitis caused by toxocariasis.

Basophils and mast cells

Basophils, a third type of polymorphonuclear leukocyte, are the bloodborne equivalent of the tissue-bound mast cell. Mast cells exist in 2 major subtypes—connective tissue and mucosal—both of which can release preformed granules and synthesize certain mediators de novo. *Connective tissue mast cells* contain abundant granules with histamine and heparin, and they synthesize prostaglandin D_2 upon stimulation. In contrast, *mucosal mast cells* require T-lymphocyte cytokine help for granule formation, and they normally contain low levels of histamine. Mucosal mast cells primarily synthesize leukotrienes after stimulation. The tissue location can alter the granule type and functional activity, but the regulation of these important differences is not well understood.

Basophils and mast cells differ from other granulocytes in several important ways. The granule contents are different from those of neutrophils and eosinophils, and mast cells express high-affinity Fc receptors for immunoglobulin E (IgE). *Fc* (from "*fragment, crystallizable*") refers to the constant region of immunoglobulin that binds cell surface receptors (see Chapter 2). Mast cells act as major effector cells in IgE-mediated, immune-triggered inflammatory reactions, especially allergy or immediate hypersensitivity. Mast cells may also participate in the induction of cell-mediated immunity, wound healing, and other functions not directly related to IgE-mediated degranulation. Other stimuli, such as complement or certain cytokines, may also trigger degranulation.

The normal human conjunctiva contains significant numbers of mast cells localized in the substantia propria but not in the epithelium. In certain atopic and allergic disease states, such as vernal conjunctivitis, not only does the number of mast cells increase in the substantia propria, but the epithelium also becomes densely infiltrated. Careful anatomical studies have shown that the choroid and anterior uveal tract also contain significant densities of connective tissue–type mast cells; the cornea has none.

Monocytes and macrophages

Monocytes, the circulating cells, and macrophages, the tissue-infiltrating equivalents, are important effectors in all forms of immunity and inflammation. Monocytes are relatively large cells (12–20 μm in suspension but up to 40 μm in tissues) that travel through many normal sites. Most normal tissues have at least 2 identifiable macrophage populations: tissue-resident and blood-derived. Although exceptions exist, in general, tissue-resident macrophages represent monocytes that migrated into a tissue during embryologic development, thereby acquiring tissue-specific properties and specific cellular markers. In many tissues, resident macrophages have been given tissue-specific names: Kupffer cells in the liver, alveolar macrophages in the lung, and microglia in the brain and retina. Blood-derived macrophages usually represent monocytes that have recently migrated from the blood into a fully developed tissue site.

Macrophages serve 3 primary functions:

- as scavengers to clear cell debris and pathogens
- as antigen-presenting cells (APCs) for T lymphocytes
- as inflammatory effector cells

In vitro studies indicate that resting monocytes can be primed through various signals into efficient APCs and, upon additional signals, activated into effector cells. Effective activation stimuli include exposure to bacterial products such as lipopolysaccharide, phagocytosis of antibody-coated or complement-coated pathogens, or exposure to mediators released during inflammation, such as IL-1 or interferon gamma.

Only on full activation do macrophages become most efficient at the synthesis and release of inflammatory mediators and the killing and degradation of phagocytosed pathogens. At some sites of inflammation, macrophages undergo a morphologic change in size and histologic features into an *epithelioid cell.* Epithelioid cells can fuse into multinucleated *giant cells.* Such cells are characteristic of the granulomatous inflammation associated with uveitic conditions such as sarcoidosis. Macrophages are extremely important effector cells in both adaptive and innate immunity. They are often detectable in acute ocular infections, even if other cell types such as neutrophils are more numerous.

Dendritic cells and Langerhans cells

Dendritic cells (DCs) are terminally differentiated, bone marrow–derived, circulating mononuclear cells that are distinct from the lineage of macrophages and monocytes. They make up approximately 0.1%–1.0% of blood mononuclear cells. However, in tissue sites, DCs become large (15–30 μm), with cytoplasmic veils that form extensions 2 to 3 times the diameter of the cell, and resemble the dendritic structure of neurons. In many nonlymphoid and lymphoid organs, DCs become a system of APCs. These sites recruit DCs by defined migration pathways, and DCs in each site share features of structure and function. DCs function as accessory cells important to the processing and presentation of antigens to T lymphocytes; the distinctive function of DCs is to initiate responses in quiescent lymphocytes. Thus, DCs may act as the most potent leukocytes for generating primary T-lymphocyte–dependent immune responses.

Epidermal Langerhans cells (LCs) are the best-characterized subset of DCs. LCs account for approximately 3%–8% of the cells in most human epithelia, including the skin, conjunctiva, nasopharyngeal mucosa, vaginal mucosa, and rectal mucosa. LCs are identified on the basis of their many dendrites, electron-dense cytoplasm, and Birbeck granules. At rest they are not active APCs, but activity develops after in vitro culture with certain cytokines. As a result, LCs transform and lose their granules and more resemble blood and lymphoid DCs. Evidence suggests that LCs can leave the skin and move along the afferent lymph vessels to draining lymphoid organs. LCs are important components of the immune system and play a role in antigen presentation, control of lymphoid cell traffic, differentiation of T lymphocytes, and induction of delayed hypersensitivity. Elimination of LCs from skin before an antigen challenge inhibits the induction of the contact hypersensitivity response. In the conjunctiva and limbus, LCs are the only cells that constitutively express major histocompatibility (MHC) class II molecules. LCs are present in the peripheral cornea, and any kind of irritation to the central cornea will result in central migration of the peripheral LCs.

Lymphocytes

Lymphocytes are small (10–20 μm) cells with large, dense nuclei also derived from stem cell precursors within the bone marrow. However, unlike other leukocytes, lymphocytes require subsequent maturation in peripheral lymphoid organs. Lymphocytes can be subdivided by the expression of specific cell-surface proteins (ie, *surface markers*). These markers are in turn related to the functional and molecular activity of individual subsets. Three broad categories of lymphocytes have been identified: T lymphocytes; B lymphocytes; and non-T, non-B lymphocytes. These subsets are discussed in greater detail in Chapter 2.

Abbas AK, Lichtman AH. *Basic Immunology: Functions and Disorders of the Immune System.* 3rd ed. Philadelphia, PA: WB Saunders; 2010.

Overview of the Innate Immune System

The innate immune response can be thought of as a "preprogrammed" reaction to recognized foreign substances within the body, such as bacterial cell wall structures or foreign proteins. The innate immune response is similar for all encountered triggers, and generates biochemical mediators and cytokines that recruit nonspecific effector cells, especially macrophages and neutrophils, to remove the offending stimulus through phagocytosis or enzymatic degradation.

The receptors of innate immunity are essentially identical among all individuals within a species. The innate immune receptors respond to conserved molecular motifs on triggering stimuli, such as specific amino acid sequences, certain lipoproteins, and certain phospholipids expressed by microbes. The innate immune response to acute infection is the classic example of this process. For example, in endophthalmitis, bacteria-derived toxins or host cell debris stimulate the recruitment of neutrophils and monocytes, leading to the production of inflammatory mediators and phagocytosis of the bacteria. These responses to *Staphylococcus* organisms are nearly identical to those mounted against any other bacteria. Nonspecific receptors that recognize families of related toxins or molecules in the environment determine this response.

Immunity Versus Inflammation

An immune response is the process for removing an offending stimulus. When this response becomes clinically apparent within a tissue, it is termed an *inflammatory response*. More precisely, an inflammatory response is a sequence of molecular and cellular events triggered by innate or adaptive immunity resulting in 5 characteristic cardinal clinical manifestations: pain, hyperemia, edema, heat, and loss of function. These clinical signs reflect 2 main physiologic changes within a tissue: cellular recruitment and altered vascular permeability. Inflammatory response is associated with the following typical pathologic findings:

- infiltration of effector cells resulting in the release of biochemical and molecular mediators of inflammation, such as cytokines (eg, interleukins and chemokines) and lipid mediators (eg, prostaglandins and platelet-activating factors)
- presence of oxygen metabolites (eg, superoxide and nitrogen radicals)
- presence of granule products as well as catalytic enzymes (eg, collagenases and elastases)
- activation of plasma-derived enzyme systems (eg, complement components and fibrin)

These effector systems are described in greater detail later in this chapter.

In practice, many clinicians use the term *immune response* to mean adaptive immunity and the term *inflammation* to imply innate immunity. However, it is important to remember that both adaptive and innate immune responses usually function physiologically at a subclinical level without overt manifestations. For example, in most persons, ocular surface allergen exposure, which occurs daily in all humans, or bacterial contamination during cataract surgery, which occurs in most eyes, is usually cleared by innate or adaptive mechanisms without overt inflammation. Similarly, both adaptive and innate immunity can trigger inflammation, and the physiologic changes induced by each form of immunity may be indistinguishable. For example, the hypopyon of bacterial endophthalmitis, which results from innate immunity against bacterial toxins, and the hypopyon of lens-associated uveitis, which presumably results from an inappropriate adaptive immune response against lens antigens, cannot be distinguished clinically or histologically.

Delves PJ, Roitt IM, Burton D, Martin S. *Roitt's Essential Immunology.* 11th ed. Malden, MA: Blackwell Publishing; 2006.

Medzhitov R, Janeway C Jr. Innate immunity. *N Engl J Med.* 2000;343(5):338–344.

Murphy K, Travers P, Walport M. *Janeway's Immunobiology.* 7th ed. London: Taylor & Francis; 2007.

Triggers of Innate Immunity

Whereas adaptive immune responses use a complex afferent and processing system to activate effector responses, innate immune responses generally use more direct triggering mechanisms. Four of the most important triggering or response mechanisms to initiate an effector response of innate immunity are reviewed here (Table 1-1).

Bacteria-Derived Molecules That Trigger Innate Immunity

Bacterial lipopolysaccharide

Bacterial lipopolysaccharide (LPS), also known as *endotoxin*, is an intrinsic component of the cell walls of most gram-negative bacteria. One of the most important triggering molecules of innate immunity, LPS consists of 3 components: lipid A, O polysaccharide, and core oligosaccharide.

Lipid A is responsible for most of the inflammatory effects of LPS. It consists of 2 glucosamine units with several attached fatty acid chains. It is capable of activating effector cells at concentrations of a few picograms per milliliter. The exact structures of lipid A, O polysaccharide, and core oligosaccharide will vary from species to species of bacteria, but all are recognized by the innate immune system. The primary receptors for LPS are toll-like receptors (TLRs), principally TLR4 and TLR2, which are expressed on macrophages, neutrotrophils, and dendritic cells, as well as B cells and T cells.

LPS is an important cause of morbidity and mortality during infections with gram-negative bacteria and is the major cause of shock, fever, and other pathophysiologic responses to bacterial sepsis. The immunoreactivity of LPS functions through the innate immune system, and does not induce antigen-specific effects per se. The pleiotropic effects of LPS include activation of monocytes and neutrophils, leading to up-regulation of genes for various cytokines (IL-1, IL-6, tumor necrosis factor [TNF]); degranulation;

Table 1-1 Effector Reactivities of the Innate Immune Response in the Eye

Bacteria-derived molecules that trigger innate immunity
Lipopolysaccharide (LPS)
Other cell wall components
Exotoxins and secreted toxins

Nonspecific soluble molecules that trigger or modulate innate immunity
Plasma-derived enzymes
Acute phase reactants
Local production of cytokines by parenchymal cells within a tissue site

Innate mechanisms for recruitment and activation of neutrophils
Cell adhesion and transmigration
Activation mechanisms
  Phagocytosis of bacteria

Innate mechanisms for recruitment and activation of macrophages
Cell adhesion and transmigration
Activation mechanisms
  Scavenging
  Priming
  Activation

activation of complement through the alternative pathway; and direct impact on the vascular endothelium. Interestingly, footpad injection of LPS in rodents results in an acute anterior uveitis; this animal model is called *experimental immune uveitis* (EIU; see Chapter 4). See Clinical Examples 1-1 and 1-2.

Other bacterial cell wall components

The bacterial cell wall and membrane are complex, with numerous polysaccharide, lipid, and protein structures that can initiate the innate immune response whether or not they act as antigens for adaptive immunity. Such toxins may include

- muramyl dipeptide
- lipoteichoic acids, in gram-positive bacteria
- lipoarabinomannan, in mycobacteria
- other poorly characterized soluble factors, such as heat shock proteins, common to all bacteria

CLINICAL EXAMPLE 1-1

Lipopolysaccharide-induced uveitis Humans are intermittently exposed to low doses of LPS that are released from the gut, especially during episodes of diarrhea and dysentery, and exposure to LPS may play a role in dysentery-related uveitis, arthritis, and reactive arthritis. Systemic administration of a low dose of LPS in rabbits, rats, and mice produces a mild acute uveitis; this effect occurs at doses of LPS lower than those that cause apparent systemic shock. In rabbits, a breakdown of the blood–ocular barrier occurs because of leakage of plasma proteins through uveal vessels and loosening of the tight junctions between the nonpigmented ciliary epithelial cells. Rats and mice develop an acute neutrophil and monocytic infiltrate in the iris and ciliary body within 24 hours.

The precise mechanism of the LPS-induced ocular effects after systemic administration is unknown. One possibility is that LPS circulates and binds to the vascular endothelium or other sites within the anterior uvea. Alternatively, LPS might cause activation of uveal macrophages or circulating leukocytes, leading them to preferentially adhere to the anterior uveal vascular endothelium. It is clear that toll-like receptor 2 (TLR2) recognizes LPS, and binding of LPS by TLR2 on macrophages results in macrophage activation and secretion of a wide array of inflammatory cytokines. Degranulation of platelets is among the first of histologic changes in LPS uveitis, probably mediated by eicosanoids, platelet-activating factors, and vasoactive amines. The subsequent intraocular generation of several mediators, especially leukotriene B_4, thromboxane B_2, prostaglandin E_2, and IL-6, correlates with the development of the cellular infiltrate and vascular leakage.

Not surprisingly, direct injection of LPS into various ocular sites can initiate a severe localized inflammatory response. For example, intravitreal injection of LPS triggers a dose-dependent infiltration of the uveal tract, retina, and vitreous with neutrophils and monocytes. Injection of LPS into the central cornea causes development of a ring infiltrate as a result of the infiltration of neutrophils circumferentially from the limbus.

CLINICAL EXAMPLE 1-2

Role of bacterial toxin production and severity of endophthalmitis The effect of toxin production by various bacterial strains on the severity of endophthalmitis has recently been evaluated in experimental studies. It has been known for nearly a century that intraocular injection of LPS is highly inflammatory and accounts for much of the enhanced pathogenicity of gram-negative infections of the eye. Using clinical isolates or bacteria genetically altered to diminish production of the various types of bacterial toxins, investigators have recently demonstrated that toxin elaboration by the living organism in gram-positive or gram-negative endophthalmitis greatly influences inflammatory cell infiltration and retinal cytotoxicity. This research suggests that sterilization with antibiotic therapy alone, in the absence of antitoxin therapy, may not prevent activation of innate immunity, ocular inflammation, and vision loss in eyes infected by toxin-producing strains.

> Booth MC, Atkuri RV, Gilmore MS. Toxin production contributes to severity of *Staphylococcus aureus* endophthalmitis. In: Nussenblatt RB, Whitcup SM, Caspi RR, Gery I, eds. *Advances in Ocular Immunology: Proceedings of the 6th International Symposium on the Immunology and Immunopathology of the Eye.* New York, NY: Elsevier; 1994:269–272.
>
> Jett BD, Parke DW 2nd, Booth MC, Gilmore MS. Host/parasite interactions in bacterial endophthalmitis. *Zentralbl Bakteriol.* 1997;285(3):341–367.

Killed lysates of many types of gram-positive bacteria or mycobacteria have been demonstrated to directly activate macrophages, making them useful as adjuvants. Some of these components have been implicated in various models for arthritis and uveitis. In many cases, the molecular mechanisms are probably similar to LPS.

Exotoxins and other secretory products of bacteria

Various bacteria are known to secrete products such as *exotoxins* into the microenvironment in which they are growing. Many of these products are enzymes that, although not directly inflammatory, can cause tissue damage that subsequently results in inflammation and tissue destruction. Examples include

- collagenases
- hemolysins such as streptolysin O, which can kill neutrophils by causing cytoplasmic and extracellular release of their granules
- phospholipases such as the *Clostridium perfringens* α-toxins, which kill cells and cause necrosis by disrupting cell membranes

For example, intravitreal injection of a purified hemolysin BL toxin derived from *Bacillus cereus* can cause direct necrosis of retinal cells and retinal detachment. In animal studies, the toxin produced by as few as 100 *Bacillus* bacteria is capable of causing complete loss of retinal function in 12 hours. In addition to being directly toxic, bacterial exotoxins can also be strong triggers of innate immune response.

Callegan MC, Jett BD, Hancock LE, Gilmore MS. Role of hemolysin BL in the pathogenesis of extraintestinal *Bacillus cereus* infection assessed in an endophthalmitis model. *Infect Immun.* 1999;67(7):3357–3366.

Medzhitov R, Janeway C. Innate immunity. *N Engl J Med.* 2000;343(5):338–344.

Murphy K, Travers P, Walport M. *Janeway's Immunobiology.* 7th ed. London: Taylor & Francis; 2007.

Other Triggers or Modulators of Innate Immunity

Various traumatic or toxic stimuli within ocular sites can trigger innate immunity. For example, trauma or toxins interacting directly with nonimmune ocular parenchymal cells, especially iris or ciliary body epithelium, retinal pigment epithelium, retinal Müller cells, or corneal or conjunctival epithelium, can result in a wide range of mediator, cytokine, and eicosanoid synthesis, and this mechanism should be considered a form of innate immunity. Thus, phagocytosis of staphylococci by corneal epithelium, microtrauma to the ocular surface epithelium by contact lenses, chafing of iris or ciliary epithelium by an intraocular lens (IOL), or laser treatment of the retina can stimulate ocular cells to produce mediators that assist in the recruitment of innate effector cells such as neutrophils or macrophages. See Clinical Example 1-3.

Innate Mechanisms for the Recruitment and Activation of Neutrophils

Neutrophils are among the most efficient effectors of innate immunity following trauma or acute infection. Neutrophils are categorized as either *resting* or *activated*, based on secretory and cell membrane activity. Cellular recruitment of resting, circulating neutrophils

---

CLINICAL EXAMPLE 1-3

Uveitis-glaucoma-hyphema syndrome One cause of postoperative inflammation following cataract surgery, uveitis-glaucoma-hyphema (UGH) syndrome is related to the physical presence of certain IOL styles. Although UGH syndrome was more common when rigid anterior chamber lenses were used during the early 1980s, it has also been reported with posterior chamber lenses. The pathogenesis of UGH syndrome appears to be related to various mechanisms for activation of innate immunity. One of the most likely mechanisms is cytokine and eicosanoid synthesis triggered by mechanical chafing or trauma to the iris or ciliary body. Plasma-derived enzymes, especially complement or fibrin, can enter the eye through vascular permeability altered by surgery or trauma and can then be activated by the surface of IOLs. Adherence of bacteria and leukocytes to the surface has also been implicated. Toxicity caused by contaminants on the lens surface during manufacturing has become rare. Nevertheless, even many noninflamed eyes with IOLs can demonstrate histologic evidence of low-grade foreign-body reactions around the haptics.

Pepose JS, Holland GN, Wilhelmus KR, eds. *Ocular Infection and Immunity.* St Louis, MO: Mosby; 1996.

by the innate immune response occurs rapidly in a tightly controlled process requiring 2 main mechanisms:

- neutrophil adhesion to the vascular endothelium through cell-adhesion molecules (CAMs) on leukocytes as well as on endothelial cells primarily in postcapillary venules
- transmigration of the neutrophils through the endothelium and its extracellular matrix, mediated by chemotactic factors

For resting neutrophils to escape from blood vessels, an essential adhesion with activated vascular endothelial cells must occur; this is triggered by various innate stimuli, such as LPS, physical injury, thrombin, histamine, or leukotriene release.

The initial phase involves *neutrophil rolling,* a process by which neutrophils bind loosely but reversibly to nonactivated endothelial cells (Fig 1-1). Involved are molecules on both cell types belonging to at least 3 sets of CAM families:

- the *selectins,* especially L-, E-, and P-selectin
- the *integrins,* especially leukocyte function–associated antigen 1 (LFA-1) and macrophage-1 antigen (Mac-1)
- molecules in the immunoglobulin superfamily, especially intercellular adhesion molecule 1 (ICAM-1) and ICAM-2

The primary events are mediated largely by members of the selectin family and occur within minutes of stimulation. Nonactivated neutrophils express L-selectin, which mediates a weak bond to endothelial cells by binding to specific selectin ligands. Upon exposure to the triggering molecules described in the previous section, endothelial cells become activated, expressing in turn at least 2 other selectins (E and P) by which they can bind to the neutrophils and help stabilize the interaction by a process called *adhesion.* Subsequently, other factors, such as platelet-activating factor (PAF), various cytokines, and bacterial products, can induce the up-regulation of the β-integrin family. As integrins are expressed, the selectins are shed, and neutrophils then bind firmly to endothelial cells through the immunoglobulin superfamily molecules.

Subsequent to adhesion, various chemotactic factors are required to induce *transmigration* of neutrophils across the endothelial barrier and extracellular matrix into the tissue site. Chemotactic factors are short-range signaling molecules that diffuse in a declining concentration gradient from the source of production within a tissue to the vessel itself. Neutrophils have receptors for these molecules, and they are induced to undergo membrane changes so they can migrate in the direction of highest concentration. A large number of such factors have been identified:

- complement products, such as C5a
- fibrin split products
- certain neuropeptides, such as substance P
- bacteria-derived formyl tripeptides, such as *N*-formyl-methionyl-leucyl-phenylalanine (fMLP)
- leukotrienes
- α-chemokines, such as IL-8

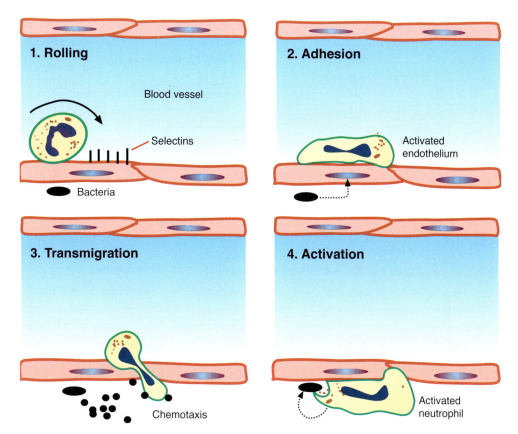

Figure 1-1 Four steps of neutrophil migration and activation. **1,** In response to innate stimuli, such as bacterial invasion of tissue, *rolling* neutrophils within the blood vessel bind loosely but reversibly to nonactivated endothelial cells by selectins. **2,** Exposure to innate activating factors and bacterial products *(dotted arrow)* activates endothelial cells, which in turn express E- and P-selectins, β-integrins, and immunoglobulin superfamily molecules to enhance and stabilize the interaction by a process called *adhesion*. **3,** Chemotactic factors triggered by the infection induce *transmigration* of neutrophils across the endothelial barrier into the extracellular matrix of the tissue. **4,** Finally, neutrophils are fully *activated* into functional effector cells upon stimulation by bacterial toxins and phagocytosis. *(Illustration by Barb Cousins, modified by Joyce Zavarro.)*

Activation of neutrophils into functional effector cells begins during adhesion and transmigration but is fully exploited upon interaction with specific signals within the injured or infected site. Perhaps the most effective triggers of activation are bacteria and their toxins, especially LPS. Other innate or adaptive mechanisms (especially complement) and chemical mediators (such as leukotrienes and PAF) can also contribute to neutrophil activation. Unlike monocytes or lymphocytes, neutrophils do not leave a tissue to recirculate but remain and die.

Phagocytosis

Phagocytosis of bacteria and other pathogens is a selective receptor-mediated process, and the 2 most important receptors are the *antibody Fc receptors* and the *complement receptors*.

Thus, pathogens in complexes with antibody or with activated complement components are specifically bound to the cell-surface-membrane–expressed Fc or complement (C) receptors and are effectively ingested. Other, less well-characterized receptors may also mediate attachment to phagocytes.

Once the offending pathogen is found by the neutrophil, the attached membrane invaginates and becomes a phagosome. Ultimately, several granules fuse with the phagosomes, a process that may occur prior to complete invagination, spilling certain granule contents outside of the phagocyte. Phagocytes are endowed with multiple means of destroying microorganisms, especially antimicrobial polypeptides that reside within cytoplasmic granules, reactive oxygen radicals generated from oxygen during the respiratory burst, and reactive nitrogen radicals. Although these mechanisms are primarily designed to destroy pathogens, released contents such as lysosomal enzymes may contribute to the amplification of inflammation and tissue damage.

Innate Mechanisms for the Recruitment and Activation of Macrophages

Monocyte-derived macrophages are the second important type of effector cell for the innate immune response following trauma or acute infection. The various molecules involved in monocyte adhesion and transmigration from blood into tissues are probably similar to those discussed in connection with neutrophils, although they have not been studied as thoroughly. However, the functional activation of macrophages is more complex. Macrophages exist in different levels or stages of metabolic and functional activity, each representing different "programs" of gene activation and synthesis of macrophage-derived cytokines and mediators:

- resting (immature or quiescent)
- primed
- activated

A fourth category of macrophages, often called *stimulated, reparative,* or *inflammatory,* is used by some immunologists to refer to those macrophages that are not quite fully activated. This multilevel model is oversimplified, but it does provide a framework for conceptualizing different levels of macrophage activation in terms of acute inflammation (Fig 1-2).

Resting and scavenging macrophages

Host cell debris is cleared from a tissue site by phagocytosis in a process called *scavenging.* Resting macrophages are the classic scavenging cell, capable of phagocytosis and uptake of the following:

- dead cell membranes
- chemically modified extracellular protein, through acetylated or oxidized lipoproteins
- sugar ligands, through mannose receptors
- naked nucleic acids as well as bacterial pathogens

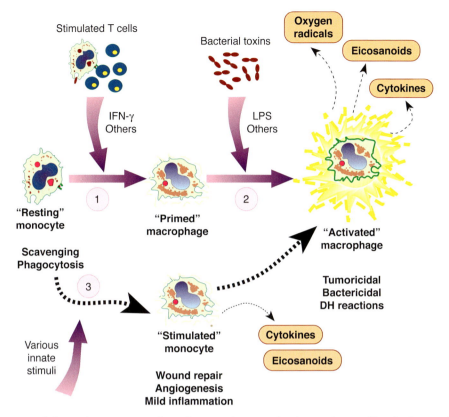

Figure 1-2 Schematic representation of macrophage activation pathway. Classically, *resting monocytes* are thought to be the principal noninflammatory scavenging phagocyte. **1,** Upon exposure to low levels of interferon gamma (IFN-γ) from T lymphocytes, monocytes become primed, up-regulating major histocompatibility complex (MHC) class II molecules and performing other functions. *Primed macrophages* function in antigen presentation. **2,** *Fully activated macrophages,* after exposure to bacterial lipopolysaccharide and interferon, are tumoricidal and bactericidal and mediate severe inflammation. **3,** *Stimulated monocytes* result from resting monocyte activation by other innate stimuli, without exposure to IFN-γ. These cells are incompletely activated, producing low levels of cytokines and eicosanoids but not reactive oxygen intermediates. These cells participate in wound healing, angiogenesis, and low-level inflammatory reactions. DH = delayed hypersensitivity, LPS = lipopolysaccharide. *(Illustration by Barb Cousins, modified by Joyce Zavarro.)*

Resting monocytes express scavenging receptors of at least 3 types but synthesize very low levels of proinflammatory cytokines. In general, scavenging can occur in the absence of inflammation. See Clinical Example 1-4.

Primed macrophages

Resting macrophages become primed by exposure to certain cytokines. Upon priming, these cells become positive for MHC class II antigen and capable of functioning as APCs to T lymphocytes (see Chapter 2). Priming implies activation of specialized lysosomal

CLINICAL EXAMPLE 1-4

Phacolytic glaucoma Mild infiltration of scavenging macrophages centered around retained lens cortex or nucleus fragments occurs in nearly all eyes with lens injury, including those subjected to routine cataract surgery. This infiltrate is notable for the *absence* of both prominent neutrophil infiltration and significant nongranulomatous inflammation. An occasional giant cell may be present, but granulomatous changes are not extensive.

Phacolytic glaucoma is a variant of scavenging macrophage infiltration in which glaucoma occurs in the setting of a hypermature cataract that leaks lens protein through an *intact* capsule. Lens protein–engorged scavenging macrophages are present in the anterior chamber, and glaucoma develops as these cells block the trabecular meshwork outflow channels. Other signs of typical lens-associated uveitis are conspicuously absent. Experimental studies suggest that lens proteins may be chemotactic stimuli for monocytes.

enzymes such as cathepsins D and E for degrading proteins into peptide fragments; up-regulation of certain specific genes, such as MHC class II, and costimulatory molecules, such as B7.1; and increased cycling of proteins between endosomes and the surface membrane. Primed macrophages thus resemble dendritic cells. They can exit tissue sites by the afferent lymphatic vessels to reenter the lymph node.

Activated and stimulated macrophages

Activated macrophages are classically defined as macrophages producing the full spectrum of inflammatory and cytotoxic cytokines; thus, they mediate and amplify acute inflammation, tumor killing, and major antibacterial activity. *Epithelioid cells* and *giant cells* represent the terminal differentiation of the activated macrophage. Activated macrophages synthesize numerous mediators to amplify inflammation:

- inflammatory or cytotoxic cytokines, such as IL-1, IL-6, and TNF-α
- reactive oxygen or nitrogen intermediates
- lipid mediators
- other products

Macrophages can be activated by many different innate stimuli, such as

- cytokines derived from T lymphocytes, as well as those derived from other cell types
- chemokines
- bacterial cell walls or toxins from gram-positive or acid-fast organisms
- complement activated through the alternative pathway
- foreign bodies composed of potentially toxic substances, such as talc or beryllium
- exposure to certain surfaces, such as some plastics

As noted above, macrophages that are partially activated to produce some inflammatory cytokines—but perhaps not fully activated to antimicrobial or tumoricidal function—are sometimes termed *stimulated* or *reparative* macrophages. Such partially activated macrophages also contribute to fibrosis and wound healing through the synthesis of mitogens such as platelet-derived growth factors (PDGFs), metalloproteinases, and other matrix degradation factors as well as to angiogenesis through synthesis of angiogenic factors such as vascular endothelial growth factor (VEGF).

Mediator Systems That Amplify Immune Responses

Although innate or adaptive effector responses may directly induce inflammation, in most cases these effectors instead initiate a process that must be amplified to produce overt clinical manifestations. Molecules generated within the host that induce and amplify inflammation are termed *inflammatory mediators,* and mediator systems include several categories of these molecules (Table 1-2). Most act on target cells through receptor-mediated processes, although some act in enzymatic cascades that interact in a complex fashion.

Plasma-Derived Enzyme Systems

Complement factors

Complement is an important inflammatory mediator in the eye. Components and fragments of the complement cascade, which account for approximately 5% of plasma protein and comprise more than 30 different proteins, represent important endogenous amplifiers of innate and adaptive immunity, as well as mediators of inflammatory responses. Both adaptive and innate immune responses can initiate complement activation pathways, which generate products that contribute to the inflammatory process (Fig 1-3). Adaptive immunity typically activates complement by the classic pathway with antigen–antibody (immune) complexes, especially those formed by IgM, IgG1, and IgG3. Innate immunity typically activates complement by the alternative pathway using certain carbohydrate moieties or LPS on the cell wall of microorganisms.

Complement serves the following 4 basic functions during inflammation:

- coats antigenic or pathogenic surfaces by C3b to enhance phagocytosis
- promotes lysis of cell membranes through pore formation by membrane attack complexes (MACs)
- recruits neutrophils and induces inflammation through generation of the anaphylatoxins C3a, C4a, and C5a
- modulates antigen-specific immune responses by complement activation products such as iC3b and MACs

---

Table 1-2 Mediator Systems That Amplify Innate and Adaptive Immune Responses

Plasma-derived enzyme systems: complement, kinins, and fibrin
Vasoactive amines: serotonin and histamine
Lipid mediators: eicosanoids and platelet-activating factors
Cytokines
Reactive oxygen intermediates
Reactive nitrogen products
Neutrophil-derived granule products

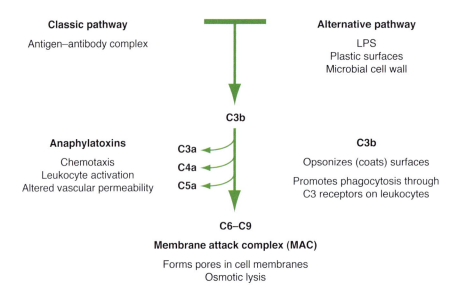

Figure 1-3 Overview of the essential intermediates of the complement pathway. LPS = lipopolysaccharide.

The anaphylatoxins, so named because they cause anaphylaxis upon systemic administration into animals, are the principal complement-derived mediators. The effects of these anaphylatoxins include chemotaxis and changes in cell adhesiveness, mediated principally by C5a, and degranulation and release of mediators from mast cells and platelets. The proinflammatory complement mediator C5a also stimulates oxidative metabolism and the production and release of toxic oxygen radicals from leukocytes, as well as the extracellular discharge of leukocyte granule contents. Complement activation products such as iC3b and MACs can also modulate antigen-specific immune responses.

Walport MT. Complement. First of two parts. *N Engl J Med.* 2001;344(14):1058–1066.
Walport MT. Complement. Second of two parts. *N Engl J Med.* 2001;344(15):1140–1144.

Fibrin and other plasma factors

Fibrin is the final deposition product of another important plasma-derived enzyme system, and its deposition during inflammation promotes hemostasis, fibrosis, angiogenesis, and leukocyte adhesion. Fibrin is released from its circulating zymogen precursor, *fibrinogen,* upon cleavage by thrombin. In situ polymerization of smaller units gives rise to the characteristic fibrin plugs or clots. Fibrin dissolution is mediated by *plasmin*, which is activated from its zymogen precursor, *plasminogen,* by plasminogen activators such as tissue plasminogen activator. Thrombin, which is derived principally from platelet granules, is released after any vascular injury that causes platelet aggregation and release.

Fibrin may be observed in severe anterior uveitis (the "plastic aqueous"). The role of fibrin deposition in the eye during uveitis is unknown, but it is thought to contribute to complications such as synechiae, cyclitic membranes, and tractional retinal detachment.

Histamine

Histamine is present in the granules of mast cells and basophils, and it is actively secreted from this source following exposure of cells to a wide range of stimuli. Histamine acts by binding to 1 of at least 3 known types of receptors that are differentially present on target cells. The best-studied pathway for degranulation is antigen cross-linking of IgE bound to mast-cell Fc IgE receptors, but many other inflammatory stimuli can stimulate secretion, including complement, direct membrane injury, and certain drugs. Classically, histamine release has been associated with allergy. The contribution of histamine to intraocular inflammation remains subject to debate.

Lipid Mediators

Two groups of lipid molecules synthesized by stimulated cells act as powerful mediators and regulators of inflammatory responses: the arachidonic acid (AA) metabolites, or *eicosanoids,* and the acetylated triglycerides, usually called *platelet-activating factors.* Both groups of molecules may be rapidly generated from the same lysophospholipid precursors by the enzymatic action of cellular phospholipases such as phospholipase A_2 (Fig 1-4).

Eicosanoids

All eicosanoids are derived from AA. AA is liberated from membrane phospholipids by phospholipase A_2, which is activated by various agonists. AA is oxidized by 2 major pathways to generate the various mediators:

- the cyclooxygenase (COX) pathway, which produces prostaglandins, thromboxanes, and prostacyclins
- the 5-lipoxygenase pathway, which produces 5-hydroperoxyeicosatetraenic acid, lipoxins, and leukotrienes

Many other important enzymes also function in eicosanoid metabolism.

The COX-derived mediators are evanescent compounds induced in virtually all cells by a variety of stimuli. In general, they act in the immediate environment of their release to directly mediate many inflammatory activities, including effects on vascular permeability, cell recruitment, platelet function, and smooth-muscle contraction.

Depending on conditions, COX-derived products can either up-regulate or down-regulate the production of cytokines, enzyme systems, and oxygen metabolites. Two forms of COX exist: COX-1 and COX-2. COX-1 is thought to be constitutively expressed in many cells, especially in cells that use prostaglandin for basal metabolic functions, such as the gastric mucosa or the renal tubular epithelium. COX-2 is inducible by many inflammatory stimuli, including other inflammatory mediators (eg, PAF and some cytokines) and innate stimuli (eg, LPS).

Prostaglandins may be the cause of cystoid macular edema (CME) in association with anterior segment surgery or inflammation. Posterior diffusion of 1 or more of the eicosanoids through the vitreous is assumed to alter capillary permeability of the perifoveal network, leading to the characteristic pattern of intraretinal fluid accumulation and cyst formation. Clinical trials in humans have indicated that topical treatment with COX

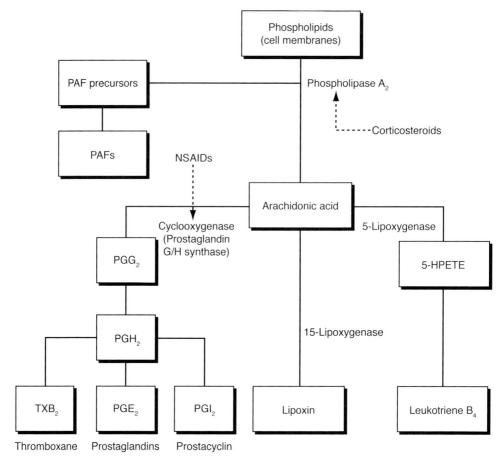

Figure 1-4 Overview of the essential intermediates of the eicosanoid and platelet-activating factor (PAF) pathways. 5-HPETE = 5-hydroperoxyeicosatetraenoic acid. *(Modified with permission from Pepose JS, Holland GN, Wilhelmus KR, eds.* Ocular Infection and Immunity. *St Louis, MO: Mosby; 1996.)*

inhibitors does diminish the onset of mild CME after cataract surgery, and both topical and systemic nonsteroidal anti-inflammatory drug (NSAID) therapy might be efficacious in the treatment of persistent CME. *Systemic NSAID therapy is effective in treating recurrent episcleritis and mild cases of scleritis.*

Prostaglandins and other eicosanoids indisputably play a major role in the physiology of the eye, reaching far beyond their putative participation as mediators of inflammation. For example, prostaglandin E_1 regulates the alternative (uveoscleral) outflow pathway for aqueous humor, perhaps explaining why intraocular pressure (IOP) is diminished in some inflamed eyes. Drugs such as latanoprost, a prostaglandin $F_{2\alpha}$ analogue, may act with a similar mechanism.

The products of the other major pathway of AA metabolism, the 5-lipoxygenase pathway, are also numerous, and some of them are extremely potent mediators of the inflammatory response. Derivatives of 5-lipoxygenase, an enzyme found mainly in granulocytes and some mast cells, have also been detected in the brain and retina. In contrast with prostaglandins, *leukotrienes* probably contribute significantly to inflammatory infiltration. One of the best characterized is leukotriene B_4, a potent chemotactic factor that also causes lysosomal enzyme release and reactive oxygen radical production by granulocytes. Some leukotrienes may have 1000 times the effect of histamine on vascular permeability. Another lipoxygenase product, lipoxin, is a potent stimulator of superoxide anion.

Platelet-activating factors

Platelet-activating factors are a family of phospholipid-derived mediators that appear to be important stimuli in the early stage of inflammation. PAFs also serve physiologic functions unrelated to inflammation, especially in reproductive biology, the physiology of secretory epithelium, and neurobiology. In these physiologic roles, a de novo biosynthetic pathway has been identified. However, the *remodeling pathway* is the one implicated in PAF inflammatory actions.

Phospholipase A_2 metabolizes phosphocholine precursors in cell membranes, releasing AA and PAF precursors, which are then acetylated into multiple species of PAF. PAF release can be stimulated by various innate triggers, such as bacterial toxins, or trauma and cytokines. PAFs not only activate platelets but also activate most leukocytes as well, which in turn produce and release additional PAFs. The PAFs function by binding to one or more guanosine triphosphate protein–associated receptors on target cells.

In vitro, PAFs induce an impressive repertoire of responses, including phagocytosis, exocytosis, superoxide production, chemotaxis, aggregation, proliferation, adhesion, eicosanoid generation, degranulation, and calcium mobilization, as well as diverse morphologic changes. PAFs seem to be a major regulator of cell adhesion and vascular permeability in many forms of acute inflammation, trauma, shock, and ischemia. PAF antagonists are being developed and tested in clinical trials. Synergistic interactions probably exist among PAFs, nitric oxide, eicosanoids, and cytokines. Intravitreal injection of PAFs in animals induces an acute retinitis. The precise role of PAFs in intraocular inflammation remains unknown.

Cytokines

Cytokines are soluble polypeptide mediators that are synthesized and released by cells for the purposes of intercellular signaling and communication. Table 1-3 lists some examples of cytokines that are associated with ocular inflammation. Cytokines can be released by a cell to signal neighboring cells at the site *(paracrine action),* to stimulate a receptor on its own surface *(autocrine action),* or in some cases to act on a distant site by release into the blood *(endocrine action).* Traditionally, investigators have subdivided cytokines into families with related activities, sources, and targets, using terms such as *growth factors, interleukins, lymphokines, interferons, monokines,* and *chemokines.* Thus, *growth factor* traditionally refers to cytokines mediating cell proliferation and differentiation. The terms *interleukin* or *lymphokine* identify cytokines thought to mediate intercellular communication among lymphocytes or other leukocytes. *Interferons* are cytokines that limit or interfere with the ability of a virus to infect a cell; *monokines* are immunoregulatory cytokines secreted by monocytes and macrophages; and *chemokines* are chemotactic cytokines.

Table 1-3 Cytokines of Relevance to Ocular Immunology

Family	Example	Major Cell Source	Major Target Cells	Major General Actions	Specific Ocular Actions
Interleukins	IL-1α	Macrophages Many others	Most leukocytes Various ocular cells	Many actions on T and B lymphocytes Systematic toxicity (fever, shock)	Altered vascular permeability Neutrophil and macrophage infiltration Langerhans migration to central cornea
	IL-6	Macrophages T lymphocytes Mast cells Mast ocular epithelium	Most leukocytes Various ocular cells	Many actions on B lymphocytes Systematic toxicity (fever, shock)	Altered vascular permeability Neutrophil infiltration High levels in many forms of uveitis and nonuveitic diseases
	IL-2	Th0 or Th1 CD4 T lymphocytes	T lymphocytes B lymphocytes NK cells	Activates CD4 and CD8 T lymphocytes Induces Th1	Detectable levels in some forms of uveitis
	IL-4	Th2 CD4 T lymphocytes Basophils, mast cells	T lymphocytes B lymphocytes	Induces Th2, blocks Th1 Induces B lymphocytes to make IgE	? Role in atopic and vernal conjunctivitis
	IL-5	Th2 CD4 T lymphocytes		Recruits eosinophils	? Role in atopic and vernal conjunctivitis
Alpha chemokines	IL-8	Many cell types	Endothelial cells Neutrophils Many others	Recruits and activates neutrophils Up-regulates CAM on endothelium	Altered vascular permeability Neutrophil infiltration
Beta chemokines	Macrophage chemotactic protein-1 (MCP-1)	Macrophages Endothelium RPE	Endothelial cells Macrophages T lymphocytes	Recruits and activates macrophages, some T lymphocytes	Recruits macrophages and T lymphocytes to eye
Tumor necrosis factors	TNF-α or -β	Macrophages (TNF-α) T lymphocytes (TNF-β)		Tumor apoptosis Macrophage and neutrophil activation Cell adhesion and chemotaxis Fibrin deposition and vascular injury Systemic toxicity (fever, shock)	Altered vascular permeability Mononuclear cell infiltration

Interferons	Interferon gamma (IFN-γ)	Th1 T lymphocytes NK cells		Activates macrophages	Neutrophil and macrophage infiltration
	IFN-α	Most leukocytes	Most parenchymal cells	Prevents viral infection of many cells Inhibits hemangioma, conjunctival intraepithelial neoplasia, and other tumors	Innate protection of ocular surface from viral infection, treatment of ocular surface neoplasms
Growth factors	Transforming growth factor β (TGF-β)	Many cells Leukocytes, T lymphocytes RPE and NPE of ciliary body Pericytes Fibroblasts	Macrophages T lymphocytes RPE Glia Fibroblasts	Suppresses T-lymphocyte and macrophage inflammatory functions Fibrosis of wounds	Regulator of immune privilege and ACAID
	Platelet-derived growth factors (PDGFs)	Platelets Macrophages RPE	Fibroblasts Glia Many others	Fibroblast proliferation	Role in inflammatory membranes, subretinal fibrosis
Neuropeptides	Substance P	Ocular nerves Mast cells	Leukocytes Others	Pain Altered vascular permeability Suppresses macrophage and T-lymphocyte inflammatory function	Altered vascular permeability Leukocyte infiltration, photophobia Role in ACAID and immune privilege
	Vasoactive intestinal peptide	Ocular nerves	Leukocytes Others		

ACAID = anterior chamber–associated immune deviation, NK = natural killer, NPE = nonpigmented epithelium, RPE = retinal pigment epithelium, Th = T helper.

However, although some cytokines are specific for particular cell types, most cytokines have such multiplicity and redundancy of source, function, and target that this focus on specific terminology is not particularly useful for the clinician. For example, activated macrophages in an inflammatory site synthesize growth factors, interleukins, interferons, and chemokines.

Both innate and adaptive responses result in the production of cytokines. T lymphocytes are the classic cytokine-producing cell of adaptive immunity, but macrophages, mast cells, and even neutrophils can synthesize a wide range of cytokines upon stimulation. Cytokine interactions can be additive, combinatorial, synergistic, or antagonistic. Elimination of the action of a single molecule may have an unpredictable outcome; for example, monoclonal antibodies directed against tumor necrosis factor α (TNF-α) result in substantial suppression of immune responses but also increase susceptibility to multiple sclerosis. Finally, not only do innate and adaptive immune responses use cytokines as mediators and amplifiers of inflammation, but cytokines also modulate the initiation of immune responses; the function of most leukocytes is altered by preexposure to various cytokines. Thus, for many cytokines, their regulatory role may be as important as their actions as mediators of inflammation.

Reactive Oxygen Intermediates

Under certain conditions, oxygen can undergo chemical modification to transform into highly reactive substances with the potential to damage cellular molecules and inhibit functional properties in pathogens or host cells. BCSC Section 2, *Fundamentals and Principles of Ophthalmology,* discusses the processes involved in greater detail in Part IV, Biochemistry and Metabolism. See especially Chapter 15, Free Radicals and Antioxidants.

Three of the most important oxygen intermediates are the superoxide anion, hydrogen peroxide, and the hydroxyl radical:

$O_2 + e^- \rightarrow O_2^-$	superoxide anion
$O_2^- + O_2^- + 2H^+ \rightarrow O_2 + H_2O_2$	superoxide dismutase catalyzes anions to form hydrogen peroxide
$H_2O_2 + e^- \rightarrow OH^- + OH\bullet$	hydroxyl anion and hydroxyl radical

Oxygen metabolites that are generated by leukocytes, especially neutrophils and macrophages, and triggered by immune responses are the most important source of free radicals during inflammation. A wide variety of stimuli can trigger leukocyte oxygen metabolism, including

- innate triggers such as LPS or fMLP
- adaptive effectors such as complement-fixing antibodies or certain cytokines produced by activated T lymphocytes
- other chemical mediator systems, such as C5a, PAF, and leukotrienes

Reactive oxygen intermediates can also be generated as part of noninflammatory cellular biochemical processes, especially by electron transport in the mitochondria, detoxification of certain chemicals, or interactions with environmental light or radiation.

Reactive intermediates are highly reactive and thus highly toxic to both living pathogens and to pathogenic mediators such as exotoxins and lipids.

Reactive Nitrogen Products

Another important pathway of host defenses and inflammation involves the toxic products of nitrogen, especially nitric oxide (NO). NO is also a highly reactive chemical species that, like reactive oxygen intermediates, is involved in various important biochemical functions in microorganisms and host cells.

The formation of NO depends on the enzyme nitric oxide synthetase (NOS), which is located in the cytosol and is dependent on NADPH (the reduced form of nicotinamide-adenine dinucleotide phosphate). NO is formed from the terminal guanidino-nitrogen atoms of L-arginine. Several types of NOS are known, including several forms of constitutive NOS and an inducible NOS. Many normal cells produce basal levels of NO, which is considered secondary to the calcium-dependent, constitutive form of the enzyme (constitutive NOS, or cNOS). Activation *induces* enhanced production of NO in certain cells, especially macrophages. This enhanced production appears to be secondary to the induced synthesis of a second, calcium-independent, form of NOS (inducible NOS, or iNOS), Many innate and adaptive stimuli modulate induction of iNOS, especially cytokines and bacterial toxins.

Neutrophil-Derived Granule Products

Neutrophils are also a source of specialized products that can amplify immune responses. A large number of biochemically defined antimicrobial polypeptides are present in many types of granules found in neutrophils. The principal well-characterized antimicrobial polypeptides found in human neutrophil granules are bactericidal/permeability-increasing protein, defensins, lysozyme, lactoferrin, and the serine proteases.

In addition to antimicrobial polypeptides, the neutrophils contain numerous other molecules that may contribute to inflammation. These include hydrolytic enzymes, elastase, metalloproteinases, gelatinase, myeloperoxidase, vitamin B_{12}–binding protein, cytochrome b_{558}, and others. Granule contents are considered to remain inert and membrane-bound when the granules are intact, but they become active and soluble when granules fuse to the phagocytic vesicles or plasma membrane.

An example of the effect of neutrophil-derived granule products is collagenase; collagenases are thought to contribute to corneal injury and liquefaction during bacterial keratitis and scleritis, especially in *Pseudomonas* infections. Collagenases also contribute to peripheral corneal melting syndromes secondary to rheumatoid arthritis–associated peripheral keratitis.

CHAPTER 2

Immunization and Adaptive Immunity: The Immune Response Arc and Immune Effectors

Unlike the innate immune response discussed in the previous chapter, the adaptive immune response is a "learned" response to specific antigens. To understand the clinically relevant features of the adaptive immune response, the reader can consider the sequence of events that follows immunization with antigen using the skin, which is the classic experimental method of introducing antigen to the adaptive immune response (see Clinical Examples 2-1). Several general immunologic concepts, especially the concept of the immune response arc, the primary adaptive immune response, and the secondary adaptive immune response, are involved in this process.

Overview of the Immune Response Arc

Interaction between antigen and the adaptive immune system at a site such as the skin can be subdivided into 3 phases:

1. afferent
2. processing
3. effector

In analogy to the neural reflex arc, the whole process is called the *immune response arc*. Each phase of this immune response arc is analogous to 1 of the 3 phases of the neural reflex arc (Fig 2-1).

In the adaptive immune response, antigen is recognized by antigen presenting cells (APCs) during the *afferent* phase of the immune response. These cells carry antigenic information via the afferent lymphatic channels to the lymph node. There, *processing* of the antigenic signal occurs, resulting in the release of immune messengers (antibodies, B lymphocytes, and T lymphocytes) into efferent lymphatic channels and venous circulation. These molecules and cells are conveyed back to the original site, where an *effector response*

CLINICAL EXAMPLES 2-1

Primary response to poison ivy toxin The first contact between the poison ivy resin urushiol and the epidermis triggers the immunologic mechanisms of poison ivy dermatitis. The *afferent phase* of this primary response begins when the toxin permeates into the epidermis, where it binds to extracellular proteins, forming a protein–toxin conjugate technically called a *hapten.* Some of the toxin is taken up by APCs, especially Langerhans cells (LCs). Over the next 4–18 hours the toxin-stimulated LCs leave the basal epidermis and migrate along afferent lymphatic channels into the draining lymph nodes. During this time, the toxin is internalized into endocytic compartments and processed by the LCs to allow recognition by helper T lymphocytes within the node. Some of the free toxin or hapten is also carried by lymph into the node.

In the lymph node, the *processing phase* begins. The urushiol-stimulated LCs interact with T lymphocytes, seeking over the next 3–5 days the rare T lymphocyte that has the correct specific antigen receptor. Once located, this naive T lymphocyte becomes primed. It is induced to undergo cell division, to acquire new functions such as cytokine secretion, and to up-regulate certain surface molecules and receptors of the plasma membrane. These primed cells ultimately either function as helper cells or become effector cells, which leave the node through efferent lymphatic channels, accumulate in the thoracic duct, and then enter venous blood, where they recirculate.

Free toxin or hapten not taken up by APCs experiences a different fate during the processing phase. It enters a zone of the lymph node populated by B lymphocytes. These naive B lymphocytes express membrane-bound antibody (IgM and IgD) that serves as an antigen receptor. If a chance encounter occurs between the correct antibody and the toxin, the B lymphocyte becomes partially activated. Completion of B-lymphocyte activation requires further interaction with helper T lymphocytes, which release cytokines, inducing B lymphocytes to undergo cell division and to increase production of antibodies, thus releasing antitoxin antibodies into the lymph fluid and ultimately the venous circulation.

The *effector phase* begins when the primed T lymphocytes, primed B lymphocytes, or antibodies leave the lymphatics and enter the peripheral site of the original antigen encounter. By 5–7 days after exposure, much of the urushiol toxin might have already been removed through nonspecific clearance mechanisms such as desquamation of exposed epidermis or washing of involved skin. When toxin-stimulated APCs do remain at the site, primed T lymphocytes become further activated into effector cells, releasing inflammatory mediators to recruit other leukocyte populations. This represents the contact hypersensitivity type of delayed hypersensitivity (DH). Rarely, if adequate free toxin is present, IgG antitoxin immune complexes can form and mediate inflammation. However, if most of the antigen has been cleared, then the primed T lymphocyte may enter the skin but become inactive, retaining memory, or the T lymphocyte may exit the skin through afferent lymphatics to reenter the lymph node. Similarly, antibodies or antibody-producing B lymphocytes may remain in the skin or reach the lymph nodes.

Secondary response to poison ivy toxin The immunologic mechanisms work much faster after the second encounter with poison ivy toxin. The initial steps of the *afferent phase* of this secondary response are identical to those of the initial exposure. However, if a memory T lymphocyte is present at the cutaneous site, then the *processing* and *effector phases* occur within 24 hours at the site, as the memory T lymphocyte becomes activated directly upon interacting with the LC. In addition, some LCs leave the skin, enter the draining node, and encounter memory T lymphocytes there.

Processing during the secondary response is much more rapid, and within 24 hours restimulated memory cells enter the circulation and migrate to the toxin-exposed cutaneous site. Because abundant toxin may remain, additional T lymphocyte–LC stimulation occurs, inducing vigorous T-lymphocyte cytokine production. The inflammatory mediators, in turn, recruit neutrophils and monocytes, leading to a severe inflammatory reaction within 12–36 hours after exposure, causing the typical epidermal blisters of poison ivy. Because the response is delayed by 24 hours, it is considered DH and, in this case, a specific form of DH called *contact hypersensitivity.*

Primary and secondary response to tuberculosis The primary and secondary immune response arcs can occur at different sites, as with the immunologic mechanisms of the first and second encounter with *Mycobacterium tuberculosis* antigens. The afferent phase of the primary response occurs after the inhalation of the live organisms, which proliferate slowly within the lung. Alveolar macrophages ingest the bacteria and transport the organisms to the hilar lymph nodes, where the processing phase begins. Over the next few days, as T and B lymphocytes are primed, the hilar nodes become enlarged because of the increased number of dividing T and B lymphocytes as well as by the generalized increased trafficking of other lymphocytes through the nodes. The effector phase begins when the primed T lymphocytes recirculate and enter the infected lung. The T lymphocytes interact with the macrophage-ingested bacteria, and cytokines are released that activate neighboring macrophages to fuse into giant cells, forming caseating granulomas. Meanwhile, some of the effector T lymphocytes home to other lymph nodes throughout the body, where they become inactive memory T lymphocytes, trafficking and recirculating throughout the secondary lymphoid tissue.

A secondary response using the immune response arc of the skin is the basis of the tuberculin skin test to diagnose tuberculosis. The afferent phase of the secondary response begins when a purified protein derivative (PPD) reagent, antigens purified from mycobacteria, is injected into the dermis, where the PPD is taken up by dermal macrophages. The secondary processing phase begins when these PPD-stimulated macrophages migrate into the draining lymph node, where they encounter memory T lymphocytes from the previous lung infection, leading to reactivation of memory T lymphocytes. The secondary effector phase commences when these reactivated memory T lymphocytes recirculate and home back into the dermis and encounter additional antigen and macrophages at the site, causing the T lymphocytes to become fully activated and release cytokines. Within 24–72 hours, these cytokines induce infiltration of additional lymphocytes and monocytes as well as fibrin clotting. This process produces the typical indurated dermal lesion of the tuberculosis skin test, called the *tuberculin form* of DH.

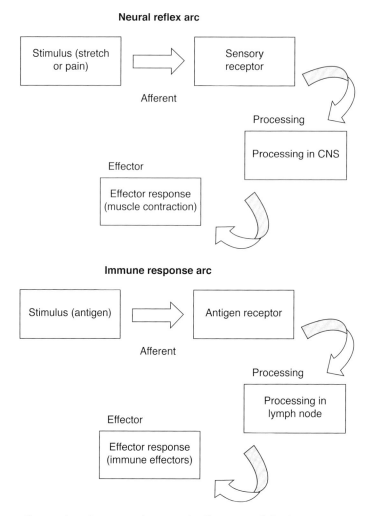

Figure 2-1 Comparison between the neural reflex arc and the immune response arc.

occurs (eg, immune complex formation or delayed hypersensitivity reaction). The following discussion covers the important aspects of each phase in more detail.

Phases of the Immune Response Arc

Afferent Phase

The initial recognition, transport, and presentation of antigenic substances to the adaptive immune system constitute the afferent phase of the immune response arc. The term *antigen* refers to substances recognized by the immune system, resulting in antibody production and development of "sensitized" T lymphocytes. The term *epitope* refers to each specific portion of an antigen to which the immune system can respond. A complex 3-dimensional protein has multiple antigenic epitopes against which antibodies with different paratopes might bind, as well as many other sites that remain invisible to the immune system. The term *paratope* refers to the epitope-specific binding site on the Fab (*fragment, antigen-binding*) portion of the antibody. In addition, antigenic proteins can be enzymatically digested into many different peptide fragments by APCs, some of which then serve as antigenic epitopes for T lymphocytes.

Afferent lymphatic channels

Also simply called *lymphatics,* afferent lymphatic channels are veinlike structures that drain extracellular fluid (ie, lymph) from a site into a regional node. Lymphatics serve 2 major purposes: to convey immune cells and to carry whole antigen from the site of inoculation to a lymph node.

Antigen-presenting cells

APCs are specialized cells that bind and phagocytize antigen at a site. Following ingestion of antigen, APCs migrate to lymph nodes, where they process the antigen, typically by intracellular proteolysis to short amino acid chains of 7 to 11 amino acids. These peptides are then combined with a groove structure in the human leukocyte antigen (HLA) molecules present on the surface of the APC, forming a unique epitope. The combination of peptide and HLA protein is recognized by T-lymphocyte receptors CD4 and CD8, thereby beginning the activation process of adaptive immunity. Different HLA molecules vary in their capacity to bind various peptide fragments within their groove, and thus the HLA type determines the repertoire of peptide antigens capable of being presented to T lymphocytes. Specific HLA alleles are important risk factors for certain forms of uveitis. See Chapter 4 for a more thorough discussion of HLA molecules and disease susceptibility.

Major histocompatibility complex (MHC) class I molecules (ie, HLA-A, -B, and -C) serve as the antigen-presenting platform for CD8 T lymphocytes (Fig 2-2). CD8 T lymphocytes include natural killer T cells and regulatory T cells. Class I molecules are present on almost all nucleated cells. In general, class I APCs are best for processing peptide antigens that have been synthesized by the host cell itself, including most tumor peptides or viral peptides after host cell invasion.

MHC class II molecules (ie, HLA-DR, -DP, and -DQ) serve as the antigen-presenting platform for CD4, or *helper,* T lymphocytes (Fig 2-3). All APCs for CD4 T lymphocytes must express the MHC class II molecule, and the antigen receptor on the helper T lymphocyte can recognize peptide antigens only if they are presented with class II molecules simultaneously. However, only certain cell types express MHC class II molecules on their plasma membrane. Macrophages and dendritic cells are the most important class II APCs. B lymphocytes can also function as class II–dependent APCs, especially within a lymph node. In general, class II–dependent APCs are the most efficient, "professional" APCs for processing extracellular protein antigens that have been endocytosed from the external environment (eg, bacterial or fungal antigens).

Processing Phase

The conversion of the antigenic stimulus into an immunologic response through priming of naive B and T lymphocytes within the lymph nodes and spleen constitutes the processing phase of the immune response arc. This is also called *activation,* or *sensitization,* of

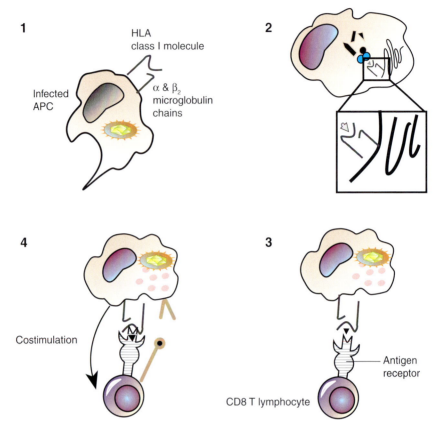

Figure 2-2 Class I–dependent antigen-presenting cells (APCs). **1,** APC is infected by a virus, which causes the cell to synthesize virus-associated peptides that are present in the cytosol. **2,** The viral antigen must be transported (through specialized transporter systems) into the endosomal compartment, where the antigen encounters class I human leukocyte antigen (HLA) molecules. The fragment is placed into the pocket formed by the α chain of the class I HLA molecule. Unlike class II molecules, the second chain, called β₂-microglobulin, is constant among all class I molecules. **3,** The CD8 T-lymphocyte receptor recognizes the fragment–class I complex. **4,** With the help of costimulatory molecules such as CD28-B7 and cytokines, the CD8 T lymphocyte becomes primed, or partially activated. A similar mechanism is used to recognize tumor antigens that are produced by cells after malignant transformation. *(Illustration by Barb Cousins, modified by Joyce Zavarro.)*

lymphocytes. Processing involves regulation of the interaction between antigen and naive lymphocytes (B lymphocytes or T lymphocytes that have not yet encountered their specific antigen), followed by their subsequent activation (Fig 2-4). The following discussion focuses on a few key concepts.

Preconditions necessary for processing

Helper T lymphocytes are the principal cell type for immune processing. Most helper T lymphocytes express CD4 molecules on their cell membrane. T lymphocytes have an antigen receptor that detects antigen only when a trimolecular complex is formed consisting of an APC-HLA molecule, a processed antigen fragment, and a T-lymphocyte antigen receptor. The CD4 molecule stabilizes binding and enhances signaling between the

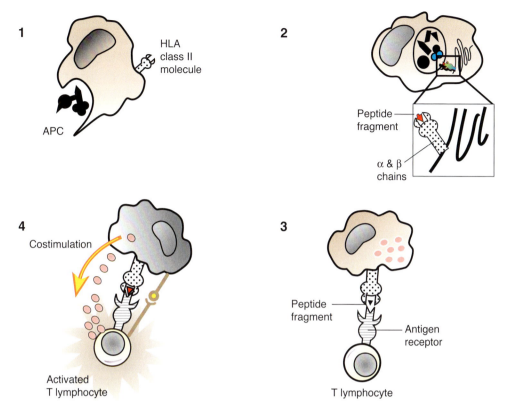

Figure 2-3 Class II–dependent antigen-processing cells (APCs). **1,** APCs endocytose exogenous antigens into the endosomal compartment. **2,** There, the antigen is digested into peptide fragments and placed into the groove formed by the α and β chains of the human leukocyte antigen (HLA) class II molecule. **3,** The CD4 T-lymphocyte receptor recognizes the fragment–class II complex. **4,** With the help of costimulatory molecules such as CD28-B7 and cytokines, the CD4 T lymphocyte becomes primed, or partially activated. *(Illustration by Barb Cousins, modified by Joyce Zavarro.)*

HLA complex and the T-lymphocyte receptor. When helper T lymphocytes specific for an antigen become primed and partially activated, they acquire new functional properties, including cell division, cytokine synthesis, and cell membrane expression of *accessory molecules* such as cell-adhesion molecules and costimulatory molecules. The synthesis and release of immune cytokines, especially interleukin-2 (IL-2), by T lymphocytes is crucial for the progression of initial activation and the functional differentiation of T lymphocytes. The primed T lymphocyte produces IL-2, a potent mitogen, inducing mitosis, with resultant autocrine stimulation.

Helper T-lymphocyte differentiation

At the stage of initial priming, CD4 T lymphocytes are usually classified as T helper-0, or Th0, cells. However, CD4 T lymphocytes can differentiate into functional subsets as a consequence of differences in gene activation and the secretion of specific panels of cytokines. One subset, T helper-1 (Th1), secretes interferon gamma (IFN-γ), tumor necrosis factor β (TNF-β), and IL-12 but *not* IL-4, IL-5, or IL-10. Another subset, T helper-2 (Th2), secretes

Immune processing

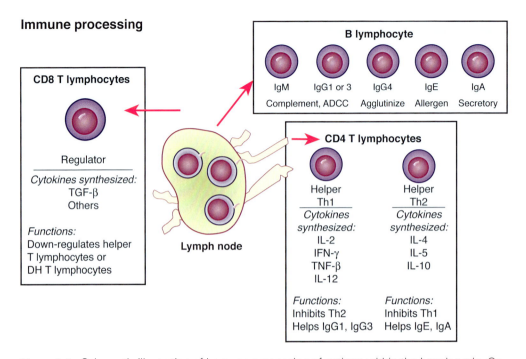

Figure 2-4 Schematic illustration of immune processing of antigen within the lymph node. On exposure to antigen and antigen-presenting cells (APCs) within the lymph node, the 3 major lymphocyte subsets—B lymphocytes, CD4 T lymphocytes, and CD8 T lymphocytes—are activated to release specific cytokines and perform specific functional activities. B lymphocytes are stimulated to produce one of the various antibody isotypes, whose functions include complement activation, antibody-dependent cellular cytotoxicity (ADCC), agglutinization, allergen recognition, and release into secretions. CD4 T lymphocytes become activated into T helper-1 (Th1) or T helper-2 (Th2) subsets. Th1 lymphocytes function to help B lymphocytes secrete immunoglobulin G1 (IgG1) and IgG3; inhibit Th2; and release cytokines such as interleukin-2 (IL-2), interferon gamma (IFN-γ), tumor necrosis factor β (TNF-β), and IL-12. Th2 lymphocytes function to help B lymphocytes secrete IgE and IgA; inhibit Th1 lymphocytes; and synthesize cytokines such as IL-4, IL-5, and IL-10. CD8 T lymphocytes become activated into regulatory T lymphocytes that function by inhibiting other CD4 T lymphocytes, often by secreting cytokines such as transforming growth factor β (TGF-β). *(Illustration by Barb Cousins, modified by Joyce Zavarro.)*

IL-4, IL-5, and IL-10 but not Th1 cytokines. In recent years, 2 additional T-cell subsets have been recognized. Th17 cells are so-named because they produce IL-17, as well as IL-21 and -22. Th17 cells have been implicated in a number of autoimmune conditions, including some forms of uveitis. T regulatory (Treg) cells form another subset of helper T cells; they are identified not by their cytokine profile but by the simultaneous surface expression of CD4, CD25, and Foxp3. Treg cells are essentially suppressor-type T cells that down-regulate other T cell populations. Treg cells appear to be generated in the thymus in development and are essential to self-tolerance, the process by which autoreactive T cells are minimized and their function down-regulated.

These subsets are important because the different cytokines produced by different cell types profoundly influence subsequent "downstream" immune processing, B-lymphocyte antibody synthesis, and cell-mediated effector responses (see the following section). For example, IFN-γ, produced by Th1 lymphocytes, blocks the differentiation and activation of Th2 lymphocytes, and IL-4, produced by Th2 lymphocytes, blocks the differentiation of Th1 lymphocytes. The process determining whether a Th1 or a Th2 response develops consequent to exposure to a particular antigen is not entirely understood, but presumed variables include cytokines preexisting in the microenvironment, the nature of the antigen, the amount of antigen, and the type of APC. For example, IL-12, which is produced by macrophage APCs, might preferentially induce Th1 responses.

Amadi-Obi A, Yu CR, Liu X, Mahdi RM, et al. Th17 cells contribute to uveitis and scleritis and are expanded by IL-2 and inhibited by IL-27/STAT1. *Nat Med.* 2007;13(6):711–718.

Caspi R. Autoimmunity in the immune privileged eye: pathogenic and regulatory T cells. *Immunol Res.* 2008;42(1–3):41–50.

von Andrien UH, Mackay CR. T-cell function and migration. Two sides of the same coin. *N Engl J Med.* 2000;343(14):1020–1034.

B-lymphocyte activation

One of the major regulatory functions for helper T lymphocytes is B-lymphocyte activation. B lymphocytes are responsible for producing antibodies, which are glycoproteins that bind to a specific antigen. B lymphocytes begin as naive lymphocytes with immunoglobulin M (IgM) and IgD on the cell surface; these serve as the B-lymphocyte antigen receptor. Through these surface antibodies, B lymphocytes can detect epitopes on intact antigens and thus do not require antigen processing by APCs. After appropriate stimulation of the B-lymphocyte antigen receptor, helper T lymphocyte–B lymphocyte interaction occurs, leading to further B-lymphocyte activation and differentiation. B lymphocytes acquire new functional properties, such as cell division, cell surface expression of accessory molecules, and the ability to synthesize and release large quantities of antibodies. Most important, activated B lymphocytes acquire the ability to change antibody class from IgM to another class (eg, to IgG1, IgA, or another immunoglobulin). This shift requires a molecular change of the immunoglobulin heavy chain class, and this is regulated by specific cytokines released by the helper T lymphocyte. For example, treatment of an antigen-primed B lymphocyte with IFN-γ induces a switch from IgM to IgG1 production. Treatment with IL-4 induces a switch from IgM to IgE production.

Role of regulatory T lymphocytes

The immunoregulatory role of regulatory (or suppressor) T lymphocytes has become partially clarified, especially through the induction of immunomodulatory cytokine synthesis by regulatory T lymphocytes. Originally, regulatory T lymphocytes were thought to express the CD8 marker and to become activated during the initial phases of processing. More recently, Treg $CD4^+$ $CD25^+$ $Foxp3^+$ T lymphocytes have also been observed to have regulatory functions. In many cases, both CD8 and CD4 regulatory T lymphocytes appear to operate by the release of immunomodulatory cytokines such as transforming growth factor β, which can inhibit or alter the effector function of other T lymphocytes. Regulatory T lymphocytes are potentially important as they may provide a means for induction of tolerance to specific antigens.

Effector Phase

During the effector phase, the adaptive immune response (eg, the elimination of offending foreign antigen) is physically carried out. Antigen-specific effectors exist in 2 major subsets:

- T lymphocytes
- B lymphocytes plus their antibodies

In general, effector lymphocytes require 2 exposures to antigen. The initial exposure, often called *priming* or *activation,* occurs in the lymph node. A second exposure, often called *restimulation,* occurs in the peripheral tissue in which the initial antigen contact occurred. This second exposure is usually necessary to fully activate the effector mechanism within a local tissue.

Subsets of effector T lymphocytes can be divided into 2 main types by functional differences in experimental assays or by differences in cell surface molecules (Fig 2-5). *Delayed hypersensitivity* (DH) T lymphocytes usually express CD4 (and so recognize antigen with MHC class II) and release IFN-γ and TNF-β. They function by homing to a tissue, recognizing antigen and APCs, becoming fully activated, and releasing cytokines and

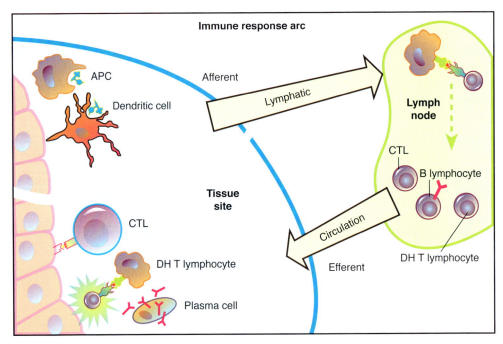

Figure 2-5 Schematic representation of effector mechanisms during adaptive immunity. Not only is the immune response initiated within the tissue site, but ultimately the immune response arc is completed when effectors encounter antigen within the tissue after release into the circulation from the lymph node. The 3 most important effector mechanisms of adaptive immunity include cytotoxic T lymphocytes (CTLs), delayed hypersensitivity (DH) T lymphocytes, and antibody-producing B lymphocytes, especially plasma cells. APC = antigen-presenting cell. *(Illustration by Barb Cousins, modified by Joyce Zavarro.)*

mediators that then recruit other nonspecific, antigen-independent effector cells such as neutrophils, basophils, or monocytes. As with helper T lymphocytes, Th1 and Th2 types of DH effector cells have been identified.

Cytotoxic T lymphocytes are the other major type of effector T lymphocyte. Cytotoxic T lymphocytes express CD8 and serve as effector cells for killing tumors or virally infected host cells through release of cytotoxic cytokines or specialized pore-forming molecules. A third subset of effector lymphocytes, grouped as non-T, non-B lymphocytes, includes natural killer cells, lymphokine-activated cells, and killer cells.

Antibodies, or *immunoglobulins,* are soluble antigen-specific effector molecules of adaptive immunity. After appropriate antigenic stimulation with T-lymphocyte help, B lymphocytes secrete IgM antibodies and, later, other isotypes, into the efferent lymph fluid draining into the venous circulation. Antibodies then mediate a variety of immune effector activities by combining with antigen in the blood or in tissues.

Immune Response Arc and Primary or Secondary Immune Response

Concept of Immunologic Memory

Immunologic memory is probably the most distinctive feature of adaptive immune responses; protective immunization is the prototypical example of this powerful phenomenon. Classically, immunologic "memory" was the concept used to explain why serum antibody production for a specific antigen began much more quickly and rose to much higher levels after reexposure to that antigen but not after exposure to a different antigen. Later it was learned that memory applied not only to antibody production by B lymphocytes but also to that by T lymphocytes.

Differences in primary and secondary responses

The idea of an *anamnestic response* posits that the second encounter with an antigen is regulated differently from the first encounter. Differences in the primary and secondary immune response arc, especially in the processing and effector phases, offer partial explanation. During the processing phase of the primary response, antigen must find the relatively rare specific B lymphocyte (perhaps 1 in 100,000) and T lymphocyte (perhaps 1 in 10,000) and then stimulate these cells from a completely resting and naive state, a sequence that requires days. The secondary processing response for T and B lymphocytes is shorter for at least 3 reasons:

- Upon removal of antigen, T and B lymphocytes activated during the primary response may gradually return to a resting state, but they retain the capacity to become reactivated within 12–24 hours of antigen exposure. They are now memory cells rather than naive cells.
- Because stimulated lymphocytes divide, the population of potential antigen-responsive T or B lymphocytes will have increased manyfold, and these cells will have migrated to other sites of potential encounters with antigen.

- In some cases, such as in mycobacterial infection, low doses of antigen may remain in the node or site, producing a chronic, low-level, continuous antigenic stimulation of T and B lymphocytes.

For antibody responses, another memory function dependent on antibody requires even less time and operates primarily at the level of the effector phase. IgM produced during the effector phase of the primary response and released into the blood is often too large a molecule (at 900 kDa molecular weight) to passively leak into a peripheral site. However, during the secondary response, antibody class switching has occurred so that IgG or other isotypes that passively leaked into a site or have been actively produced there can immediately combine with an antigen, causing the secondary response triggered by antibody to be very rapid *(immediate hypersensitivity)*.

Homing

Memory also requires that lymphocytes demonstrate a complex migratory pattern called *homing*. Thus, lymphocytes pass from the circulation into various tissues, from which they subsequently depart, and then pass by way of lymphatics to reenter the circulation. Homing involves the dynamic interaction between lymphocytes and endothelial cells using multiple cell-adhesion molecules. Usually, the major types of lymphocytes that migrate into tissue sites are memory lymphocytes that express higher levels of certain cell-adhesion molecules, such as the integrins, than do naive cells. In contrast, naive lymphocytes tend to migrate to lymphoid tissues, where they have the chance of meeting their cognate antigen. Inflammation, however, changes the rules and serves to break down homing patterns. At inflammatory sites, the volume of lymphocyte migration is far greater and selection much less precise, although migration of memory cells or activated lymphocytes still exceeds that of naive cells.

Effector Reactivities of Adaptive Immunity

Although most adaptive (or innate) immune responses are protective and occur subclinically, when adaptive immune responses do cause inflammation, these responses have classically been called *immune hypersensitivity reactions.* The traditional classification for describing the 4 mechanisms of adaptive immune-triggered inflammatory responses—namely, anaphylaxis, cytotoxic antibodies, immune complex reactions, and cell-mediated reactions—was elaborated by Coombs and Gell in 1962, and a fifth category, *stimulatory hypersensitivity,* was added later (Table 2-1). This system is of historical importance and familiarity with it is important in interpretation of much older literature. However, this

Table 2-1 Types of Hypersensitivity (Coombs and Gell)

Type I	Anaphylaxis
Type II	Cytotoxic antibodies
Type III	Immune complex reactions
Type IV	Cell-mediated reactions
Type V	Stimulatory hypersensitivity

classification was developed before T lymphocytes had been discovered, in a time when understanding was limited to antibody-triggered mechanisms. In addition, it is unlikely that any effector mechanism in a disease process represents only 1 type of response. For example, all antibody-dependent mechanisms require a processing phase using helper T lymphocytes, which may also contribute to effector responses. Finally, the term *hypersensitivity* may obscure the concept that many of these same mechanisms are often protective and noninflammatory.

Delves PJ, Martin S, Burton D, Roitt IM. *Roitt's Essential Immunology.* 11th ed. Malden, MA: Blackwell; 2006.

Goldsby RA, Kindt TJ, Osborne BA, Kuby J. *Immunology.* 5th ed. New York, NY: WH Freeman; 2003.

Male DK, Cooke A, Owen M, Trowsdale J, Champion B. *Advanced Immunology.* 3rd ed. St Louis, MO: Mosby; 1996.

Antibody-Mediated Immune Effector Responses

Structural and functional properties of antibody molecules

Structural features of immunoglobulins Five major classes (M, G, A, E, and D) of immunoglobulin exist in 9 different subclasses, or isotypes (IgG1, IgG2, IgG3, IgG4, IgM, IgA1, IgA2, IgE, and IgD). The basic immunoglobulin structure is composed of 4 covalently bonded glycoprotein chains that form a monomer of approximately 150,000–180,000 daltons (Fig 2-6). Each antibody monomer contains 2 identical light chains, either kappa (κ) or lambda (λ), and 2 identical heavy chains from 1 of the 9 structurally distinct subclasses

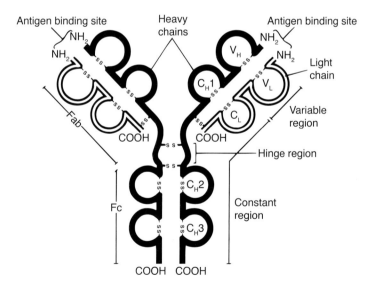

Figure 2-6 Schematic representation of an immunoglobulin molecule. The *solid lines* indicate the identical 2 heavy chains; the *open lines* indicate the identical light chains; *-s-s-* indicates intrachain and interchain covalent disulfide bonds. *(Reprinted with permission from* Dorland's Illustrated Medical Dictionary. *28th ed. Philadelphia, PA: WB Saunders; 1994:824.)*

of immunoglobulins. Thus, the heavy chain type defines the specific isotype (Table 2-2). IgM can form pentamers or hexamers in vivo, and IgA can form dimers in secretions, so the molecular size of these 2 classes in vivo is much larger than that of the others.

Each monomer has analogous regions called *domains*. Certain domains carry out specific functions of the antibody molecule. In particular, the Fab region on each molecule contains the antigen recognition-combining domain, called the *hypervariable region*. The opposite end of the molecule, on the heavy chain portion, contains the attachment site for effector cells (the *Fc portion*); it also contains the site of other effector functions, such as complement activation (for IgG3) or binding to the secretory component so it can be transported through epithelia and secreted into tears (for IgA). Table 2-2 summarizes the important structural differences among immunoglobulin isotypes.

Functional properties of immunoglobulins The immunoglobulin isotypes do not all mediate the effector functions of antibody activity equally. For example, human IgM and IgG3 are good complement activators, but IgG4 is not. Only IgA1 and IgA2 can bind the secretory component and thus be actively passed into mucosal secretions after transport through the epithelial cell from the subepithelial location, where they are synthesized by B lymphocytes. Other isotypes must remain in the subepithelial tissue. The importance of these differences is that 2 antibodies with the identical capacity to bind to an antigen, but of different isotype, will produce different effector and inflammatory outcomes.

Terminology

Clonality Each B cell creates, via genetic recombination, a unique Fab fragment that will recognize a unique antigen. B cells can therefore react to a particular protein or antigen, and different B cells responding to different epitopes produce antibodies specific to that epitope. The reactivity of all the antibodies in a serum is termed the *polyclonal response*. Modern molecular biologic techniques allow the amplification of a single B-cell clone and production of large amounts of a single, molecularly clonal, antibody. Such antibodies are called *monoclonal*. "Biologic" drugs such as infliximab, daclizumab, adalimumab, and rituximab are recombinant monoclonal antibodies.

Idiotypes Various regions of an antibody can themselves be antigenic. These antigenic sites are called *idiotopes,* as distinguished from *epitopes,* the antigenic sites on foreign molecules. Antibodies to idiotopes are called *idiotypes*. Anti-idiotypic antibodies might be important feedback mechanisms for immune regulation. For example, infliximab is a monoclonal humanized antibody to tumor necrosis factor α (TNF-α) and is used to treat some forms of uveitis. Efficacy of this drug may be limited by the development of anti-idiotype antibodies that neutralize the antigen binding site for TNF-α.

Infiltration of B lymphocytes into tissues and local production of antibody

B-lymphocyte infiltration B lymphocytes can infiltrate the site of an immunologic reaction in response to persistent antigenic stimulus, leading to a clinical picture of moderate to severe inflammation. If the process becomes chronic, plasma cell formation occurs, representing fully differentiated B lymphocytes that have become dedicated to antibody synthesis. In both of these cases, local production of antibody specific for the inciting antigen(s) occurs within the site. If the antigen is known, as for certain presumed infections, local antibody formation can be used as a diagnostic test.

Table 2-2 Structural and Functional Properties of Immunoglobulin Isotypes

Immunoglobulin Isotype (Heavy Chain)	% of Total Serum Igs	Structural Properties		Functional Properties		
		Relative Size	Other Structural Features	Activates Complement	Fc Receptor Binding Preferences	Other Functions
IgD δ	<1%	Monomer	Mostly on surface of B lymphocytes	No		B-lymphocyte antigen receptor
IgM μ	5%	Pentamer or hexamer	Mostly on B lymphocytes or intravascular	Strong (classic pathway)		B-lymphocyte antigen receptor, agglutinization, neutralization, intravascular cytolysis
IgG1 γ	50%	Monomer	Intravascular, in tissues, crosses placenta	Moderate (classic pathway)	Monocytes	Cytolysis
IgG2 γ	18%	Monomer	Same as IgG1	Weak (classic pathway)	Neutrophil monocytes, killer lymphocytes	ADCC
IgG3 γ	6%	Monomer	Same as IgG1	Strong (classic pathway)	Neutrophil monocytes, killer lymphocytes	ADCC, agglutinization, cytolysis
IgG4 γ	3%	Monomer	Same as IgG1	No		Neutralization
IgE ε	<<1%	Monomer	Mostly in skin or mucosa, bound to mast cells	No	Mast cells	Mast-cell degranulation
IgA1 α	15%	Mostly monomer in serum, dimer in secretions	In mucosal secretions, binds secretory component in subepithelial tissues for transepithelial transport and protection from proteolysis	Moderate (alternative pathway)		Mucosal immunity, neutralization
IgA2 α	3%	Same as IgA1	Same as IgA1	Same as IgA1		

ADCC = antibody-dependent cellular cytotoxicity.

Differentiation between local production of antibody and passive leakage from the blood involves calculation of the *Goldmann-Witmer (GW) coefficient,* which is generated by comparison of the ratio of intraocular fluid to serum antibody concentration for the specific antibody in question to the intraocular fluid to serum ratio of total immunoglobulin levels. Theoretically, a coefficient above 1.0 would indicate local production of antibodies within the eye. In practice, however, positive quotients above 3.0 are used most often to improve specificity and positive predictive value. See Clinical Example 2-2.

Local antibody production within a tissue and chronic inflammation Persistence of antigen within a site, coupled with infiltration of specific B lymphocytes and local antibody formation, can produce a chronic inflammatory reaction with a complicated histologic pattern, often demonstrating lymphocytic infiltration, plasma cell infiltration, and granulomatous features. This process is sometimes called the *chronic Arthus reaction.* This mechanism may contribute to the pathophysiology of certain chronic autoimmune disorders, such as rheumatoid arthritis, which feature formation of pathogenic antibodies.

Foster CS, Streilein JW. Immune-mediated tissue injury. In: Albert DM, Jakobiec FA, Azar DT, Gragoudas ES, eds. *Principles and Practice of Ophthalmology.* 2nd ed. Philadelphia, PA: WB Saunders; 2000:74–82.

Lymphocyte-Mediated Effector Responses

Delayed hypersensitivity T lymphocytes

Delayed hypersensitivity (Coombs and Gell type IV) represents the prototypical adaptive immune mechanism for lymphocyte-triggered inflammation. It is especially powerful in secondary immune responses. Previously primed DH CD4 T lymphocytes leave the lymph node, home into local tissues where antigen persists, and become activated by further restimulation with the specific priming antigen and MHC class II–expressing

---

CLINICAL EXAMPLE 2-2

Identification of rubella virus reactivity in Fuchs heterochromic iridocyclitis
Fuchs heterochromic iridocyclitis (FHI) is a unilateral chronic anterior uveitis that frequently features elevated intraocular pressure, early cataract, and iris atrophy leading to heterochromia. By sampling aqueous at time of cataract surgery, Quentin and Rieber were able to demonstrate markedly elevated intraocular IgG titers to rubella virus in 52 eyes of patients with FHI compared with that found in 50 control subjects. The average GW coefficient (local antibody titer) was 20.6 in patients with FHI compared with less than 1.4 in control subjects. The authors found that a cutoff of 1.5 identified all subjects with FHI and no control subjects (although studies of other diseases suggest a cutoff of 3.0 may have better specificity).

Quentin CD, Reiber H. Fuchs heterochromic cyclitis: rubella virus antibodies and genome in aqueous humor. *Am J Ophthalmol.* 2004; 138(1):46–54.

APCs. Fully activated DH T lymphocytes secrete mediators and cytokines, leading to the recruitment and activation of macrophages or other nonspecific leukocytes (Fig 2-7). The term *delayed* for this type of hypersensitivity refers to the fact that the reaction becomes maximal 12–48 hours after antigen exposure.

Analysis of experimental animal models and the histologic changes of human inflammation suggest that different subtypes of DH might exist. One of the most important determinants of the pattern of DH reaction is the subtype of DH CD4 effector T cells that

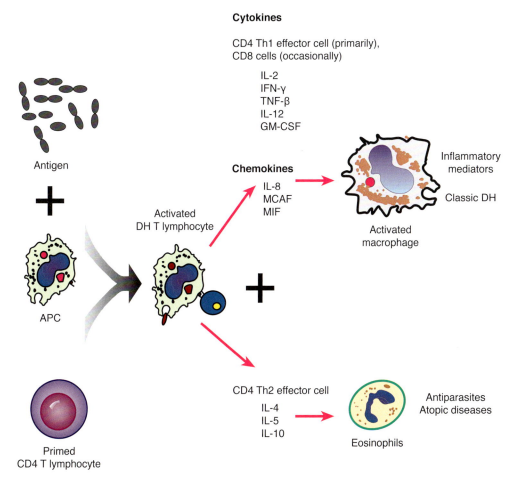

Figure 2-7 Schematic representation of the 2 major forms of delayed hypersensitivity (DH). CD4 T lymphocytes, having undergone initial priming in the lymph node, enter the tissue site, where they again encounter antigen-presenting cells (APCs) and antigen. Upon restimulation, they become activated into either T helper-1 (Th1) or T helper-2 (Th2) effector cells. Th1 lymphocytes are the classic DH effector cells, which are associated with most severe forms of inflammation. Th2 lymphocytes are thought to be less intensively inflammatory, but they have been associated with parasite-induced granulomas and atopic diseases. IFN = interferon, IL = interleukin, GM-CSF = granulocyte-macrophage colony-stimulating factor, MCAF = monocyte chemotactic and activating factor, MIF = macrophage migration inhibiting factor, TNF = tumor necrosis factor. *(Illustration by Barb Cousins, modified by Joyce Zavarro.)*

mediate the reaction. Just as helper T lymphocytes can be differentiated into 2 groups—Th1 and Th2 subsets—according to the spectrum of cytokines secreted, DH T lymphocytes can also be grouped by the same criteria. Experimentally, the Th1 subset of cytokines, especially IFN-γ (also known as *macrophage-activating factor*) and TNF-β, activates macrophages to secrete inflammatory mediators and kill pathogens, thus amplifying inflammation. Th1-mediated DH mechanisms, therefore, are thought to produce the following:

- the classic DH reaction (eg, the PPD skin reaction)
- immunity to intracellular infections (eg, to mycobacteria or *Pneumocystis* organisms)
- immunity to fungi
- most forms of severe T-lymphocyte–mediated autoimmune diseases
- chronic transplant rejection

Table 2-3 summarizes ocular inflammatory diseases thought to require a major contribution of Th1 DH effector mechanisms.

The Th2 subset of DH cells secretes IL-4, IL-5, and other cytokines. IL-4 can induce B lymphocytes to synthesize IgE, and IL-5 can recruit and activate eosinophils within a site. IL-4 can also induce macrophage granulomas in response to parasite-derived antigens. Thus, Th2-mediated DH mechanisms are thought to play a major role in the following:

- response to parasite infections
- late-phase responses of allergic reactions
- asthma
- atopic dermatitis or other manifestations of atopic diseases

The persistence of certain infectious agents, especially bacteria within intracellular compartments of APCs or certain extracellular parasites, can cause destructive induration

Table 2-3 Ocular Inflammatory Diseases Thought to Require a Major Contribution of Th1-Mediated DH Effector Mechanisms

Site	Disease	Presumed Antigen
Conjunctiva	Contact hypersensitivity to contact lens solutions	Thimerosal or other chemicals
	Giant papillary conjunctivitis	Unknown
	Phlyctenulosis	Bacterial antigens
Cornea and sclera	Chronic allograft rejection	Histocompatibility antigens
	Marginal infiltrates of blepharitis	Bacterial antigens
	Disciform keratitis after viral infection	Viral antigens
Anterior uvea	Acute anterior uveitis	Uveal autoantigens, bacterial antigens
	Sarcoidosis-associated uveitis	Unknown
	Intermediate uveitis	Unknown
Retina and choroid	Sympathetic ophthalmia	Retinal or uveal autoantigens
	Vogt-Koyanagi-Harada syndrome	Retinal or uveal autoantigens
	Birdshot retinochoroidopathy	Unknown
Orbit	Acute thyroid orbitopathy	Unknown
	Giant cell arteritis	Unknown

with granuloma formation and giant cells, termed the *granulomatous* form of DH. However, immune complex deposition and innate immune mechanisms in response to heavy metal or foreign-body reactions can also cause granulomatous inflammation, in which the inflammatory cascade (resulting in DH) is triggered in the absence of specific T lymphocytes. Unfortunately, for most clinical entities in which T-lymphocyte responses are suspected, especially autoimmune disorders such as multiple sclerosis or rheumatoid arthritis, the precise immunologic mechanism remains highly speculative. See Clinical Examples 2-3.

Cytotoxic lymphocytes

Cytotoxic T lymphocytes Cytotoxic T lymphocytes (CTLs) are a subset of antigen-specific T lymphocytes, usually bearing the CD8 marker, that are especially good at killing tumor cells and virus-infected cells. CTLs can also mediate graft rejection and some types of autoimmunity. In most cases, the ideal antigen for CTLs is an intracellular protein that either occurs naturally or is produced as a result of viral infection. CTLs appear to require help from CD4 helper T-lymphocyte signals to fully differentiate. Primed *precursor* CTLs leave the lymph node and migrate to the target tissue, where they are restimulated by the interaction of the CTL antigen receptor and foreign antigens within the antigen pocket of MHC class I molecules (HLA-A, -B, or -C) on the target cell. Additional CD4 T lymphocytes help at the site, and expression of other accessory costimulatory molecules on the target is often required to obtain maximal killing.

CTLs kill cells in 1 of 2 ways: assassination or suicide induction (Fig 2-8). *Assassination* refers to CTL-mediated lysis of targets; a specialized pore-forming protein called *perforin,* which puts pores, or holes, into cell membranes, causes osmotic lysis of the cell. *Suicide induction* refers to the capability of CTLs to stimulate programmed cell death of target cells, called *apoptosis,* using the CD95 ligand (the FasL) to activate its receptor on targets. Alternatively, CTLs can release cytotoxic cytokines such as TNF to induce apoptosis. CTLs produce low-grade lymphocytic infiltrate within tumors or infected tissues and usually kill without causing significant inflammation.

Natural killer cells Natural killer (NK) cells are a subset of non-T, non-B lymphocytes. They also kill tumor cells and virus-infected cells, but unlike CTLs, NK cells do not have a specific antigen receptor. Instead, they are triggered by a less well-characterized NK cell receptor. Once triggered, however, NK cells kill target cells using the same molecular mechanisms as CTLs. Because NK cells are not antigen-specific, they theoretically have the advantage of not requiring the time delay caused by induction of the adaptive, antigen-specific CTL immune response. However, NK cells do seem to require some of the same effector activation signals at the tissue site, especially cytokine stimulation. Thus, NK cells are probably most effective in combination with adaptive effector responses.

Combined Antibody and Cellular Effector Mechanisms

Antibody-dependent cellular cytotoxicity

An antibody can combine with a cell-associated antigen such as a tumor or viral antigen, but if the antibody is not a subclass that activates complement, it may not induce any apparent cytotoxicity. However, because the Fc tail of the antibody is externally exposed,

CLINICAL EXAMPLES 2-3

***Toxocara* granuloma (Th2 DH)** *Toxocara canis* is a nematode parasite that infects up to 2% of all children worldwide and may occasionally produce inflammatory vitreoretinal manifestations. Although the ocular immunology of this disorder is not clearly delineated, animal models and a study of the immunopathogenesis of human nematode infections at other sites suggest the following scenario. The primary immune response begins in the gut after ingestion of viable eggs, which mature into larvae within the intestine. The primary processing phase produces a strong Th2 response, leading to a primary effector response that includes production of IgM, IgG, and IgE antibodies, as well as Th2-mediated DH T lymphocytes. Accidental avoidance of immune effector mechanisms may result in hematogenous dissemination of a few larvae to the choroid or retina, followed by invasion into the retina and/or vitreous. There, a Th2-mediated T-lymphocyte effector response recognizes larva antigens and releases Th2-derived cytokines to induce eosinophil and macrophage infiltration, causing the characteristic eosinophilic granuloma seen in the eye. In addition, antilarval B lymphocytes can infiltrate the eye and are induced to secrete various immunoglobulins, especially IgE. Finally, eosinophils, in part by attachment through Fc receptors, can recognize IgE or IgG bound to parasites and release cytotoxic granules containing the antiparasitic cationic protein directly in the vicinity of the larvae, using a mechanism similar to antibody-dependent cellular cytotoxicity.

> Grencis RK. Th2-mediated host protective immunity to intestinal nematode infections. *Philos Trans R Soc Lond Biol Sci.* 1997;352(1359): 1377–1384.

Sympathetic ophthalmia (Th1 DH) Sympathetic ophthalmia is a bilateral panuveitis that follows penetrating trauma to 1 eye (see Chapter 6 for a more detailed discussion). This disorder represents one of the few human diseases in which autoimmunity can be directly linked to an initiating event. In most cases, penetrating injury activates the afferent phase. It is unclear whether the injury causes a de novo primary immunization to self-antigens, perhaps because of externalization of sequestered uveal antigens through the wound and exposure to the afferent immune response arc of the conjunctiva or extraocular sites, or if it instead somehow changes the immunologic microenvironment of the retina, retinal pigment epithelium (RPE), and uvea so that a secondary afferent response is initiated that serves to alter preexisting tolerance to retinal and uveal self-antigens.

It is generally thought that the inflammatory effector response is dominated by a Th1-mediated DH mechanism generated in response to uveal or retinal antigens. CD4 T lymphocytes predominate early in the disease course, although CD8, or suppressor, T lymphocytes can be numerous in chronic cases. Activated macrophages are also numerous in granulomas, and Th1 cytokines have been identified in the vitreous or produced by T lymphocytes recovered from the eyes of affected patients. Although the target antigen for sympathetic ophthalmia is unknown, cutaneous immunization in experimental animals with certain retinal antigens (arrestin, rhodopsin, interphotoreceptor retinoid–binding protein), RPE-associated antigens, and melanocyte-associated tyrosinase can induce autoimmune uveitis with physiology or features suggestive of sympathetic ophthalmia. Th1-mediated DH is thought to mediate many forms of ocular inflammation. Table 2-3 lists other examples.

Boyd SR, Young S, Lightman S. Immunopathology of the noninfectious posterior and intermediate uveitides. *Surv Ophthalmol.* 2001;46(3): 209–233.

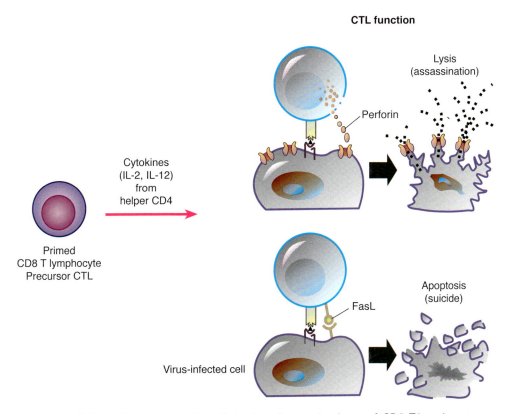

Figure 2-8 Schematic representation of the 2 major mechanisms of CD8 T-lymphocyte cytotoxicity. CD8 T lymphocytes, having undergone initial priming in the lymph node, enter the tissue site, where they again encounter antigen in the form of infected target cells. Upon restimulation, usually requiring CD4 helper T-lymphocyte factors, they become activated into fully cytolytic T lymphocytes. Cytotoxic lymphocytes (CTLs) can kill by lysing the infected cell using a pore-forming protein called perforin or by inducing programmed cell death, or *apoptosis*, using either FasL or cytokine-mediated mechanisms. *(Illustration by Barb Cousins, modified by Joyce Zavarro.)*

various leukocytes can recognize the Fc domain of the antibody molecule and be directed to the cell through the antibody. When this happens, binding to the antibody activates various leukocyte cytotoxic mechanisms, including degranulation and cytokine production.

Because human leukocytes can express various types of Fc receptors—IgG subclasses have 3 different Fcg receptors, IgE has 2 different Fce receptors, and so on—leukocyte subsets differ in their capacity to recognize and bind different antibody isotypes. Classically, *antibody-dependent cellular cytotoxicity* (ADCC) was observed to be mediated by a special subset of large granular (non-T, non-B) lymphocytes, called *killer cells,* that induce cell death in a manner similar to CTLs. The killer cell itself is nonspecific but gains antigen specificity through interaction with specific antibody. Macrophages, NK cells, certain T lymphocytes, and neutrophils can also participate in ADCC using other Fc receptor types. An IgE-dependent form of ADCC might also exist for eosinophils.

ADCC is presumed to be important in tumor surveillance, antimicrobial host protection, graft rejection, and certain autoimmune diseases such as cutaneous systemic lupus erythematosus. However, this effector mechanism probably does not play an important role in uveitis, although it might contribute to corneal graft rejection and antiparasitic immunity.

Acute IgE-mediated mast-cell degranulation

Mast cells can bind IgE antibodies to their surface through a high-affinity Fc receptor specific for IgE molecules, positioning the antigen-combining site of the bound IgE externally (Fig 2-9). The combining of 2 adjacent IgE antibody molecules with a specific allergen (see Clinical Examples 2-4) causes degranulation of the mast cell and release of mediators within minutes, producing an acute inflammatory reaction called *immediate hypersensitivity* (Coombs and Gell type I), which is characterized by local plasma leakage

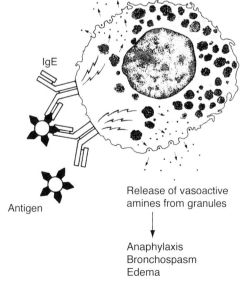

Figure 2-9 Schematic representation of IgE-mediated mast cell degranulation.

IgE

Antigen

Release of vasoactive amines from granules

Anaphylaxis
Bronchospasm
Edema

and itching. When severe, this response can produce a systemic reaction called *anaphylaxis*, which ranges in severity from generalized skin lesions such as erythema, urticaria, or angioedema to severely altered vascular permeability with plasma leakage into tissues that causes airway obstruction or hypotensive shock.

CLINICAL EXAMPLES 2-4

Allergic conjunctivitis Allergic conjunctivitis is an atopic (out of place or inappropriate) immune response to a family of antigens called *allergens,* ordinarily harmless and tolerated by most humans, that induce predominantly an acute IgE–mast-cell effector response in individuals genetically destined to be "allergic" to such substances. The primary response presumably has occurred during a prior exposure to the allergen, often within the nasopharynx, during which afferent and processing phases were initiated. During this primary response, allergen-specific B lymphocytes were distributed to specialized areas in various mucosa-associated lymphoid tissue (MALT) sites. At these sites, the B lymphocytes, with T-lymphocyte help, switch from IgM-antiallergen production to IgE-antiallergen production. IgE released at the site then combines with the Fc receptors of mast cells, thereby "arming" the mast cells with a specific allergen receptor (ie, the antigen-recognizing Fab portion of the IgE). Thus, 1 mast cell may have bound IgE specific for numerous different allergens.

When reexposure to allergen occurs, it must permeate beyond the superficial conjunctival epithelium to the subepithelial region, where the antigen binds allergen-specific IgE on the surface of mast cells. Degranulation occurs within 60 minutes, leading to the release of mediators, most particularly histamine, causing chemosis and itching. A late response, within 4–24 hours, is characterized by the recruitment of lymphocytes, eosinophils, and neutrophils. The role of Th2 DH or helper T lymphocytes in the effector response has not been confirmed for allergic conjunctivitis, but presumably both play a role, especially in B-lymphocyte differentiation, because the IgE is thought to be produced locally within the conjunctiva.

Atopic keratoconjunctivitis Atopic keratoconjunctivitis (AKC) is a complex, vision-threatening ocular allergy with chronic inflammation of the palpebral and bulbar conjunctiva with both immediate and delayed cell-mediated inflammation (see BCSC Section 8, *External Disease and Cornea*). Analysis of biopsy specimens reveals the inflammatory infiltration to consist of mast cells and eosinophils, as well as activated CD4 T lymphocytes and B lymphocytes. Although the immunopathogenesis is not clearly defined, a mechanism similar to that of atopic dermatitis can be inferred, combining poorly understood genetic mechanisms, chronic mast-cell degranulation, and features of Th2-type DH. The immunopathogenesis of vernal conjunctivitis and giant papillary conjunctivitis is probably also similar. The eosinophil, with its highly toxic cytokines, eosinophil major basic protein and eosinophil cationic protein, is the effector cell most responsible for corneal damage and vision loss in patients with AKC.

CHAPTER 3

Ocular Immune Responses

Regional Immunity and Immunologic Microenvironments

Regional Immunity

The idea that each organ and tissue site has its own particular immune response arc, which may vary significantly from the classic cutaneous response, is called *regional immunity*. Regional immunity of the tissue site can characterize all 3 phases—afferent, processing, and effector—of the responses involved. For instance, the immune response arc for oral immunization (eg, polio vaccine) differs from that for intramuscular immunization (eg, mumps/measles/rubella vaccine), which differs from that for cutaneous vaccination (eg, bacille Calmette-Guérin vaccine). Regional immunity also affects the transplantation of donor tissue, such as a kidney or cornea. Such transplantations require the recipient to produce afferent, processing, and effector responses to the transplant, all modified by the unique location.

Just as regional differences in immune responses occur because of differences in the immunologic microenvironments of various tissue sites, regional differences can be identified for specific locations within and around the eye. Immune responses in health and disease are affected by differences in the immunologic microenvironment (Table 3-1) in such areas as the

- conjunctiva
- anterior chamber, anterior uvea (iris and ciliary body), and vitreous
- cornea and sclera
- retina, retinal pigment epithelium (RPE), and choriocapillaris
- choroid

Immune Responses of the Conjunctiva

Features of the Immunologic Microenvironment

The conjunctiva shares many of the features typical of mucosal sites. It is composed of 2 layers: an epithelial layer and a connective tissue layer called the *substantia propria*. The conjunctiva is well vascularized and has good lymphatic drainage to preauricular and submandibular nodes. The tissue is richly invested with Langerhans cells, other dendritic cells, and macrophages that serve as potential antigen-presenting cells (APCs). Conjunctival

Table 3-1 Comparison of Immune Microenvironments in Various Normal Ocular Sites

	Conjunctiva	Cornea, Sclera	Anterior Chamber, Anterior Uvea, Vitreous	Subretina, RPE, Choroid
Anatomical features	Lymphatics, follicles	Lymphatics at limbus, none centrally Macromolecules diffuse through stroma	No lymphatics, antigen clearance through trabecular meshwork Partial blood–uveal barrier	No lymphatics Blood–retina barrier Uveal circulation permeable
Resident APCs	Dendritic and Langerhans cells, macrophages	Langerhans cells at limbus No APCs in central cornea No APCs in sclera Epithelium/endothelium can be induced to express class II MHC	Many dendritic cells and macrophages in iris and ciliary body Hyalocytes are macrophage-derived	Microglia in the retina Dendritic cells and macrophages in choriocapillaris RPE can be induced to express class II MHC
Specialized immune compartments for localized immune processing	?? Follicles	None	None	None
Resident effector cells	Mast cells, T lymphocytes, B lymphocytes, plasma cells, rare neutrophils	Centrally—none Sclera—none	Rare to no T lymphocytes or B lymphocytes, rare mast cells	Retina—normally no lymphocytes Choroid—mast cells, some lymphocytes
Resident effector molecules	All antibody iso-types, especially IgE, IgG sub-classes, IgA in tears Complement and kininogen precursors present	Peripherally—Igs but minimal IgM Centrally—minimal antibody, some complement present Sclera—low antibody concentration, minimal IgM	Kallikrein but not kininogen precursors Some complement present, but less than in blood Minimal Igs in iris, some IgG in ciliary body and aqueous humor	Retina—minimal to no Igs Choroid—IgG and IgA
Immunoregulatory systems	Mucosa-associated lymphoid tissue	Immune privilege—Fas ligand, avascularity, lack of central APCs	Immune privilege—anterior chamber-associated immune deviation, immunosuppressive factors in aqueous, Fas ligand	Immune privilege— ?? mechanisms

APC = antigen-presenting cell.

follicles that enlarge after certain types of ocular surface infection or inflammation represent collections of T lymphocytes, B lymphocytes, and APCs. By analogy with similar sites, such as Peyer patches of the intestine, these follicles are likely a site for localized immune processing of antigens that permeate through the thin overlying epithelium.

The conjunctiva, especially the substantia propria, is richly infiltrated with potential effector cells, predominately mast cells. All antibody isotypes are represented, and presumably local production as well as passive leakage occurs. IgA is the most abundant antibody in the tear film. Soluble molecules of the innate immune system are also represented, especially complement. The conjunctiva appears to support most adaptive and innate immune effector responses, especially antibody-mediated and lymphocyte-mediated responses, although IgE-mediated mast-cell degranulation is one of the most common and important. See also Part IV of BCSC Section 8, *External Disease and Cornea*.

Immunoregulatory Systems

The most important immunoregulatory system for the conjunctiva is called *mucosa-associated lymphoid tissue* (MALT). The MALT concept refers to the interconnected network of mucosal sites (the epithelial lining of the respiratory tract, gut, and genitourinary tract and the ocular surface and its adnexae) that share certain specific immunologic features:

- rich investment of APCs
- specialized structures for localized antigen processing (eg, Peyer patches and tonsils)
- unique effector cells (eg, intraepithelial T lymphocytes and abundant mast cells)

However, the most distinctive aspect of MALT is the distribution and homing of effector T and B lymphocytes induced by immunization at 1 mucosal site to all MALT sites because of the shared expression of specific cell-adhesion molecules on postcapillary venules of the mucosal vasculature. MALT immune response arcs tend to favor T helper-2 (Th2)–dominated responses that result in the production of predominantly IgA and IgE antibodies. Immunization of soluble antigens through MALT, especially in the gut sites, often produces oral tolerance, presumably by activating Th2-like regulatory T lymphocytes that suppress T helper-1 (Th1)–delayed hypersensitivity (DH) effector cells.

Clinical Example 3-1 gives an example of an immune response to conjunctivitis.

Immune Responses of the Anterior Chamber, Anterior Uvea, and Vitreous

Features of the Immunologic Microenvironment

Numerous specialized anatomical features of the anterior region of the eye affect ocular immune responses. The anterior chamber is a fluid-filled cavity; circulating aqueous humor provides a unique medium for intercellular communication among cytokines,

CLINICAL EXAMPLE 3-1

Immune response to viral conjunctivitis Conjunctivitis caused by adenovirus infection is a common ocular infection (see BCSC Section 8, *External Disease and Cornea*). Although precise details of the immune response after conjunctival adenovirus infection are still being discovered, they can be inferred from knowledge of viral infection at other mucosal sites and from animal studies. After infection with adenovirus, the epithelial cells begin to die within 36 hours. Innate immune mechanisms that can assist in limiting infection become activated soon after infection. For example, infected cells produce cytokines such as interferons that limit spread of the infectious virus and recruit nonspecific effector cells such as macrophages and neutrophils.

However, the adaptive immune response to adenovirus infection is considered more important in viral clearance. The primary adaptive response begins when macrophages and dendritic cells become infected or take up cell debris and viral antigens. Both APCs and extracellular antigenic material are conveyed to the preauricular and submandibular nodes along lymphatic channels, where helper T-lymphocyte and antibody responses are activated, producing characteristic lymphadenopathy. Local immune processing may also occur within the follicle if virus invades the epithelial capsule. During the early effector phase of the primary B-lymphocyte response, IgM antibodies are released into the blood that will *not* be very effective in controlling surface infection, although they will combat widespread viremia. However, IgM-bearing B lymphocytes eventually infiltrate the conjunctival stroma and may release antibodies locally in the conjunctiva. Later, during the primary effector response, class switching to IgG or IgA may occur to mediate local effector responses, such as neutralization or complement-mediated lysis of infected cells.

The most active effector response later in acute viral infection comes from CD8-positive natural killer cells and cytotoxic T lymphocytes (CTLs), which kill infected epithelium. However, adenovirus can block the expression of major histocompatiblility complex (MHC) class I on infected cells and thereby escape being killed by CTLs. Adaptive immunity can also activate macrophages by antiviral DH mechanisms later during infection. DH response to viral antigens is thought to contribute to the development of the corneal subepithelial infiltrates that occur in some patients late in adenovirus infection.

The secondary response of the conjunctiva, assuming a prior primary exposure to the same virus at some other mucosal site, differs in that antibody-mediated effector mechanisms dominate. Because of MALT, antivirus IgA is present not only in blood but also in tears as a result of differentiated IgA-secreting B lymphocytes in the lacrimal gland, the substantia propria, and follicles. Thus, recurrent infection is often prevented by preexisting neutralizing antibodies that had disseminated into tears or follicles following the primary infection. However, if the inoculum of recurrent virus overwhelms this antibody barrier, or if the virus has mutated its surface glycoproteins recognized by antibodies, then epithelial infection does occur. Additional immune processing can occur in the follicle and draining nodes. Specific memory effector CTLs are effective in clearing infection within a few days.

Hendricks RL. Immunopathogenesis of viral ocular infections. *Chem Immunol.* 1999;73:120–136.

Nathanson N. *Viral Pathogenesis and Immunity.* 2nd ed. London: Academic Press; 2007.

immune cells, and resident tissue cells of the iris, ciliary body, and corneal endothelium. Although aqueous humor is relatively protein-depleted compared to serum (it contains about 0.1%–1.0% of the total serum protein concentration), even normal aqueous humor contains a complex mixture of biological factors, such as immunomodulatory cytokines, neuropeptides, and complement inhibitors, that can influence immunologic events within the eye.

A partial blood–ocular barrier is present. Fenestrated capillaries in the ciliary body allow a size-dependent concentration gradient of plasma macromolecules to permeate the interstitial tissue; smaller plasma-derived molecules are present in higher concentration than are larger molecules. The tight junctions between the pigmented and the nonpigmented ciliary epithelium provide a more exclusive barrier, preventing interstitial macromolecules from permeating directly through the ciliary body into the aqueous humor. Nevertheless, low numbers of plasma macromolecules bypass the nonpigmented epithelium barrier and may permeate by diffusion anteriorly through the uvea to enter the anterior chamber through the anterior iris surface.

The inner eye does not contain well-developed lymphatic channels. Rather, clearance of soluble substances depends on the aqueous humor outflow channels; clearance of particulates depends on endocytosis by trabecular meshwork endothelial cells or macrophages. Nevertheless, antigen inoculation into the anterior chamber results in efficient communication with the systemic immune response. Intact soluble antigens gain entrance to the venous circulation, where they communicate with the spleen.

The iris and ciliary body contain significant numbers of macrophages and dendritic cells that serve as APCs and possible effector cells. Immune processing is unlikely to occur locally, but APCs leave the eye by the trabecular meshwork and migrate to the spleen (a process known as *homing*), where processing occurs. Few resident T lymphocytes and some mast cells are present in the normal anterior uvea; B lymphocytes, eosinophils, and neutrophils are normally not present. Very low concentrations of IgG and complement components occur in normal aqueous humor.

The vitreous has not been studied as carefully as the anterior chamber, but likely manifests most of the same properties, with several notable exceptions. The vitreous gel can electrostatically bind charged protein substances and may thus serve as an antigen depot as well as a substrate for leukocyte cell adhesion. Because the vitreous contains type II collagen, it may serve as a depot of potential autoantigen as well.

Immunoregulatory Systems

Relatively mild degrees of inflammation that would be harmless in the skin, for example, can cause severe vision loss if they occur in the eye. Several immunoregulatory mechanisms have arisen to modulate intraocular immune responses. In aggregate, these mechanisms are called *immune privilege.* The modern concept of immune privilege refers to the observation that tumor implants or allografts survive better within an immunologically privileged region, whereas a similar implant or graft is rapidly rejected by immune mechanisms within the skin or other nonprivileged sites. Other immune-privileged sites are the subretinal space, the brain, and the testes. Although the nature of the antigen involved is probably important, immune privilege of the anterior uvea has been observed with a wide variety of antigens, including alloantigens (eg, transplantation antigens), tumor antigens, haptens, soluble proteins, autoantigens, bacteria, and viruses.

The best studied mechanism of immune privilege in the eye is called *anterior chamber–associated immune deviation*, or ACAID. Whereas immunization with antigen in the skin elicits a strong delayed-type sensitivity, immunization of the anterior chamber with identical antigen results in a robust antibody response, but with a virtual absence of delayed-type hypersensitivity. Indeed, preexisting delayed-type hypersensitivity can be suppressed by the ACAID response. Following injection of antigen into the anterior chamber, the afferent phase begins when specialized macrophages residing in the iris recognize and take up the antigen. The APC function of these uveal macrophages has been altered by exposure to immunoregulatory cytokines normally present within aqueous humor and uveal tissue, especially transforming growth factor β_2 (TGF-β_2). The TGF-β_2–exposed antigen-stimulated ocular macrophages leave by the trabecular meshwork and the Schlemm canal to enter the venous circulation, where they preferentially migrate to the spleen. Here, the antigen signal is processed, with activation of not only helper T lymphocytes and B lymphocytes but also regulatory T lymphocytes. Splenectomy eliminates ACAID, demonstrating the importance of this site for generation of immune deviation. The CD8 regulatory cells serve to alter CD4 helper T-lymphocyte responses in the spleen and to down-regulate CD4 T-lymphocyte DH responses to the specific immunizing antigen at all body sites. Thus, the resulting effector response is characterized by a selective suppression of antigen-specific DH and a selectively diminished production of complement-fixing isotypes of antibodies.

ACAID represents an attenuated effector arc. Additionally, the eye is protected from severe inflammation by *effector blockade.* Th1 T lymphocytes, cytotoxic T lymphocytes, natural killer cells, and complement activation appear to function less effectively in the anterior uvea than elsewhere. For instance, the anterior uvea is *relatively* resistant to induction of a secondary purified protein derivative DH response after primary immunization with mycobacteria in the skin. There are several mechanisms of effector blockade, but one of the most important and best studied involves the *Fas ligand* (FasL, or CD95 ligand). The FasL is constitutively expressed on the iris and corneal endothelium. This protein is a potent trigger of programmed cell death, or *apoptosis,* of lymphocytes expressing the Fas receptor. Thus, even if an immune response develops to an ocular antigen, the inflammation can be down-regulated by this mechanism of effector blockade.

Foster CS, Streilein JW. Basic immunology. In: Foster CS, Vitale AT, eds. *Diagnosis and Treatment of Uveitis*. Philadelphia, PA: WB Saunders; 2002:34–78.

Niederkorn JY. The induction of anterior chamber-associated immune deviation. *Chem Immunol Allergy*. 2007;92:27–35.

Sugita S, Ng TF, Lucas PJ, Gress RE, Streilein JW. B7$^+$ iris pigment epithelium induce CD8$^+$T regulatory cells; both suppress CTLA-4$^+$ T cells. *J Immunol*. 2006;176(4):118–127.

Immune Responses of the Cornea

Features of the Immunologic Microenvironment

The cornea is unique in that the periphery and the central portions of the tissue represent distinctly different immunologic microenvironments (Fig 3-1). In normal eyes, only the limbus is vascularized. Whereas the limbus is richly invested with Langerhans cells, the paracentral and central cornea are normally devoid of APCs. However, various stimuli, such as mild trauma, certain cytokines (eg, interleukin-1), or infection, can recruit APCs to the central cornea. Plasma-derived enzymes such as complement, IgM, and IgG are present in moderate concentrations in the periphery, but only low levels of the IgM are present centrally.

Corneal cells also appear to synthesize various antimicrobial and immunoregulatory proteins. Effector cells are absent or scarce in the normal cornea, but neutrophils, monocytes, and lymphocytes can readily migrate through the stroma if appropriate chemotactic stimuli are activated. Lymphocytes, monocytes, and neutrophils can also adhere to the endothelial surface during inflammation, giving rise to keratic precipitates or the classic Khodadoust line of endothelial rejection (Fig 3-2). Localized immune processing probably does not occur in the cornea. See also BCSC Section 8, *External Disease and Cornea*.

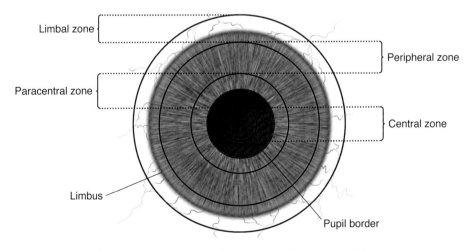

Figure 3-1 Topographic zones of the cornea. *(Illustration by Christine Gralapp.)*

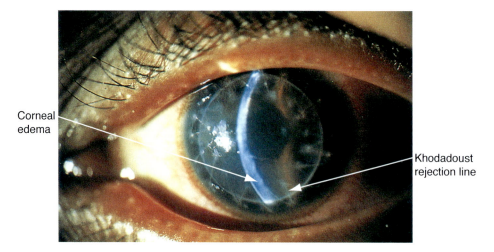

Corneal edema

Khodadoust rejection line

Figure 3-2 Endothelial graft rejection with stromal and epithelial edema on the trailing aspect of the migrating Khodadoust line.

Immunoregulatory Systems

The cornea also demonstrates a form of immune privilege different from that observed in the anterior uvea. Immune privilege of the cornea is multifactorial. Normal limbal physiology is a major component, especially the maintenance of avascularity and lack of APCs in the mid- and central cornea. The absence of APCs and lymphatic channels partially inhibits afferent recognition in the central cornea, and the absence of postcapillary venules centrally can limit the efficiency of effector recruitment, although both effector cells and molecules can ultimately infiltrate even avascular cornea. Another factor is the presence of intact immunoregulatory systems of the anterior chamber (eg, ACAID), to which the corneal endothelium is exposed. Finally, effector blockade likely provides relative immune privilege to the cornea. Allografts tolerated between different strains of wild-type mice are rejected when mice genetically lack either Fas or FasL.

See Clinical Example 3-2.

Immune Responses of the Retina, RPE, Choriocapillaris, and Choroid

Features of the Immunologic Microenvironment

The immunologic microenvironments of the retina, RPE, choriocapillaris, and choroid have not been well described. The retinal circulation demonstrates a blood–ocular barrier at the level of tight junctions between adjacent endothelial cells. The vessels of the choriocapillaris are highly permeable to macromolecules and allow transudation of most plasma macromolecules into the extravascular spaces of the choroid and choriocapillaris. The tight junctions between the cells of the RPE probably provide the true physiologic barrier between the choroid and the retina. Well-developed lymphatic channels are absent, although both the retina and the choroid have abundant potential APCs. In the retina,

CLINICAL EXAMPLE 3-2

Corneal allograft rejection Penetrating keratoplasty, or the transplantation of corneal allografts, enjoys an extremely high success rate (>90%) even in the absence of systemic immunomodulation. This rate is substantially superior to acceptance rates after transplantation of other donor tissues. The mechanisms of corneal graft survival have been attributed to immune privilege. In experimental models, factors contributing to rejection include the following:

- presence of central corneal vascularization
- induction of MHC molecule expression by the stroma, which is normally quite low
- contamination of the donor graft with donor-derived APCs prior to transplantation
- MHC disparity between the host and the donor
- preimmunization of the recipient to donor transplantation antigens

In addition, loss of the immunoregulatory systems of the anterior chamber can influence corneal allograft immunity, and the expression of FasL on corneal endothelium has been observed to be essential for allograft protection in animal models. Rapid replacement of donor epithelium by host epithelium removes this layer as an antigenic stimulus. Once activated, however, antibody-dependent DH and CTL-related mechanisms can target transplantation antigens in all corneal layers.

Klebe S, Coster DJ, Williams KA. Rejection and acceptance of corneal allografts. *Curr Opin Organ Transplant.* 2009;14(1):4–9.

resident microglia (bone marrow–derived cells related to dendritic cells) are interspersed within all layers and can undergo physical changes and migration in response to various stimuli. The choriocapillaris and choroid are richly invested with certain potential APCs, especially macrophages and dendritic cells.

The RPE can be induced to express MHC class II molecules, suggesting that the RPE may also interact with T lymphocytes. The presence of T lymphocytes or B lymphocytes within the normal posterior segment has not been carefully studied, but effector cells appear to be absent from the normal retina. The density of mast cells is moderate in the choroid, especially around the arterioles, but lymphocytes are present only in very low density. Eosinophils and neutrophils appear to be absent. Under various clinical or experimental conditions, however, high densities of T lymphocytes, B lymphocytes, macrophages, and neutrophils can infiltrate the choroid, choriocapillaris, and retina. The RPE and various cell types within the retina and the choroid (eg, pericytes) can synthesize many different cytokines (eg, TGF-β) that may alter the subsequent immune response. Local immune processing does not appear to occur. See also BCSC Section 12, *Retina and Vitreous.*

Streilein JW, Ma N, Wenkel H, Ng TF, Zamiri P. Immunobiology and privilege of neuronal retina and pigment epithelium transplants. *Vision Res.* 2002;42(4):487–495.

Wenkel H, Streilein JW. Evidence that retinal pigment epithelium functions as an immune-privileged tissue. *Invest Ophthalmol Vis Sci.* 2000;41(11):3467–3473.

Immunoregulatory Systems

Recently, it has been demonstrated that a form of immune privilege is present after sub-retinal injection of antigen. The mechanism is unclear but is probably similar to ACAID. This observation may be important because of growing interest in retinal transplantation, stem cell therapies, and gene therapy. (See Clinical Examples 3-3.) The capacity of the

---

CLINICAL EXAMPLES 3-3

Retinal transplantation Transplantation of retina, RPE, or embryonic stem cell–derived retinal tissue is being investigated as a method for restoring retinal function in various disorders. In experimental animal models, sub-retinal transplantation of fetal retinal tissue or various kinds of RPE allografts often show longer survival than the same grafts implanted elsewhere, even without systemic immunomodulation. The afferent phase recognition of al-loantigens is likely performed by retinal microglia or recruited blood-derived macrophages from the choriocapillaris.

The subretinal cytokine environment is likely altered in the setting of retinal diseases, such as retinitis pigmentosa or macular degeneration, due to changes in the blood–retina barrier arising from retinal cell and RPE in-jury. However, injured RPE can still synthesize either immunomodulatory or inflammatory cytokines. The site of immune processing is unknown, but the spleen or some other secondary compartment outside of the eye is likely involved. In mice with fetal retinal grafts, immune rejection occurs by an unusual, slowly progressive cytotoxic mechanism not involving typical antibody-mediated cytolysis or DH T lymphocytes. In humans and nonhu-man primates, rejection of RPE allografts has occurred in both subacute and chronic forms.

Retinal gene therapy Retinal gene therapy is the intentional transfection of photoreceptors or RPE with a replication-defective virus that has been ge-netically altered to carry a replacement gene of choice. This gene becomes expressed in any cell infected by the virus. Immune clearance of the virus has been shown to cause loss of expression of the transferred gene in other body sites. Two applications of gene therapy in primates (including humans!) have been successfully completed. In one, an adeno-associated viral vector was used to replace the defective *RPE65* gene responsible for Leber congeni-tal amaurosis. In this case, the target tissue was RPE. The presence of virus in this site outside the blood–retina barrier raises the possibility of chronic inflammation, and so immunomodulatory therapy is given along with the gene therapy. In the second, dichromatic New World monkeys underwent cone photoreceptor gene therapy with an adeno-associated virus encoding the missing cone gene, which resulted in the new cone pigment being ex-pressed in photoreceptors. As photoreceptors are within the privileged site of the retina, no additional immunomodulation is necessary.

Mancuso K, Hauswirth WW, Li Q, et al. Gene therapy for red-green colour blindness in adult primates. *Nature.* 2009;461(7265):784–787.

choriocapillaris and choroid to function as unique environments for the afferent or effector phases has not yet been evaluated.

Anand V, Duffy B, Yang Z, Dejneka NS, Maguire AM, Bennett J. A deviant immune response to viral proteins and transgene product is generated on subretinal administration of adenovirus and adeno-associated virus. *Mol Ther.* 2002;5(3):125–132.

Stein-Streilein J, Streilein JW. Anterior chamber-associated immune deviation (ACAID): regulation, biological relevance, and implications for therapy. *Int Rev Immunol.* 2002;21(2–3): 123–152.

CHAPTER 4

Special Topics in Ocular Immunology

Animal Models of Human Uveitis

Experimental Autoimmune Uveitis

Experimental autoimmune uveitis (EAU) is the animal model of human uveitis that most closely resembles sympathetic ophthalmia; it is the most widely used and well-studied uveitis model. In the original form of the model, a retinal extract was prepared and used to immunize rats and rabbits. Following intradermal immunization with Freund complete adjuvant, the animals develop a panuveitis approximately 1–2 weeks later. Features of EAU include inflammation of the anterior segment cell, vitreous, and choroid. Refinements of the model over time have included immunization with purified arrestin (also called *S-antigen*), and application to mice with immunization of interphotoreceptor retinoid-binding protein (IRBP)–derived peptides. EAU has been induced in a wide variety of species from rodents to primates. The model has given substantial insight into the mechanisms of human uveitis, and has been useful for evaluating potential drugs for treatment of uveitis.

Experimental Immune Uveitis

Experimental immune uveitis (EIU) is a more transient uveitis model induced by footpad injection of small amounts of lipopolysaccharide in mice and rats (see Chapter 1). Sixteen to 48 hours after administration, mice develop a transient, marked anterior uveitis. This model has been especially useful for studies of the dynamics of leukocyte function in the anterior chamber. It is not clear how this model correlates with human disease.

Equine Recurrent Uveitis

This spontaneous uveitis occurs in horses. It is typically a bilateral uveitis featuring anterior and posterior segment inflammation. The disease affects up to 10% of horses. Immunologic studies have indicated the presence of autoantibodies and autoreactive T cells in this disease.

AIRE-Deficient Mice

AIRE deficiency represents the sole spontaneous mouse model of uveitis. AIRE (for *autoimmune regulator*) is a transcription factor used by the thymus in the process of thymic tolerance. Early in life, the thymus expresses many cell-type–specific proteins; T-cell clones reactive to these proteins are deleted. This is an important mechanism in the development of self-tolerance. Mice lacking AIRE do not express these proteins during development, and spontaneously develop a posterior uveitis. Recent work has suggested that the major antigen targeted in this autoimmune uveitis is IRBP—the same protein used to generate mouse models of EAU.

Caspi RR, Silver PB, Luger D, et al. Mouse models of experimental autoimmune uveitis. *Ophthalmic Res.* 2008;40(3–4):169–174.

DeVoss J, Hou Y, Johannes K, et al. Spontaneous autoimmunity prevented by thymic expression of a single self-antigen. *J Exp Med.* 2006;203(12):2727–2735.

HLA Associations and Disease

Normal Function of HLA Molecules

All animals with white blood cells express a family of cell-surface glycoproteins called *major histocompatibility complex* (MHC) proteins. In humans, the MHC proteins are called *human leukocyte antigen* (HLA) molecules. As discussed in Chapter 2, 6 different families of HLA molecules have been identified:

- 3 MHC class I: HLA-A, -B, -C
- 3 MHC class II: HLA-DR, -DP, -DQ

A seventh category, HLA-D, does not exist as a specific molecule but instead represents a functional classification as determined by an in vitro assay. MHC class III molecules and minor MHC antigens have also been identified, but they are not discussed here.

The important role MHC molecules play in immunologic function is discussed in Chapter 2. HLAs are also considered to be human immune response genes, because the HLA type determines the capacity of the antigen-presenting cell (APC) to bind peptide fragments and thus determines T-lymphocyte immune responsiveness.

Allelic Variation

Many different alleles or polymorphic variants of each of the 6 HLA types exist within the population: more than 25 alleles for HLA-A, 50 for HLA-B, 10 for HLA-C, 100 for HLA-DR, and so on. Because there are 6 major HLA types and each individual has a pair of each HLA type, or 1 *haplotype,* from each parent, an APC expresses 6 pairs of MHC molecules. Thus, with the exception of identical twins, only rarely will all 12 potential haplotypes match in 2 individuals.

Allelic diversity may be designed to provide protection through *population-wide immunity.* Each HLA haplotype theoretically covers a set of antigens to which a particular individual can respond adaptively. Thus, in theory, the presence of many different HLA alleles within a population should ensure that the adaptive immune system in at least some individuals in the whole group will be able to respond to a wide range of potential pathogens. The converse also holds true: some individuals may be at increased risk for immunologic diseases, because of either aberrantly strong immune response to a benign pathogen, or autoimmune disease arising from inappropriate recognition of host peptides in the context of a particular HLA as foreign. See Clinical Example 4-1.

Clinical detection and classification of different alleles

Traditionally, the different alleles of HLA-A, -B, -C, and -DQ were detected by reacting lymphocytes with special antisera standardized by International HLA Workshops sponsored by the World Health Organization (WHO). HLA-DP and HLA-DR typing requires specialized T-lymphocyte culture assays. More recently, molecular techniques have been developed to characterize the nucleic acid sequence of various MHC alleles. HLA molecules are composed of 2 chains: α and β chains for class II, and the α chain and the β_2-microglobulin chain for class I. Because subtle differences in molecular structure can be easily missed using antisera-based assays, molecular genotyping is a more precise method to determine MHC types. Thus, the genotype specifies the chain, the major genetic type,

---

CLINICAL EXAMPLE 4-1

HLA-B27–associated acute anterior uveitis Approximately 50% of patients with acute anterior uveitis (AAU) express the HLA-B27 haplotype, and many of these patients also experience other immunologic disorders, such as reactive arthritis, ankylosing spondylitis, inflammatory bowel disease, and psoriatic arthritis (see Chapter 6). Although the immunopathogenesis remains unknown, various animal models permit some informed speculation. Many cases of uveitis or reactive arthritis follow gram-negative bacillary dysentery or chlamydial infection. The possible role of bacterial lipopolysaccharide and innate mechanisms was discussed in Chapter 1. Experiments in rats and mice genetically altered to express human HLA-B27 molecules seem to suggest that bacterial infection of the gut predisposes rats to arthritis and a reactive arthritis–like syndrome, although uveitis is uncommon.

It has been suggested that chronic intracellular chlamydial infection of a joint, and presumably the eye, might stimulate an adaptive immune response using the endogenous (class I) antigen-processing pathway of the B27 molecule, invoking a CD8 T-lymphocyte effector mechanism activated to kill the microbe but indirectly injuring the eye. Others have suggested that B27 amino acid sequences might present *Klebsiella* peptide antigens to CD8 T lymphocytes, but how a presumed exogenous bacterial antigen would be presented through the class I pathway is unknown. Another hypothesis posits that molecular mimicry may exist between bacterial antigens and some amino acid sequences of HLA-B27. Analysis of human AAU fluids and various animal models of AAU and arthritis suggests that anterior uveitis might be a CD4 Th1-mediated DH response, possibly in response to bacteria-derived antigens (such as bacterial cell wall antigens or heat shock proteins trapped in the uvea) or to endogenous autoantigens of the anterior uvea (possibly melanin-associated antigens, type I collagen, or myelin-associated proteins). How a CD4-predominant mechanism would relate to a class I immunogenetic association is unclear.

and the specific minor molecular variant subtype. For example, genotype DRB1*0408 refers to the HLA-DR4 molecule β chain with the "–08" minor variant subtype. Haplotypes currently recognized as a single group will continue to be subdivided into new categories or new subtypes. For example, at least 2 different A29 subtypes and 8 different HLA-B27 subtypes have been recognized.

Disease Associations

In 1973, the first association between an HLA haplotype and a disease—ankylosing spondylitis—was identified. Since then, more than 100 other disease associations have been made, including several for ocular inflammatory diseases (Table 4-1). In general, an HLA–disease association is defined as the statistically increased frequency of an HLA haplotype in persons with that disease as compared to the frequency in a disease-free population. The ratio of these 2 frequencies is called *relative risk,* which is the simplest method for expressing the magnitude of an HLA–disease association. Nevertheless, several caveats must be kept in mind:

- The HLA association identifies individuals at risk, but it is not a diagnostic marker. The associated haplotype is not necessarily present in all people affected with the specific disease, and its presence in a person does not ensure the correct diagnosis.
- The association depends on the validity of the haplotyping. Older literature often reflects associations based on HLA classifications (some provisional) that might have changed.

Table 4-1 HLA Associations and Ocular Inflammatory Disease

Disease	HLA Association	Relative Risk (RR)
Uveitic diseases with strong HLA associations		
Tubulointerstitial nephritis and uveitis (TINU) syndrome	HLA-DRB1*0102	RR = 167
Birdshot retinochoroidopathy	HLA-A29, -A29.2	RR = 80–158, for North Americans and Europeans
Reactive arthritis	HLA-B27	RR = 60
Acute anterior uveitis	HLA-B27	RR = 8
Uveitic diseases with weaker HLA associations		
Juvenile idiopathic arthritis	HLA-A2, -DR5, -DR8, -DR11, -DP2.1	Acute systemic disease
Behçet disease	HLA-B51	RR = 4–6; Japanese and Middle Eastern descent
Intermediate uveitis	HLA-B8, -B51, -DR2, -DR15	RR = 6, possibly the DRB1*1501 genotype
Sympathetic ophthalmia	HLA-DR4	
Vogt-Koyanagi-Harada syndrome	HLA-DR4	RR = 2, Japanese and North Americans
Sarcoidosis	HLA-B8	Acute systemic disease
	HLA-B13	Chronic systemic disease but not for eye
Multiple sclerosis	HLA-B7, -DR2	
Retinal vasculitis	HLA-B44	Britons

- The association is only as strong as the clinical diagnosis. Diseases that are difficult to diagnose on clinical features may obscure real associations.
- The concept of *linkage disequilibrium* proposes that if 2 genes are physically near on the chromosome, they may be inherited together rather than undergo genetic randomization in a population. Thus, HLA may be coinherited with an unrelated disease gene, and sometimes 2 HLA haplotypes can occur together more frequently than predicted by their independent frequencies in the population.

It is important to remember that HLA–disease associations are simply that—associations between an MHC molecule and a clinical condition. Testing for HLA can provide supportive evidence for a particular diagnosis but cannot make a definitive diagnosis. For example, approximately 8% of the white population in the United States is HLA-A29 positive, but fewer than 1 in 10,000 US residents have birdshot retinochoroidopathy (although nearly all patients with birdshot retinochoroidopathy are HLA-A29 positive). Thus, the vast majority of individuals who are HLA-A29 positive will never have birdshot retinochoroidopathy.

Several explanations have been offered for HLA–disease associations. The most direct theory postulates that HLA molecules act as peptide-binding molecules for etiologic antigens or infectious agents. Thus, individuals bearing a specific HLA molecule might be predisposed to processing certain antigens, such as an infectious agent that cross-reacts with a self-antigen, and other individuals, lacking that haplotype, would not be so predisposed. Specific variations or mutations in the peptide-binding region would greatly influence this mechanism; these variations can be detected only by molecular typing. Preliminary data in support of this theory have been provided for patients with type 1 diabetes.

A second theory proposes molecular mimicry between bacterial antigens and an epitope of an HLA molecule (ie, an antigenic site on the molecule itself). An appropriate antibacterial effector response might inappropriately initiate a cross-reaction effector response with an epitope of the HLA molecule. A third theory suggests that the T-lymphocyte antigen receptor (gene) is really the true susceptibility factor. Because a specific T-lymphocyte receptor uses a specific HLA haplotype, a strong correlation would exist between an HLA and the T-lymphocyte antigen receptor repertoire.

Levinson RD. Immunogenetics of ocular inflammatory disease. *Tissue Antigens.* 2007;69(2): 105–112.

PART II

Intraocular Inflammation and Uveitis

CHAPTER 5

Clinical Approach to Uveitis

The uvea consists of the middle, pigmented, vascular structures of the eye and includes the iris, ciliary body, and choroid. *Uveitis* is broadly defined as inflammation (ie, *-itis*) of the uvea (from the Latin *uva*, meaning "grape"). The study of uveitis is complicated by the myriad causes of inflammatory reaction of the inner eye that can be broadly categorized into infectious and noninfectious etiologies. In addition, processes that may only secondarily involve the uvea, such as ocular toxoplasmosis, a disease that primarily affects the retina, may cause a marked inflammatory spillover into the choroid and vitreous.

Because uveitis is frequently associated with systemic disease, a careful, thorough history and review of systems is an essential first step in elucidating the cause of a patient's inflammatory disease. Next, a thorough physical examination of the eye and pertinent organ systems must be done to determine the type of inflammation present. Each patient demonstrates only some of the possible symptoms and signs of uveitis. After the physician has used the information obtained from the history and physical examination to determine the anatomical classification of uveitis, he or she can use several associated (historical and physical) factors to further subcategorize, which leads in turn to choosing the laboratory studies. Laboratory studies can help determine the etiology of the intraocular inflammation, which then leads to the selection and administration of therapeutic options. However, laboratory studies are never a substitute for a thorough history and physical examination.

This text uses an etiologic division of uveitic entities into noninfectious (autoimmune) and infectious conditions. These conditions are then further subcategorized and described using the anatomical classification of uveitis.

Albert DM, Jakobiec FA, eds. *Principles and Practice of Ophthalmology.* 2nd ed. Philadelphia, PA: WB Saunders; 1999.

Foster CS, Vitale AT. *Diagnosis and Treatment of Uveitis.* Philadelphia, PA: WB Saunders; 2002.

Michelson JB. *Color Atlas of Uveitis.* 2nd ed. St Louis, MO: Mosby; 1991.

Nussenblatt RB, Whitcup SM. *Uveitis: Fundamentals and Clinical Practice.* 3rd ed. Philadelphia, PA: Mosby; 2004.

Rao NA, Forster DJ, Augsburger JJ. *The Uvea: Uveitis and Intraocular Neoplasms.* New York, NY: Gower Medical Publishing; 1992.

Classification of Uveitis

Several schemes for the classification of uveitis currently exist. These are based on anatomy (the portion of the uvea involved), clinical course (acute, chronic, or recurrent), etiology (infectious or noninfectious), and histology (granulomatous or nongranulomatous). The rapid expansion of published clinical information on various uveitic entities from a myriad of global sources using different classification and grading systems and the undeniable need for multicenter, randomized clinical trials to better understand the course, prognosis, and treatment of various uveitic entities led the Standardization of Uveitis Nomenclature (SUN) Working Group in 2005 to develop an anatomical classification system, descriptors, standardized grading systems, and terminology. This system was adopted by leading uveitis specialists from all over the world. Discussion in this book divides uveitic entities into etiologic categories (infectious or noninfectious) and then follows this basic anatomical classification into 4 groups (Table 5-1):

- anterior uveitis
- intermediate uveitis
- posterior uveitis
- panuveitis

The SUN Working Group further refined this anatomical classification of uveitis by also defining descriptors based on clinical onset, duration, and course (Table 5-2); in addition, they recommended specific terminology for grading and following uveitic activity (Table 5-3).

The Standardization of Uveitis Nomenclature (SUN) Working Group. Standardization of uveitis nomenclature for reporting clinical data. Results of the First International Workshop. *Am J Ophthalmol.* 2005;140(3):509–516.

Table 5-1 The SUN Working Group Anatomical Classification of Uveitis

Type	Primary Site of Inflammation	Includes
Anterior uveitis	Anterior chamber	Iritis Iridocyclitis Anterior cyclitis
Intermediate uveitis	Vitreous	Pars planitis Posterior cyclitis Hyalitis
Posterior uveitis	Retina or choroid	Focal, multifocal, or diffuse choroiditis Chorioretinitis Retinochoroiditis Retinitis Neuroretinitis
Panuveitis	Anterior chamber, vitreous, and retina or choroid	

Reprinted with permission from The Standardization of Uveitis Nomenclature (SUN) Working Group. Standardization of nomenclature for reporting clinical data. Results of the First International Workshop. *Am J Ophthalmol.* 2005;140(3):510.

Table 5-2 The SUN Working Group Descriptors in Uveitis

Category	Descriptor	Comment
Onset	Sudden	
	Insidious	
Duration	Limited	≤3 months' duration
	Persistent	>3 months' duration
Course	Acute	Episode characterized by sudden onset and limited duration
	Recurrent	Repeated episodes separated by periods of inactivity without treatment ≥3 months' duration
	Chronic	Persistent uveitis with relapse in <3 months after discontinuing treatment

Reprinted with permission from The Standardization of Uveitis Nomenclature (SUN) Working Group. Standardization of nomenclature for reporting clinical data. Results of the First International Workshop. *Am J Ophthalmol.* 2005;140(3):511.

Table 5-3 The SUN Working Group Activity of Uveitis Terminology

Term	Definition
Inactive	Grade 0 cells (anterior chamber)
Worsening activity	2-step increase in level of inflammation (eg, anterior chamber cells, vitreous haze) or increase from grade 3+ to 4+
Improved activity	2-step decrease in level of inflammation (eg, anterior chamber cells, vitreous haze) or decrease to grade 0
Remission	Inactive disease for ≥3 months after discontinuing all treatments for eye disease

Reprinted with permission from The Standardization of Uveitis Nomenclature (SUN) Working Group. Standardization of nomenclature for reporting clinical data. Results of the First International Workshop. *Am J Ophthalmol.* 2005;140(3):513.

Anterior Uveitis

The anterior chamber is the primary site of inflammation in anterior uveitis. Anterior uveitis can have a range of presentations, from a quiet white eye with low-grade inflammatory reaction apparent only on close examination to a painful red eye with moderate or severe inflammation. Inflammation confined to the anterior chamber is called *iritis;* if it spills over into the retrolental space, it is called *iridocyclitis;* if it involves the cornea, it is called *keratouveitis;* and if the inflammatory reaction involves the sclera and uveal tract, it is called *sclerouveitis.* Chapter 6 discusses anterior uveitis in greater detail. See Table 5-4.

Intermediate Uveitis

In intermediate uveitis the major site of inflammation is the vitreous. Inflammation of the middle portion (posterior ciliary body, pars plana) of the eye manifests primarily as floaters affecting vision; the eye frequently appears quiet externally. Visual loss is primarily a result of chronic cystoid macular edema (CME) or, less commonly, cataract formation. See Chapter 7 of this volume for discussion, as well as Table 5-4.

Table 5-4 Flowchart for Evaluation of Uveitis Patients

Type of Inflammation	Associated Factors	Suspected Disease	Laboratory Tests, Imaging
		Panuveitis	
	See entities described below: sarcoidosis, toxoplasmosis, toxocariasis, endophthalmitis, VKH syndrome, sympathetic ophthalmia, syphilis, cysticercosis		
		Anterior Uveitis	
Acute/sudden onset, severe with or without fibrin membrane or hypopyon	Arthritis, back pain, GI/GU symptoms Aphthous ulcers	Seronegative spondyloarthropathies Behçet disease	HLA-B27, sacroiliac films HLA-B5, -B51 (not essential, rarely obtained)
	Postsurgical, posttraumatic None	Infectious endophthalmitis Idiopathic	Vitreous culture, vitrectomy Possibly HLA-B27
Moderate severity (red, painful)	Shortness of breath, African descent	Sarcoidosis	Serum ACE, lysozyme; chest x-ray; gallium scan; biopsy
	Posttraumatic Increased IOP Poor response to steroids	Traumatic iritis Glaucomatocyclitic crisis, herpetic iritis Syphilis	RPR, VDRL (screening); FTA-ABS (confirmatory)
	Post–cataract extraction None	Low-grade endophthalmitis, IOL-related iritis Idiopathic	Consider vitrectomy, culture
Chronic; minimal redness, pain	Child, especially with arthritis Heterochromia, diffuse KP, unilateral Postsurgical	JIA-related iridocyclitis Fuchs heterochromic iridocyclitis Low-grade endophthalmitis (eg, *Propionibacterium acnes*); IOL-related	ANA, ESR, rheumatoid factor None Consider vitrectomy, capsulectomy with culture
	None	Idiopathic	
		Intermediate Uveitis	
Mild to moderate	Shortness of breath, African descent Tick exposure, erythema chronicum migrans rash	Sarcoidosis Lyme disease	As above ELISA
	Neurologic symptoms Over age 50 None	Multiple sclerosis Intraocular lymphoma Pars planitis	MRI of brain Vitrectomy, cytology

	Clinical features	Diagnosis	Workup
Chorioretinitis *with* vitritis			
Focal	Adjacent scar; raw meat ingestion	Toxoplasmosis	ELISA
	Child; history of geophagia	Toxocariasis	ELISA
	HIV infection	CMV retinitis	
Multifocal	Shortness of breath	Sarcoidosis	As above
		Tuberculosis	PPD, chest x-ray
	Peripheral retinal necrosis	Acute retinal necrosis (ARN)	VZV, HSV titers (ELISA), possibly vitrectomy/retinal biopsy
		Progressive outer retinal necrosis (PORN) if immunocompromised	
	AIDS	Syphilis, toxoplasmosis	As above
	IV drug use, hyperalimentation, immunosuppression	*Candida, Aspergillus* infection	Blood, vitreous cultures
	Visible intraocular parasite; from Africa or Central/South America	Cysticercosis	
	Over age 50	Onchocerciasis	As above
	None	Intraocular lymphoma	HLA-A29, fluorescein angiography (FA)
		Birdshot retinochoroidopathy	Rule out TB, sarcoidosis, syphilis
		Multifocal choroiditis with panuveitis	
Diffuse	Dermatologic/CNS symptoms; serous RD	Vogt-Koyanagi-Harada (VKH) syndrome	FA, lumbar puncture to document CSF pleocytosis
	Postsurgical/traumatic, bilateral	Sympathetic ophthalmia	FA
	Postsurgical/traumatic, unilateral	Infectious endophthalmitis	As above
	Child; history of geophagia	Toxocariasis	As above
Chorioretinitis *without* vitritis			
Focal	None; history of carcinoma	Neoplastic	Metastatic workup
Multifocal	Ohio/Mississippi Valley	Ocular histoplasmosis	FA if macula involved
	Lesions confined to posterior pole	White dot syndromes (eg, APMPPE, MEWDS, PIC)	FA
	Geographic (maplike) pattern of scars	Serpiginous choroiditis	FA
Diffuse	From Africa, Central/South America	Onchocerciasis	
Vasculitis			
	Aphthous ulcers, hypopyon	Behçet disease	As above
	Malar rash, female, arthralgias	Systemic lupus erythematosus (SLE)	ANA
	Chronic sinusitus with hemorrhagic rhinorrhea, dyspnea, renal insufficiency, purpura	Wegener granulomatosis	c-ANCA (anti-proteinase 3)

Posterior Uveitis

Posterior uveitis is defined as intraocular inflammation primarily involving the retina and/or choroid. Inflammatory cells may be observed diffusely throughout the vitreous cavity, overlying foci of active inflammation, or on the posterior vitreous face. Ocular examination reveals focal, multifocal, or diffuse areas of retinitis or choroiditis, with varying degrees of vitreous cellular activity, the clinical appearances of which may be similar for different entities. Certain posterior uveitic syndromes present either as a focal or multifocal retinitis, whereas others localize predominantly to the choroid in a similar distribution, involving the retina secondarily, with or without vitreous cells and/or involvement of the retinal vasculature (Tables 5-5 through 5-8). Macular edema, retinal vasculitis, and retinal or choroidal neovascularization are structural complications of certain uveitic entities and not considered essential to the anatomical classification of posterior uveitis. Chapters 6 and 7 discuss noninfectious and infectious posterior uveitis in greater detail.

Panuveitis

The primary sites of inflammation in panuveitis (diffuse uveitis) are the anterior chamber, vitreous, and retina or choroid. Many systemic infectious and noninfectious diseases

Table 5-5 **Posterior Uveitis With Retinitis**

Focal Retinitis	Multifocal Retinitis
Toxoplasmosis	Syphilis
Onchocerciasis	HSV
Cysticercosis	VZV
Masquerade syndromes	CMV
	DUSN
	Candida infection
	Sarcoidosis
	Cat-scratch disease
	Masquerade syndromes

CMV = cytomegalovirus, DUSN = diffuse unilateral subacute neuroretinitis, HSV = herpes simplex virus, VZV = varicella-zoster virus.

Adapted with permission from Foster CS, Vitale AT. *Diagnosis and Treatment of Uveitis*. Philadelphia, PA: WB Saunders; 2002.

Table 5-6 **Posterior Uveitis With a Focal (Solitary) Chorioretinal Lesion**

With Vitreal Cells	Without Vitreal Cells
Toxocariasis	Tumor
Sarcoidosis	Serpiginous choroiditis
Tuberculosis	
Nocardia	
Cat-scratch disease	

Adapted with permission from Foster CS, Vitale AT. *Diagnosis and Treatment of Uveitis*. Philadelphia, PA: WB Saunders; 2002.

Table 5-7 Posterior Uveitis With Multifocal Chorioretinal Lesions

With Vitreal Cells	Without Vitreal Cells
Birdshot retinochoroidopathy	OHS
MCP	PIC
SFU syndrome	PORT
Sympathetic ophthalmia	Acute retinal pigment epitheliitis
VKH syndrome	Subacute sclerosing panencephalitis
Sarcoidosis	Serpiginous choroiditis*
West Nile virus	
Cat-scratch disease	
Malignant masquerade syndromes	
Rubella measles*	
MEWDS*	
APMPPE*	

*Usually.

APMPPE = acute posterior multifocal placoid pigment epitheliopathy, MCP = multifocal choroiditis and panuveitis, MEWDS = multiple evanescent white dot syndrome, OHS = ocular histoplasmosis syndrome, PIC = punctate inner choroiditis, PORT = punctate outer retinal toxoplasmosis, SFU = subretinal fibrosis and uveitis, VKH = Vogt-Koyanagi-Harada.

Adapted with permission from Foster CS, Vitale AT. *Diagnosis and Treatment of Uveitis*. Philadelphia, PA: WB Saunders; 2002.

Table 5-8 Posterior Uveitis With Retinal Vasculitis

Primarily Arteritis	Primarily Phlebitis	Arteritis and Phlebitis
Systemic lupus erythematosus	Sarcoidosis	Toxoplasmosis
Polyarteritis nodosa	Multiple sclerosis	Relapsing polychondritis
Syphilis	Behçet disease	Wegener granulomatosis
HSV (ARN/BARN)	Birdshot retinochoroidopathy	Crohn disease
VZV (PORN)	HIV paraviral syndrome	Frosted branch angiitis
IRVAN	Eales disease	
Churg-Strauss syndrome		

ARN = acute retinal necrosis; BARN = bilateral acute retinal necrosis; HIV = human immunodeficiency virus; HSV = herpes simplex virus; IRVAN = idiopathic retinal vasculitis, aneurysms, and neuroretinitis; PORN = progressive outer retinal necrosis; VZV = varicella-zoster virus

Adapted with permission from Foster CS, Vitale AT. *Diagnosis and Treatment of Uveitis*. Philadelphia, PA: WB Saunders; 2002.

associated with uveitis may produce diffuse intraocular inflammation with concomitant iridocyclitis and posterior uveitis. Chapters 6 and 7 discuss noninfectious and infectious panuveitis in greater depth, and Chapter 8 covers endophthalmitis. See also Table 5-4.

Categorization by Clinical Course

Uveitis may be subcategorized as acute, chronic, or recurrent: *acute* is generally the term used to describe episodes of sudden onset and limited duration that usually resolve within a few weeks to months, whereas *chronic uveitis* is persistent, with relapse in less than 3 months after discontinuing treatment. *Recurrent uveitis* is characterized by repeated episodes separated by periods of inactivity without treatment 3 months or longer in duration.

Whether the inflammation is severe or low grade can influence categorization and prognosis. The inflammatory process may occur in 1 or both eyes, or it may alternate between them. The distribution of ocular involvement—focal, multifocal, or diffuse—is also helpful to note when classifying uveitis.

Chronic uveitis can be further characterized histologically as being either granulomatous or nongranulomatous. *Nongranulomatous* inflammation typically has a lymphocytic and plasma cell infiltrate, whereas *granulomatous* reactions also include epithelioid and giant cells. Discrete granulomas are characteristic of sarcoidosis; diffuse granulomatous inflammation appears in Vogt-Koyanagi-Harada (VKH) syndrome and sympathetic ophthalmia. Zonal granulomatous disease can be seen with lens-induced uveitis. However, the physician should be aware that the *clinical* appearance of uveitis as granulomatous or nongranulomatous may not necessarily correlate with the *histologic* description and may instead be related to the stage in which the disease is first seen, the amount of presenting antigen, or the host's state of immunocompromise (eg, a patient being treated with corticosteroids).

Symptoms of Uveitis

Symptoms produced by uveitis depend on which part of the uveal tract is inflamed, the rapidity of onset (sudden or insidious), the duration of the disease (limited or persistent), and the course of the disease (acute, chronic, or recurrent) (Table 5-9).

Acute-onset anterior uveitis (iridocyclitis) causes pain, photophobia, redness, and blurred vision. Pain usually results from the acute onset of inflammation in the region of the iris, as in acute iritis, or from secondary glaucoma. The pain associated with ciliary spasm in iritis may be a referred pain that seems to radiate over the larger area served by cranial nerve V (the trigeminal nerve). Epiphora, redness, and photophobia are usually present when inflammation involves the iris, cornea, or iris–ciliary body.

In contrast, chronic iridocyclitis in patients with juvenile idiopathic arthritis (JIA) may not be associated with any symptoms at all. However, with chronic iridocyclitis,

---

Table 5-9 Symptoms of Uveitis

Redness
Pain
Photophobia
Epiphora
Visual disturbances
  Diffuse blur, caused by:
    Myopic or hyperopic shift
    Inflammatory cells
    Cataract
  Scotomata (central or peripheral)
  Floaters

blurred vision may develop as a result of calcific band keratopathy, cataract, or CME. Recurrent anterior uveitis is marked by periods of inactivity of 3 or more months off medications followed by a return of symptoms.

Intermediate uveitis produces symptoms of floaters and blurred vision. Floaters result from the shadows cast by vitreous cells and snowballs on the retina. Blurred vision may be caused by CME or vitreous opacities in the visual axis.

Presenting symptoms in patients with posterior uveitis include painless decreased visual acuity, floaters, photopsia, metamorphopsia, scotomata, nyctalopia, or a combination of these. This blurred vision may be caused by the primary effects of uveitis, such as retinitis and/or choroiditis directly affecting macular function, or to the complications of inflammation such as CME, epiretinal membrane, retinal ischemia, and choroidal neovascularization. Blurred vision may also result from refractive error such as a myopic or hyperopic shift associated with macular edema, hypotony, or a change in lens position. Other possible causes of blurred vision include opacities in the visual axis from inflammatory cells, fibrin, or protein in the anterior chamber; keratic precipitates (KPs); secondary cataract; vitreous debris; macular edema; and retinal atrophy.

Signs of Uveitis

Part I of this volume reviews the basic concepts of immunology, which can be used to understand the symptoms and signs of inflammation in uveitis. An inflammatory response to infectious, traumatic, neoplastic, or autoimmune processes produces the signs of uveitis (Table 5-10). Chemical mediators of the acute stage of inflammation include serotonin, complement, and plasmin. Leukotrienes, kinins, and prostaglandins modify the second phase of the acute response through antagonism of vasoconstrictors. Activated complement is a leukotactic agent. Polymorphonuclear leukocytes, eosinophils, and mast cells may all contribute to signs of inflammation. However, the lymphocyte is by far the predominant inflammatory cell in the inner eye in uveitis. These chemical mediators result in vascular dilation (ciliary flush), increased vascular permeability (aqueous flare), and chemotaxis of inflammatory cells into the eye (aqueous and vitreous cellular reaction).

Anterior Segment

Signs of uveitis in the anterior portion of the eye include

- keratic precipitates (Figs 5-1, 5-2)
- inflammatory cells
- flare (Fig 5-3)
- fibrin
- hypopyon
- pigment dispersion
- pupillary miosis
- iris nodules (Fig 5-4)
- synechiae, both anterior and posterior (Fig 5-5)
- band keratopathy (seen with long-standing uveitis)

Table 5-10 Signs of Uveitis

Eyelid and skin Vitiligo Nodules	**Intraocular pressure** Hypotony Secondary glaucoma
Conjunctiva Perilimbal or diffuse injection Nodules	**Vitreous** Inflammatory cells (single/clumped) Traction bands
Corneal endothelium Keratic (cellular) precipitates (diffuse or gravitational) Fibrin Pigment (nonspecific)	**Pars plana** Snowbanking **Retina** Inflammatory cells
Anterior/posterior chamber Inflammatory cells Flare (proteinaceous influx) Pigment (nonspecific)	Inflammatory cuffing of blood vessels Edema Cystoid macular edema Retinal pigment epithelium: hypertrophy/clumping/loss Epiretinal membranes
Iris Nodules Posterior synechiae Atrophy Heterochromia	**Choroid** Inflammatory infiltrate Atrophy Neovascularization
Angle Peripheral anterior synechiae Nodules Vascularization	**Optic Nerve** Edema (nonspecific) Neovascularization

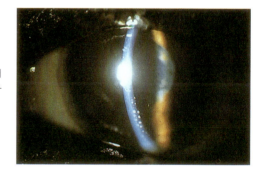

Figure 5-1 Keratic precipitates (medium and small) with broken posterior synechiae. *(Courtesy of H. Jane Blackman, MD.)*

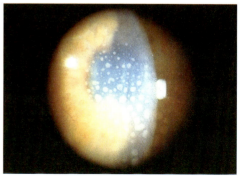

Figure 5-2 Large "mutton-fat" keratic precipitates in a patient with sarcoidosis. Large keratic precipitates such as these generally indicate a granulomatous disease process. *(Courtesy of David Forster, MD.)*

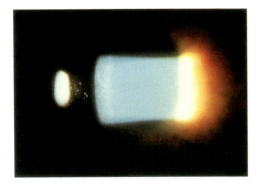

Figure 5-3 Aqueous flare (4+) in a patient with acute iritis.

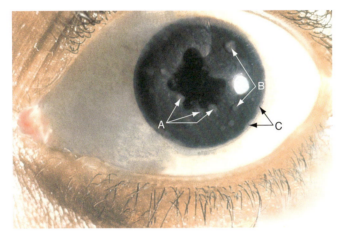

Figure 5-4 Posterior synechiae and iris nodules in a patient with sarcoidosis. Note the 3 types of iris nodules: **A,** Koeppe nodules (pupillary border); **B,** Busacca nodules (midiris); and **C,** Berlin nodules (iris angle). *(Courtesy of David Forster, MD.)*

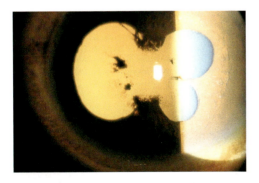

Figure 5-5 Multiple posterior synechiae preventing complete dilation of the pupil. *(Courtesy of David Forster, MD.)*

Keratic precipitates are collections of inflammatory cells on the corneal endothelium. When newly formed, they tend to be white and smoothly rounded, but they then become crenated (shrunken), pigmented, or glassy. Large, yellowish KPs are described as *mutton-fat KPs;* these are usually associated with granulomatous types of inflammation (see the discussion earlier in this chapter on the distinction between granulomatous and nongranulomatous inflammation). The SUN group (see Classification of Uveitis earlier in the chapter) is working to establish photographic guidelines for describing KPs.

Perilimbal vascular engorgement (ciliary flush) or diffuse injection of the conjunctiva, episclera, or both is typical with acute anterior uveitis. With increased capillary permeability, the anterior chamber reaction can be described as

- serous (aqueous flare caused by protein influx)
- purulent (polymorphonuclear leukocytes and necrotic debris causing hypopyon)
- fibrinous (plasmoid, or intense fibrinous exudate)
- sanguinoid (inflammatory cells with erythrocytes manifested by hypopyon mixed with hyphema)

The SUN group also specifically developed an updated method of grading anterior chamber cells and flare. The intensity of the cellular reaction in the anterior chamber is graded according to the number of inflammatory cells seen in a 1-mm × 1-mm high-powered beam at full intensity at a 45°–60° angle (Table 5-11).

Flare may also be graded similarly, and the SUN group described flare intensity as it had been described previously by Hogan et al (Table 5-12).

Iris involvement may manifest as either anterior or posterior synechiae, iris nodules (Koeppe nodules at the pupillary border, Busacca nodules within the iris stroma, and Berlin nodules in the angle; see Fig 5-4), iris granulomas, heterochromia (eg, Fuchs heterochromic iridocyclitis), or stromal atrophy (eg, herpetic uveitis).

Table 5-11 The SUN Working Group Grading Scheme for Anterior Chamber Cells

Grade	Cells in Field (High-Intensity 1 × 1-mm Slit Beam)
0	<1
0.5+	1–5
1+	6–15
2+	16–25
3+	26–50
4+	>50

Reprinted with permission from The Standardization of Uveitis Nomenclature (SUN) Working Group. Standardization of nomenclature for reporting clinical data. Results of the First International Workshop. *Am J Ophthalmol.* 2005;140(3):512.

Table 5-12 The SUN Working Group Grading Scheme for Anterior Chamber Flare

Grade	Description
0	None
1+	Faint
2+	Moderate (iris and lens details clear)
3+	Marked (iris and lens details hazy)
4+	Intense (fibrin or plasmoid aqueous)

Reprinted with permission from The Standardization of Uveitis Nomenclature (SUN) Working Group. Standardization of nomenclature for reporting clinical data. Results of the First International Workshop. *Am J Ophthalmol.* 2005;140(3):512.

With uveitic involvement of the ciliary body and trabecular meshwork, intraocular pressure (IOP) is often low secondary to decreased aqueous production or increased alternative outflow, but IOP may increase precipitously if the meshwork becomes clogged by inflammatory cells or debris or if the trabecular meshwork itself is the site of inflammation (trabeculitis). Pupillary block with iris bombé and secondary angle closure may also lead to an acute rise in IOP.

Hogan MJ, Kimura SJ, Thygeson P. Signs and symptoms of uveitis. I. Anterior uveitis. *Am J Ophthalmol.* 1959;47(5, part 2):155–170.

Intermediate Segment

Signs in the intermediate anatomical area of the eye include vitreal inflammatory cells, which are graded from 0 to 4+ in density:

Grade	Number of cells
0	No cells
0.5+	1–10
1+	11–20
2+	21–30
3+	31–100
4+	>100

The SUN group did not achieve consensus regarding a grading system for vitreous cells. However, the National Institutes of Health (NIH) grading system for vitreous haze, which has now been adopted by the SUN group, grades both vitreous cells and flare and may be a better indicator of disease activity than cell counts alone. With this method, standardized photographs are used for comparison to ultimately arrive at the level of vitreous haze. Additional uveitic changes may be seen in the vitreous, namely:

- *snowball opacities,* which are common with sarcoidosis or intermediate uveitis
- exudates over the pars plana *(snowbank).* Active snowbanks have a fluffy or shaggy appearance. If pars planitis becomes inactive, the pars plana appears gliotic or fibrotic and smooth; thus, these changes are not referred to as *snowbanks.*
- vitreal strands

Chronic uveitis may be associated with cyclitic membrane formation, secondary ciliary body detachment, and hypotony.

Posterior Segment

Signs in the posterior segment of the eye include

- retinal or choroidal inflammatory infiltrates
- inflammatory sheathing of arteries or veins
- exudative, tractional, or rhegmatogenous retinal detachment
- retinal pigment epithelial hypertrophy or atrophy*
- atrophy or swelling of the retina, choroid, or optic nerve head*

- preretinal or subretinal fibrosis*
- retinal or choroidal neovascularization*

The *asterisk* indicates structural complications. Retinal and choroidal signs may be unifocal, multifocal, or diffuse. Uveitis can be diffuse throughout the eye (panuveitis) or appear dispersed with spillover from 1 area to another, as with toxoplasmosis primarily involving the retina but spilling over to the anterior chamber inflammation as well.

Review of the Patient's Health and Other Associated Factors

Many aspects of the patient's medical history other than ocular symptoms and signs can help in the classification or identification of uveitis (Table 5-13). A comprehensive history and review of systems is of paramount importance in helping to elucidate the cause of uveitis. In this regard, a diagnostic survey for uveitis as shown in the appendix can be very helpful. The age, gender, sexual practices, and racial background of the patient are important elements in some uveitic syndromes.

Although ocular inflammation may be an isolated process involving only the eye, it can also be associated with a systemic condition. However, ocular inflammation frequently does not correlate with the inflammatory activity elsewhere in the body, so it is important for the clinician to carefully review systems. In some cases, the uveitis may actually precede the development of inflammation at other body sites. Immunocompromise, use of intravenous drugs, hyperalimentation, and the patient's occupation are just a few risk factors that can direct the investigation.

Table 5-13 Medical History Factors in Diagnosis of Uveitis

Modifying Factors	Associated Factors Suggesting Systemic Conditions
Time course of disease	Immune system status
Acute	Systemic medications
Recurrent	Trauma history
Chronic	Travel history
Severity	Social history
Severe	Eating habits
Inactive	Pets
Distribution of uveitis	Sexual practices
Unilateral	Occupation
Bilateral	Drug use
Alternating	
Focal	
Multifocal	
Diffuse	
Patient's sex	
Patient's age	
Patient's race	

Differential Diagnosis of Uveitic Entities

The differential diagnosis of uveitis is broad and includes infectious agents (viruses, bacteria, fungi, protozoa, and helminths), noninfectious entities of presumed immunologic or allergic origin, masquerade syndromes such as endophthalmitis and neoplastic disease, and unknown or idiopathic causes. Large cell lymphoma (previously called *reticulum cell sarcoma*), retinoblastoma, leukemia, and malignant melanoma may all be mistaken for uveitis. In addition, juvenile xanthogranuloma, pigment dispersion syndrome, retinal detachment, retinitis pigmentosa, and ocular ischemia syndrome all must be considered in the differential diagnosis of uveitis.

Although pattern recognition alone is frequently sufficient to establish a definitive diagnosis, accurate biomicroscopic and funduscopic descriptions of posterior segment inflammatory conditions are extremely helpful in performing the differential diagnosis and in distinguishing individual entities, because their distribution and evolution may be quite characteristic. However, many patients do not present with the classic signs and symptoms of a particular disease. Some patients require ongoing monitoring, as the clinical appearance may be unclear or change with time and treatment. The presentation of a disease can also be modified by previous therapy or by a delay in seeing the physician.

Once a comprehensive history has been taken and physical examination performed, the most likely causes are ranked in a list based on how well the individual patient's uveitis "fits" with the various known uveitic entities. This *naming-meshing system* first classifies the type of uveitis based on anatomical criteria and associated factors (eg, acute versus chronic, unilateral versus bilateral) and then matches the pattern of uveitis exhibited by the patient with a list of potential uveitic entities that share similar characteristics. One such system for helping to identify a possible cause for a particular patient's uveitis is outlined in Table 5-4.

Epidemiology of Uveitis

Although uveitis causes 10% of cases of all blindness in the United States, its incidence is only about 15 new cases/100,000 persons per year. Prevalence varies by geographic location, age of study population, academic center, and study date. For example, sarcoidosis has replaced Behçet disease as the most common identifiable cause of uveitis in Japan. A recent epidemiologic study of uveitis in northern California suggests an incidence of 52.4/100,000 person-years, threefold higher than previously reported in studies from the United States. In addition, the incidence and prevalence were lowest in the pediatric age groups (prevalence of 30/100,000) and highest in those over age 65 (prevalence of 151.3/100,000). Females are slightly more commonly affected. Most cases are chronic and bilateral with significant complication rates. Table 5-14 summarizes the data from several surveys, comparing the prevalence of various types of uveitis in both university/referral-based and community-based populations from around the world. This distribution is generally similar: anterior involvement is most common, followed by panuveitis, then

Table 5-14 Epidemiology of Uveitis

Study	Anatomical Distribution of Uveitis, %*				
	Anterior	Intermediate	Posterior	Panuveitis	Indeterminate
Smith et al (2009) United States (N=527; pediatric only)	44.6%	28.1%	14.4%	12.9%	
Rathinam and Namperumalsalmy (2007) India (n=8759)	57.4%	9.5%	10.6%	22.4%	
Yang et al (2005) China (N=1752)	45.6%	6.1%	6.8%	41.5%	
Sengun et al (2005) Turkey (N=300)	43.6%	9%	26.6%	20.6%	
Gritz and Wong (2004) United States (n=382; new cases only)	70.2%	2.9%	2.1%	5.0%	18.0%
Singh et al (2004) India (N=1233)	49.2%	16.1%	20.2%	14.7%	
Wakefield and Chang (2007) Combined data from 24 international studies (1990–2007)	13%–92%	0%–17%	2%–48%	4%–69%	

*The variability of data is due to nomenclature, referral bias, geographic location, and the year when the study was performed. The SUN classification system has been more widely used since 2005 and should result in more meaningful information from these types of studies.

posterior uveitis, and finally intermediate uveitis. Most university/referral-based studies probably overestimate the prevalence of intermediate and posterior uveitis compared to cases actually seen in the community.

In general, idiopathic causes are more frequently found in anterior uveitis and infectious causes are more common in posterior uveitis. Behçet disease is highly prevalent in Turkey and in China, whereas birdshot retinochoroidopathy is more common in western Europe. VKH syndrome is clearly more common among patients with identifiable causes of uveitis in China. Tuberculosis and leptospirosis remain the main causes of infectious uveitis in India. Viral uveitis followed by toxoplasmosis is predominant in the Middle East and in France.

Bodaghi B, Cassoux N, Wechsler B, et al. Chronic severe uveitis: etiology and visual outcome in 927 patients from a single center. *Medicine (Baltimore)*. 2001;80(4):263–270.

Goto H, Mochizuki M, Yamaki K, Kotake S, Usui M, Ohno S. Epidemiological survey of intraocular inflammation in Japan. *Jpn J Ophthalmol*. 2007;51(1):41–44.

Gritz DC, Wong IG. The incidence and prevalence of uveitis in Northern California. The Northern California Epidemiology of Uveitis Study. *Ophthalmology*. 2004;111(3):491–500.

Nagpal A, Leigh JF, Acharya NR. Epidemiology of uveitis in children. *Int Ophthalmol Clin*. 2008;48(3):1–7.

Rathinam SR, Namperumalsamy P. Global variation and pattern changes in epidemiology of uveitis. *Indian J Ophthalmol*. 2007;55(3):173–183.

Sengun A, Karadag R, Karakurt A, Saricaoglu MS, Abdik O, Hasiripi H. Causes of uveitis in a referral hospital in Ankara, Turkey. *Ocul Immunol Inflamm*. 2005;13(1):45–50.

Singh R, Gupta V, Gupta A. Patterns of uveitis in a referral eye clinic in north India. *Indian J Ophthalmol.* 2004;52(2):121–125.

Smith JA, Mackensen F, Sen HN, et al. Epidemiology and course of disease in childhood uveitis. *Ophthalmology.* 2009;116(8):1544–1551.

Yang P, Zhang Z, Zhou H, et al. Clinical patterns and characteristics of uveitis in a tertiary center for uveitis in China. *Curr Eye Res.* 2005;30(11):943–948.

Wakefield D, Chang JH. Epidemiology of uveitis. *Int Ophthalmol Clin.* 2005;45(2):1–13.

Laboratory and Medical Evaluation

Medical history, review of systems, thorough ophthalmologic and general physical examination, and formulation of a working differential diagnosis are cornerstones of the workup of a patient with uveitis and should precede any laboratory testing. Laboratory testing is not a substitute for a thorough, hands-on clinical evaluation.

Identification of the underlying cause of the disease may require laboratory and medical evaluation guided by the history and physical examination. *There is no one standardized battery of tests that needs to be ordered for all patients with uveitis.* Rather, a tailored approach should be taken based on the most likely causes for each patient. Once a list of differential diagnoses is compiled, appropriate laboratory tests can be ordered. Many patients require only 1 or a few diagnostic tests. When the history and physical examination do not clearly indicate the cause, most uveitis specialists will employ a few studies—purified protein derivative (PPD) skin test; serum angiotensin-converting enzyme (ACE), lysozyme, and syphilis serologies; and chest radiograph or chest computed tomography—to rule out the most common causes, which include syphilis, sarcoidosis, and tuberculosis. Tables 5-4 and 5-15 list some of the laboratory tests and their indications. These laboratory tests are discussed further in the chapters that follow, which cover the various types of uveitis.

In the evaluation of patients with certain types of uveitis, ancillary testing can also be extremely helpful:

- *Fluorescein angiography (FA)* is an essential imaging modality for evaluating eyes with chorioretinal disease and structural complications caused by posterior uveitis. FA frequently provides critical information not obtainable from biomicroscopic or fundus examination and is useful both diagnostically and in monitoring the patient's response to therapy. CME (Fig 5-6); retinal vasculitis; secondary choroidal or retinal neovascularization; and areas of optic nerve, retinal, and choroidal inflammation can all be detected angiographically. Several of the retinochoroidopathies, or white dot syndromes, have characteristic appearances on FA.
- *Fundus autofluorescence imaging* is an emerging noninvasive modality that utilizes the fluorescent properties of lipofuscin to assess the viability of the retinal pigment epithelium (RPE)–photoreceptor complex in inflammatory chorioretinopathies that involve the outer retina, RPE, and inner choroid.
- *Indocyanine green angiography* may show 2 patterns of hypofluorescence in the presence of inflammatory choroidal vasculopathies. Type 1, which represents more selective inflammatory choriocapillaropathies, demonstrates early and late multifocal areas of hypofluorescence and may be seen in multiple evanescent white dot

Table 5-15 **Laboratory tests and imaging studies with indications**

Test	Indications
Hematologic tests	
CBC	Immunomodulatory therapy (IMT), leukemia, lymphoma, immune status (neutropenia, etc)
ESR	Giant cell arteritis
Quantiferon gold	Latent and active tuberculosis
T-cell subsets	Opportunistic infection, HIV
Serologic tests	
Liver function tests (SGPT, SGOT)	IMT, sarcoidosis, hepatitis
BUN, creatinine	IMT (cyclosporine, sirolimus), glomerulonephritis
Angiotensin-converting enzyme	Sarcoidosis
Calcium	Sarcoidosis
ANA (antinuclear antibody)	Connective tissue disease, juvenile idiopathic arthritis
Antiphospholipid antibodies	Vascular occlusion
Rheumatoid factor, anticitrullinated antibodies	Rheumatoid arthritis, juvenile idiopathic arthritis
HLA testing	
HLA-B27	Seronegative spondyloarthropathy
HLA-A29	Birdshot retinochoroidopathy
HLA-B51 (rarely obtained and of limited value)	Behçet disease
ANCA testing—c-ANCA (proteinase 3) and p-ANCA (myeloperoxidase)	Systemic vasculitides
VDRL/RPR (nontreponemal tests)	Syphilis
FTA-ABS/MHA-TP (treponoma-specific tests)	Syphilis
Lyme disease serology	Lyme disease
Brucella serology	Brucellosis
Toxoplasma antibodies	Toxoplasmosis
Fungal serology (complement fixation)	Histoplasmosis, coccidioidomycosis
Bartonella quintana and *Bartonella henselae* serology	Cat-scratch disease
EBV, HSV, VZV, CMV serology	Viral uveitis (little benefit unless negative)
HIV serology/Western blot	HIV/AIDS, opportunistic infections
CSF studies	
Protein, glucose, CSF VDRL cytology, cultures, Gram stain	APMPPE, VKH syndrome, infection, malignancy, syphilis, lymphoma
Urinalysis	Vasculitis, IMT (cyclophosphamide toxicity)
Radiographic studies	
Chest radiograph	Tuberculosis, sarcoidosis, Wegener granulomatosis
Sacroiliac joint films	HLA-B27–associated ankylosing spondylitis
CT of chest	Sarcoidosis
CT/MRI—brain and orbits	Sarcoidosis, CNS lymphoma, toxoplasmosis, multiple sclerosis
Intraocular fluid analysis and tissue biopsy	
Intraocular fluid analysis (aqueous/vitreous tap)	
Local antibody production	Local antibody production: HSV, VZV, CMV, *Toxoplasma* organisms

(Continued)

Table 5-15 *(continued)*

Test	Indications
PCR	PCR available for: Viridae: HSV-1, HSV-2, VZV, CMV, EBV Bacteria: *Staphylococcus, Bacillus, Streptococcus, Pseudomonas,* and *Nisseria* species *Mycobacterium tuberculosis* and nontuberculous mycobacteria (65-kDA sAg) *Borrelia burgdorferi* (41-kDa flagellin gene) *Bartonella henselae* *Propionibacterium* (Pa1, rPa2, rPa3 antigens) *Tropheryma whipplei* (16S rRNA gene) *Treponema pallidum* Protozoa: *Toxoplasma gondii, Onchocerca volvulus* Fungi: *Candida albicans, Aspergillus* species (28S rRNA gene) Intraocular lymphoma (IgH gene)
Endoretinal, subretinal, choroidal biopsy	Necrotizing retinitis, neoplasia (CNS lymphoma)
Skin, conjunctival, lacrimal biopsy	Sarcoidosis, infection
Stool for ova and parasites	Parasitic diseases

APMPPE = acute posterior multifocal placoid pigment epitheliopathy, c-ANCA = cytoplasmic antineutrophil cytoplasmic antibody, CMV = cytomegalovirus, EBV = Epstein-Barr virus, FTA-ABS = fluorescent treponemal antibody absorption test, HSV = herpes simplex virus, MHA-TP = microhemagglutination assay for *Treponema pallidum,* p-ANCA = perinuclear ANCA, PCR = polymerase chain reaction, RPR = rapid plasma reagin test, VDRL = Venereal Disease Research Laboratory test, VZV = varicella-zoster virus.

syndrome (MEWDS). Type 2 represents stromal inflammatory vasculopathies of the choroid and demonstrates areas of early hypofluorescence and late hyperfluorescence and may be seen in sarcoidosis, sympathetic ophthalmia, birdshot retinochoroidopathy, and VKH syndrome.

- *Ultrasonography* can be useful in demonstrating vitreous opacities, choroidal thickening, retinal detachment, or cyclitic membrane formation, particularly if media opacities preclude a view of the posterior segment.
- *Electroretinography* can be used along with visual fields to follow progression of birdshot retinochoroidopathy and, occasionally, to rule out retinitis pigmentosa as a uveitis masquerade.
- *Optical coherence tomography* (OCT) and *spectral-domain OCT* (SD-OCT) are cross-sectional imaging methods using coherent light to develop a low-coherence interferometric image of the posterior segment. OCT has become a standard of care for the objective measurement of uveitic CME (Fig 5-7), retinal thickening, subretinal fluid associated with choroidal neovascularization, and serous retinal detachments. It can be useful in eyes with smaller pupils but can be limited by

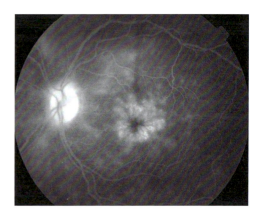

Figure 5-6 Late transit phase fluorescein angiogram of the left eye of a patient with sarcoid-associated anterior uveitis and cystoid macular edema (CME). *(Courtesy of Ramana S. Moorthy, MD.)*

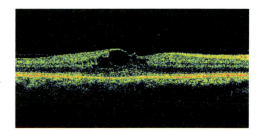

Figure 5-7 Optical coherence tomographic image of the macula of the same eye as seen in Figure 5-6, showing cystoid spaces in the parafoveal outer plexiform layer. *(Courtesy of Ramana S. Moorthy, MD.)*

media opacities. OCT can be valuable in observing patients with uveitic glaucoma. SD-OCT provides a "never-before-seen" virtual histologic analysis of the retina that is helpful in elucidating morphologic changes in many posterior uveitic and pan-uveitic entities.

- *Anterior chamber paracentesis:* Aqueous humor may be analyzed for diagnostic purposes following anterior chamber paracentesis, which is performed using sterile techniques at the slit lamp or with the patient supine on a treatment gurney or chair. Topical anesthetic drops should be instilled. The eye is prepared with topical beta-dine solution, and a lid speculum is placed if the patient is supine. A tuberculin (1-mL) syringe is attached to a sterile 30-gauge needle, which is then advanced under direct or slit-lamp visualization into the anterior chamber through the temporal limbus or clear cornea parallel to the iris plane. As much aqueous is aspirated as is safely possible (usually 0.1–0.2 mL), avoiding the iris and lens. The needle is then withdrawn, and topical antibiotic drops are instilled. Compared with diagnostic vitrectomy, this procedure is much simpler to perform in an office setting. If in-fection is suspected, the aqueous specimen should be processed for microbiologic evaluation, such as with a Gram stain. Histologic evaluation may be useful if leuke-mia or lymphoma is suspected, as in the case of a hypopyon–hyphema combination that may occur with acute myelogenous leukemic infiltration of the uveal tract. Polymerase chain reaction (PCR) evaluation may be useful if specific entities, such as herpes simplex virus types 1 or 2 (HSV-1 or -2), varicella-zoster virus (VZV), cy-tomegalovirus (CMV), or *Toxoplasma* species, are suspected. If the sample volume is large enough, the clinical appearance can often narrow the differential diagnosis and reduce the number of organisms for which to assess by PCR. Recent studies suggest similar diagnostic sensitivity (81%) and specificity (97%) of aqueous and vitreous samples, particularly in uveitis caused by HSV-1 and -2, VZV, and CMV. Evaluation of aqueous antibody production based on the Goldmann-Witmer (GW) coefficient is considered the gold standard for the diagnosis of toxoplasmosis in Europe. Diagnostic yield is increased when PCR and the GW coefficient are combined, especially in viral infections. Complications of aqueous paracentesis may include anterior chamber hemorrhage, endophthalmitis, and damage to the iris or lens. When the differential diagnosis of the uveitic entity is broader and a larger ocular fluid sample is required, vitreous biopsy should be considered.

- *Vitreous biopsy* in selected patients, with carefully planned cytologic, cytofluorographic, and microbiologic examination of vitreous fluid, can be an effective means of confirming a clinical diagnosis. The procedure is performed via a standard 3-port pars plana vitrectomy (see BCSC Section 12, *Retina and Vitreous*). If diagnostic vitrectomy (vitreous biopsy) could potentially alter the management of uveitis, it must be considered. The most common indications for this include suspected endophthalmitis, primary intraocular lymphoma or other intraocular malignancy, or infectious etiologies of posterior uveitis or panuveitis. (Endophthalmitis is discussed in detail in Chapter 8, and intraocular lymphoma in Chapter 9.) In addition, chronic uveitis that has an atypical presentation, an inconclusive systemic workup, or an inadequate response to conventional therapy may warrant a diagnostic vitrectomy. In all these scenarios, undiluted vitreous specimens are typically required for testing. It is possible to obtain 0.5–1.0 mL of undiluted vitreous for evaluation using standard vitrectomy techniques. PCR studies may also be performed on undiluted vitreous if an infectious posterior uveitis or panuveitis is suspected, but the differential diagnosis must be narrowed to a few causes because "global" PCR testing, even if it were available, would be of little value. However, many different infectious agents may be detected by PCR (see Table 5-15). Specific primers for *Toxoplasma gondii*, HSV, VZV, and CMV are readily available. Combined with the clinical picture, the presence of DNA from specific pathogens can be very sensitive and specific in establishing an etiology. Complications of diagnostic vitrectomy in uveitic eyes can include retinal tears or detachment, suprachoroidal or vitreous hemorrhage, and worsening of cataract or inflammation. Although vitreous surgery can be therapeutic and diagnostic in cases of uveitis, the pharmacokinetics of delivered intravitreal agents are markedly different in eyes that have undergone pars plana vitrectomy; the half-life of intravitreal corticosteroids, for example, is markedly reduced in vitrectomized eyes.
- *Chorioretinal biopsy*, a more technically challenging procedure, may be useful when the diagnosis cannot be confirmed on the basis of clinical appearance or other laboratory investigations. Rapidly progressive posterior uveitic or panuveitic entities, such as necrotizing retinitis in which the etiology is unknown and the therapeutic regimen is undetermined, may require chorioretinal biopsy. Suspected intraocular lymphoma confined to the subretinal space is also an indication for a chorioretinal biopsy. This procedure is performed only after all other less-invasive measures, such as serologic, radiologic, and aqueous and vitreous sample testing, have failed

to make the diagnosis. It is associated with a high rate of complications and must be performed only by vitreoretinal surgeons with extensive experience with these techniques.

Details of these methods are beyond the scope of this text.

Ciardella AP, Prall FR, Borodoker N, Cunningham ET Jr. Imaging techniques for posterior uveitis. *Curr Opin Ophthalmol.* 2004;15(6):519–530.

Davis JL, Miller DM, Ruiz P. Diagnostic testing of vitrectomy specimens. *Am J Ophthalmol.* 2005;140(5):822–829.

de Groot-Mijnes JDF, Rothova A, van Loon AM, et al. Polymerase chain reaction and Goldmann-Witmer coefficient analysis are complementary for the diagnosis of infectious uveitis. *Am J Ophthalmol.* 2006;141(2):313–318.

Harper TW, Miller D, Schiffman JC, Davis JL. Polymerase chain reaction analysis of aqueous and vitreous specimens in the diagnosis of posterior segment infectious uveitis. *Am J Ophthalmol.* 2009;147(1):140–147.

Matos K, Muccioli C, Belfort R Jr, Rizzo LV. Correlation between clinical diagnosis and PCR analysis of serum, aqueous, and vitreous samples in patients with inflammatory eye disease. *Arq Bras Oftalmol.* 2007;70(1):109–114.

Quentin CD, Reiber H. Fuchs heterochromic cyclitis: rubella virus antibodies and genome in aqueous humor. *Am J Ophthalmol.* 2004;138(1):46–54.

Sowmya P, Madhavan HN. Diagnostic utility of polymerase chain reaction on intraocular specimens to establish the etiology of infectious endophthalmitis. *Eur J Ophthalmol.* 2009;19(5):812–817.

Therapy

Many patients with mild, self-limiting anterior uveitis need no referral to a uveitis specialist. However, in uveitis with a chronic or downwardly spiraling course, referral to a uveitis specialist may be helpful not only in eliciting the cause and determining the therapeutic regimen but also in reassuring the patient that all avenues are being explored. Treatment may require coordination with other medical or surgical consultants and detailed informed consent. Discussion with the patient and other specialists about the prognosis and complications of uveitis helps to determine the appropriate therapy. Therapy for uveitis ranges from simple observation to complex medical or surgical intervention.

Medical Management of Uveitis

The goal of medical management of uveitis is to effectively control inflammation so as to eliminate or reduce the risk of vision loss from structural and functional complications that result from uncontrolled inflammation, namely cataracts, glaucoma, CME, and hypotony. Generally, medical therapy includes topical cycloplegics, topical or systemic nonsteroidal anti-inflammatory drugs, and topical or systemic corticosteroids. Corticosteroids are the best agents to control inflammation as quickly as possible. Route and dose are tailored as specifically as possible to the patient, taking into account his or her systemic involvement and other factors, such as age, immune status, tolerance for side effects, and response to treatment. As these initial agents are tapered, the dosage at which disease recrudescence occurs determines which, if any, second-line immunomodulatory agents are then used. The choice of a second-line agent also requires consideration of multiple patient factors. If second-line therapy fails, there are few treatment guidelines, and combination therapy with multiple second-line agents may be considered.

Mydriatic and Cycloplegic Agents

Topical mydriatic and cycloplegic agents are beneficial for breaking or preventing the formation of posterior synechiae and for relieving photophobia secondary to ciliary spasm. The stronger the inflammatory reaction, the stronger or more frequent the dosage of the cycloplegic. Short-acting drops such as cyclopentolate hydrochloride 1% or long-acting drops such as atropine may be used. Most cases of acute anterior uveitis require only short-acting cycloplegics; these allow the pupil to remain mobile and permit rapid recovery when they are discontinued. Patients with chronic uveitis and moderate flare in the anterior chamber (eg, JIA-associated iritis) may need to be maintained on short-acting agents (eg, tropicamide) for the long term to prevent posterior synechiae.

Nonsteroidal Anti-Inflammatory Drugs

Nonsteroidal anti-inflammatory drugs (NSAIDs) work by inhibiting cyclooxygenase (COX) isoforms 1 and 2 or 2 alone and reduce the synthesis of prostaglandins that mediate inflammation. COX-1 is present in nearly all cells and appears to be involved in cellular metabolic events such as gastric cytoprotection, platelet aggregation, and renal function, whereas COX-2 seems to mediate inflammation. The first selective COX-2 inhibitors were introduced in the late 1990s. They had less effect on platelet function and reduced the risk of secondary gastrointestinal damage; however, rofecoxib and valdecoxib were removed from the market because numerous studies identified increased risks of adverse cardiovascular events. Celecoxib was thought to have the same dangers although it is still available, with significant warnings on the package insert. Because of this cardiovascular risk and controversy, the use of COX-2 inhibitors in the treatment of ocular inflammatory diseases has been somewhat limited. Traditional NSAIDs are still utilized for the treatment of mild to moderate forms of nonnecrotizing anterior scleritis. Several studies have shown that systemic NSAIDs may be efficacious in the treatment of chronic iridocyclitis (eg, JIA-associated iridocyclitis) and possibly CME, and may allow the patient to be maintained on a lower dose of topical corticosteroids. Potential complications of prolonged systemic NSAID use include myocardial infarction, hypertension, and stroke (especially with selective COX-2 inhibitors); gastric ulceration; gastrointestinal bleeding; nephrotoxicity; and hepatotoxicity. COX-2 inhibitors should be used with caution, if no alternative agents are effective; detailed informed consent must be obtained. See also BCSC Section 1, *Update on General Medicine,* Chapter 8.

Topical NSAIDs play an even smaller role in ocular inflammatory disease; they may be used in the treatment of very mild cases of diffuse episcleritis. These agents are also useful in the treatment of postoperative pseudophakic CME. They are not useful for treating noninfectious anterior uveitis. Ketorolac and 2 newer agents, bromfenac and nepafenac, may be used for the treatment of CME. In rare cases, severe corneal problems such as keratitis and corneal perforations may occur with the use of topical NSAIDs. Most occurred with a generic formulation of diclofenac that is no longer available. Nongeneric formulations of ketorolac and diclofenac have also been implicated. Patients who have severe dry eye and rheumatoid arthritis may be more prone to such complications.

Finckh A, Aronson MD. Cardiovascular risk of cyclooxygenase inhibitors: where we stand now. *Ann Intern Med.* 2005;142(3):212–214.

Topol EJ. Arthritis medicines and cardiovascular events—"house of coxibs." *JAMA.* 2005;293: 366–368.

Corticosteroids

Corticosteroids are the mainstay of uveitis therapy. Because of their potential side effects (Table 5-16), however, they should be reserved for specific indications:

- treatment of active inflammation in the eye
- prevention or treatment of complications such as CME
- reduction of inflammatory infiltration of the retina, choroid, or optic nerve

Complications of corticosteroid therapy are numerous and can be seen with any mode of administration. Therefore, these agents should be used only when the benefits of therapy outweigh the risks of the medications themselves. Corticosteroids are not always indicated in patients with chronic flare or for the therapy of specific diseases such as Fuchs heterochromic iridocyclitis or pars planitis without macular edema, or with a peripheral toxoplasmic lesion (ie, that does not threaten the optic disc or macula).

The dose and duration of corticosteroid therapy must be individualized. It is generally preferable to begin therapy with a high dose of corticosteroids (topical or systemic) and taper it as the inflammation subsides, rather than beginning with a low dose that may have to be progressively increased to control the inflammation. To reduce the complications of therapy, patients should be maintained on the minimum dosage needed to control the inflammation. Corticosteroids must be tapered gradually (over days to weeks) and not stopped abruptly if utilized for longer than 2–3 weeks to prevent disease relapse. If surgical intervention to treat uveitis or its complications is required, the dosage may need to be increased to prevent postoperative exacerbation of the uveitis. The relative potencies of various corticosteroid preparations are summarized in Table 5-16.

Topical administration

Topical corticosteroid drops are effective primarily for anterior uveitis, although they may have beneficial effects on vitritis or macular edema in patients who are pseudophakic or aphakic. These drops are given in time intervals ranging from once daily to hourly. They can also be given in an ointment form for nighttime use or if preservatives in the eyedrops are not well tolerated. Difluprednate 0.05%, a fluorinated corticosteroid, is highly potent and has the same efficacy as the every-2-hour dosage of prednisolone when given just 4 times daily. Clinical studies suggest a similar side effect profile as prednisolone. Of the

Table 5-16 **Corticosteroids Frequently Used in Uveitis Therapy and Their Complications**

Route of Administration	Relative Anti-Inflammatory Activity*	Complications
Topical		Cataract (posterior subcapsular), elevation of IOP/glaucoma, exacerbation of external infection (eg, keratitis), corneal and scleral thinning or melting, delayed wound healing
Prednisolone acetate 1%	2.3	
Prednisolone sodium phosphate 1%	2.3	
Fluorometholone 0.1%	21	
Dexamethasone phosphate 0.1%	24	
Rimexolone 1%		
Loteprednol etabonate 0.5% or 0.2%		
Difluprednate 0.05%		
Periocular		Same complications as topical above and: Ptosis, scarring of conjunctiva/Tenon capsule, worsening of infectious uveitis, scleral perforation, hemorrhage
Long-acting		
Methylprednisolone acetate	5.0	
Triamcinolone acetonide	5.0	
Triamcinolone diacetate	5.0	
Short-acting		
Hydrocortisone sodium succinate	1.0	
Betamethasone	25	
Intraocular		Same complications as topical above and: Endophthalmitis (sterile or infectious), vitreous hemorrhage, retinal detachment
Triamcinolone (preservative-free) 4 mg/0.1 mL	5.0	
Systemic		Same complications as topical above and: Increased appetite, weight gain, peptic ulcers, sodium and fluid retention, osteoporosis/bone fractures, aseptic necrosis of hip, hypertension, diabetes mellitus, menstrual irregularities, mental status changes, exacerbation of systemic infections, impaired wound healing, acne, many others
Prednisone	4.0	
Triamcinolone	5.0	
Dexamethasone	25	
Methylprednisolone	5.0	

*Numbers represent relative anti-inflammatory activity compared to that of hydrocortisone.

topical preparations, rimexolone, loteprednol, and fluorometholone have been shown to produce a smaller ocular hypertensive effect than other medications and may be particularly useful in patients who are corticosteroid responders. However, these agents are not as effective as prednisolone in controlling uveitis that is more intense than mild to moderate. Some generic forms of prednisolone may have less of an anti-inflammatory effect than brand-name products; this should be considered when patients do not respond adequately to topical corticosteroid therapy. Differences in efficacy may be a result of differences in particle size among various suspensions and may necessitate more vigorous agitation of the drug before instillation.

> Korenfeld MS, Silverstein SM, Cooke DL, Vogel R, Crockett RS, and the Difluprednate Ophthalmic Emulsion 0.05% (Durezol) Study Group. Difluprednate ophthalmic emulsion 0.05% for postoperative inflammation and pain. *J Cataract Refract Surg.* 2009;35(1):26–34.

Periocular administration

Periocular corticosteroids are generally given as depot injections when a more posterior effect is needed or when a patient is noncompliant with or unresponsive to topical or systemic administration. They are often preferred for patients with intermediate or posterior uveitis or CME, because they deliver a therapeutic dose of medication close to the site of inflammation. Periocular corticosteroids can cause systemic side effects similar to oral corticosteroids. Triamcinolone acetonide (40 mg) and methylprednisolone acetate (40–80 mg) are the most commonly used agents.

Periocular injections can be performed using either a transseptal or a sub-Tenon (Nozik technique) approach (Fig 5-8). With a sub-Tenon injection, a 25-gauge, ⅝-inch needle is used. If the injection is given in the superotemporal quadrant (the preferred location), the upper eyelid is retracted and the patient is instructed to look down and nasally. After anesthesia is applied with a cotton swab soaked in proparacaine or tetracaine, the

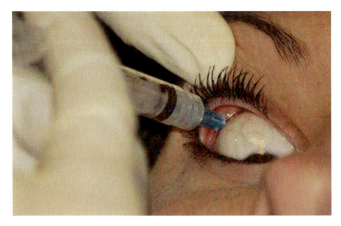

Figure 5-8 Posterior sub-Tenon injection of triamcinolone acetonide demonstrating correct position of the operator's hands and the needle. The needle is advanced to the hub with a side-to-side motion to detect any scleral engagement and directed caudad and nasally prior to injection of the corticosteroid. The positioning of the tip of the needle in its ideal location between the Tenon capsule and the sclera. *(Courtesy of Ramana S. Moorthy, MD.)*

needle is placed bevel-down against the sclera and advanced through the conjunctiva and Tenon capsule using a side-to-side movement, which allows the physician to determine whether the needle has entered the sclera or not. As long as the globe does not torque with the side-to-side movement of the needle, the physician can be reasonably sure that the needle has not penetrated the sclera. Once the needle has been advanced to the hub, the corticosteroid is injected into the sub-Tenon space. Complications of the superotemporal approach include upper lid ptosis, periorbital hemorrhage, and globe perforation.

Although sub-Tenon injections are typically given in the superotemporal quadrant, the inferotemporal approach can also be performed in a similar fashion. However, the inferior approach using the Nozik technique can be awkward to perform. The transseptal route of delivery is preferred for the inferior approach and is performed by using a short 27-gauge needle, usually on a 3-mL syringe containing the drug (Fig 5-9). The index finger may be used to push the temporal lower lid posteriorly and locate the equator of the globe. The needle is inserted inferior to the globe through the skin of the eyelid, and directed straight back through the orbital septum into the orbital fat to the hub of the needle. The needle is aspirated, and if there is no blood reflux, the corticosteroid is injected. Complications of the inferior approach can include periorbital and retrobulbar hemorrhage, lower lid retractor ptosis, orbital fat prolapse with periorbital festoon formation, orbital fat atrophy, and skin discoloration. This transseptal approach can be more painful than the sub-Tenon injection if a 25-gauge needle is used; pain can be reduced with a 27-gauge needle.

Periocular injections should not be used in cases of infectious uveitis (eg, toxoplasmosis) and should also be avoided in patients with necrotizing scleritis, because scleral thinning and perforation may result. The physician should be aware that periocular corticosteroid injections have the potential to raise the IOP precipitously or for a long time, particularly with the longer-acting agents (triamcinolone or methylprednisolone). In such cases, the periocular steroid should be surgically removed, especially if it had been given anterior to the septum or in a subconjunctival space, although subconjunctival administration is generally not performed because of the risk of subconjunctival migration of the steroid vehicle.

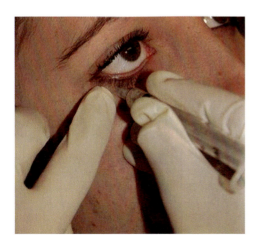

Figure 5-9 Inferior transseptal injection of triamcinolone acetonide in the right eye. A 27-gauge, ¹/₂-inch needle on a 3-mL syringe is inserted through the skin of the lower eyelid and the inferior orbital septum. By using the index finger of the opposite hand, the physician can determine the location of the equator of the globe to prevent perforation and to place the depot corticosteroid as posteriorly as possible. *(Courtesy of Ramana S. Moorthy, MD.)*

Systemic administration

Oral or intravenous therapy may supplement or replace other routes of administration. Systemic corticosteroids are used for vision-threatening chronic uveitis when topical corticosteroids are insufficient or when systemic disease also requires therapy; if they are used, the dosing and taper should be individualized to the patient. Many oral corticosteroid formulations are available; prednisone is the most commonly used. The readily available packages of methylprednisolone that are used over 1 week or less have little or no role in the treatment of uveitis. Treatment with corticosteroids may last for 3 months. If corticosteroid therapy is required for longer than 3 months, immunomodulatory therapy (IMT) is indicated.

Most patients require 1–2 mg/kg/day of oral prednisone, which is gradually tapered every 1 to 2 weeks until the disease is quiescent. The lowest possible dose that will control the ocular inflammation and minimize side effects is desired. This dose should be no more than 5–10 mg/day. If a dose greater than 5–10 mg/day is required, corticosteroid-sparing IMT must be used.

In cases of an explosive onset of severe noninfectious posterior uveitis or panuveitis, intravenous, high-dose, pulse methylprednisolone (1 g/day infused over 1 hour) therapy may be administered for 3 days, followed by a gradual taper of oral prednisone starting at 1.0–1.5 mg/kg/day. Although this approach may control intraocular inflammation, side effects are numerous and can be life-threatening. These can include psychological disturbances, hypertension, and elevated glucose levels. This therapy should be performed only in a hospital setting by those experienced with this approach and its potential side effects.

The many side effects of both short-term and long-term systemic corticosteroid use must be discussed with patients, and their general health must be closely monitored, often with the assistance of an internist. Patients with a propensity toward or manifest diabetes mellitus; those with hypertension, peptic ulcer, or gastroesophageal reflux disease; those who are immunocompromised (from acquired or congenital causes); and those with psychiatric conditions are at high risk for corticosteroid-induced exacerbations of their conditions. Corticosteroids should be avoided, if at all possible, in these patients.

Patients on high-dose oral corticosteroids should be placed on histamine-2 receptor blockers or proton pump inhibitors to prevent gastric and peptic ulcers. The risk of gastric ulcer is particularly high in patients who are concomitantly taking systemic NSAIDs. Patients maintained on long-term corticosteroid therapy, particularly aging adults and postmenopausal women, should supplement their diet with calcium and vitamin D to lessen the chances of osteoporosis. The following tests may be used to evaluate patients at risk for corticosteroid-induced bone loss:

- serial height measurements
- serum calcium and phosphorus levels
- serum 25-hydroxycholecalciferol levels (if vitamin D stores are uncertain)
- follicle-stimulating hormone and testosterone levels (if gonadal status is uncertain)
- bone mineral density screening (for anyone receiving corticosteroid therapy for more than 3 months)

The US Food and Drug Administration (FDA) has approved several agents for prevention and treatment of corticosteroid-induced osteoporosis in men and women. These may be administered to at-risk patients receiving 7.5 mg or more of daily prednisone equivalent.

Involvement of the patient's internist and/or rheumatologist is essential in the treatment of individuals on systemic corticosteroids, so that the complications of therapy may be quickly identified and treated.

Reed JB, Morse LS, Schwab IR. High-dose intravenous pulse methylprednisolone hemisuccinate in acute Behçet retinitis. *Am J Ophthalmol.* 1998(3);125:409–411.

Sasamoto Y, Ohno S, Matsuda H. Studies on corticosteroid therapy in Vogt-Koyanagi-Harada disease. *Ophthalmologica.* 1990;201(3):162–167.

Wakefield D, Jennings A, McCluskey PJ. Intravenous pulse methylprednisolone in the treatment of uveitis associated with multiple sclerosis. *Clin Experiment Ophthalmol.* 2000;28(2): 103–106.

Intravitreal administration

Intravitreal injections of triamcinolone acetonide have been used extensively in the treatment of uveitic conditions. Published literature on intravitreal triamcinolone suggests a definite treatment benefit, although of limited duration, for recalcitrant uveitic CME.

Single trans–pars plana intravitreal injections of 4 mg (0.1 mL) of triamcinolone may produce sustained visual acuity improvements for 3 to 6 months in nonvitrectomized eyes. CME may recur after 3 to 6 months. Multiple injections increase the risk of cataract formation in phakic patients, and IOP elevation may occur transiently in more than one-half of patients. Up to 25% of patients may require topical medications to control IOP, and 1%–2% may require filtering surgery. Complications such as "sterile endophthalmitis" may occur in 1%–6% of patients, but the incidence has dramatically declined since the introduction of FDA-approved, preservative-free intravitreal triamcinolone (Triescence, Alcon). Infectious endophthalmitis and rhegmatogenous retinal detachment may occur, but these are rare when proper technique is used. Long-term clinical efficacy and outcome studies are under way. This method of treatment is not curative of chronic uveitic conditions and should be used judiciously as its effects are relatively short-lived.

The sustained-release fluocinolone implant was approved by the FDA in 2005 for the treatment of chronic noninfectious posterior uveitis. Multicenter, controlled clinical studies have shown that the 0.59-mg implant is effective for a median of 30 months with a mean time of 38 months to first recurrence. At 34 weeks after implantation, inflammation was well controlled in nearly all eyes, and recurrence rates decreased by 90%, with 77% of patients able to discontinue systemic therapy and 96% able to discontinue local corticosteroid injections. However, nearly all phakic eyes developed cataract within 2 years after implantation. Glaucoma necessitating topical therapy developed in nearly 75% of patients after 3 years, and 37% required filtering surgery. Postoperative complications such as endophthalmitis, wound leaks, hypotony, vitreous hemorrhage, and retinal detachments have been reported. Reimplantation may be performed. The fluocinolone implant is being compared to standard systemic therapy in the Multicenter Uveitis Steroid Treatment (MUST) trial, which has enrolled 255 patients over 3 years. Results are pending.

A new biodegradable intraocular implant containing 700 µg of dexamethasone is currently under active investigation for the treatment of uveitis, but currently is approved by the FDA only for the treatment of macular edema caused by retinal vein occlusion. Preliminary studies suggest efficacy in the treatment of uveitic CME.

Androudi S, Letko E, Meniconi M, Papadaki T, Ahmed M, Foster CS. Safety and efficacy of intravitreal triamcinolone acetonide for uveitic macular edema. *Ocul Immunol Inflamm.* 2005;13(2–3):205–212.

Goldstein DA, Godfrey DG, Hall A, et al. Intraocular pressure in patients with uveitis treated with fluocinolone acetonide implants. *Arch Ophthalmol.* 2007;125(11):1478–1485.

Jaffe GJ. Reimplantation of a fluocinolone acetonide sustained drug delivery implant for chronic uveitis. *Am J Ophthalmol.* 2008;145(4):667–675.

Jaffe GJ, Martin DF, Callanan D, Pearson PA, Levy B, Comstock T, and the Fluocinolone Acetonide Uveitis Study Group. Fluocinolone acetonide implant (Retisert) for noninfectious posterior uveitis. Thirty-four-week results of a multicenter randomized clinical study. *Ophthalmology.* 2006;113(6):1020–1027.

Jaffe GJ, McCallum RM, Branchaud B, Skalak C, Butuner Z, Ashton P. Long-term follow-up results of a pilot trial of a fluocinolone acetonide implant to treat posterior uveitis. *Ophthalmology.* 2005;112(7):1192–1198.

Kupperman BD, Blumenkranz MS, Haller JA, et al, and the Dexamethasone DDS Phase II Study Group. Randomized controlled study of an intravitreous dexamethasone drug delivery system in patients with persistent macular edema. *Arch Ophthalmol.* 2007;125(3):309–317.

The Multicenter Uveitis Steroid Treatment Trial Research Group. The Multicenter Uveitis Steroid Treatment trial: rationale, design, and baseline characteristics. *Am J Ophthalmol.* 2010;149(4):550–561.

Stepien KE, Eaton AM, Jaffe GJ, Davis JL, Raja J, Feuer W. Increased incidence of sterile endophthalmitis after intravitreal triamcinolone acetonide in Spring 2006. *Retina.* 2009;29(2):207–213.

Immunomodulatory Medications

The addition of immunomodulatory (sometimes referred to as "immunosuppressive") medications may greatly benefit patients with severe, sight-threatening uveitis or those who are resistant to or cannot tolerate corticosteroids. These agents are thought to work by killing the rapidly dividing clones of lymphocytes that are responsible for the inflammation (see Part I, Ocular Immunology). As more evidence accumulates about the complications associated with long-term systemic corticosteroid use, IMT is being used with increasing frequency to permit corticosteroid sparing. Although the early use of IMT is indicated in certain diseases (see the following section), these drugs should also be considered in patients who require chronic corticosteroid therapy (longer than 3 months) at doses greater than 5–10 mg/day. The use of IMT can also be considered in patients with chronic topical corticosteroid dependence and those requiring multiple periocular corticosteroid injections.

Indications

The following considerations generally apply to the therapeutic use of IMT in uveitis:

- vision-threatening intraocular inflammation
- reversibility of the disease process

- inadequate response to corticosteroid treatment
  - failure of therapy
- corticosteroids contraindicated because of systemic problems or intolerable side effects
  - unacceptable corticosteroid side effects
  - chronic corticosteroid dependence

Corticosteroids are the mainstay of initial therapy, but certain specific uveitic entities also warrant the early use of IMT for treatment of intraocular inflammation, including ocular cicatricial pemphigoid, serpiginous choroiditis, Behçet disease, sympathetic ophthalmia, VKH syndrome, and necrotizing scleritis associated with systemic vasculitis. Although these disorders may initially respond well to corticosteroids, the initial treatment of these entities with IMT has been shown to improve the long-term prognosis and to lessen visual morbidity.

Relative indications for these agents include conditions that do not respond adequately to initial corticosteroid treatment and cases in which patients develop serious corticosteroid-induced side effects. Examples include intermediate uveitis (pars planitis), retinal vasculitis, panuveitis, and chronic iridocyclitis.

Treatment

Before initiating IMT, the physician should ensure that there is

- absence of infection
- absence of hepatic and hematologic contraindications
- meticulous follow-up available from a physician who is, by virtue of training and experience, qualified to prescribe and safety monitor such medications and personally manage their potential toxicities
- objective longitudinal evaluation of the disease process
- informed consent

Several classes of immunomodulatory medications exist. These include antimetabolites, inhibitors of T-cell signaling, alkylating agents, and biologic response modifiers. These agents are listed in Table 5-17, along with their mechanisms of action, dosages, and potential complications. It should be noted that no therapeutic response may occur for several weeks after initiation of IMT; therefore, most patients need to be maintained on corticosteroids until the immunomodulatory agent begins to take effect, at which time the corticosteroid dose may be gradually tapered.

Because of the potentially serious complications associated with the use of IMT, patients must be monitored closely by a practitioner who is experienced with their use. Blood monitoring, including complete blood count and liver and renal function tests, should be performed regularly. Serious complications include renal and hepatic toxicity, bone marrow suppression, and increased susceptibility to infection. In addition, alkylating agents may cause sterility and were associated in earlier studies with an increased risk of future malignancies such as leukemia or lymphoma. A recent retrospective study of 7957 patients (66,802 patient-years) with noninfectious uveitis treated with IMT showed, however, that patients who took azathioprine, methotrexate, mycophenolate mofetil, cyclosporine, systemic corticosteroids, or dapsone had overall and cancer mortality rates

Table 5-17 Immunomodulatory Medications in the Treatment of Uveitis

Medication	Mechanism of Action	Dosage	Potential Complications
Antimetabolites			
Methotrexate	Folate analogue; inhibits dihydrofolate reductase	7.5–25.0 μg/week PO or SQ	GI upset, fatigue, hepatotoxicity, pneumonitis
Azathioprine	Alters purine metabolism	100–250 mg/d PO	GI upset, hepatotoxicity
Mycophenolate mofetil	Inhibits purine synthesis	1–3 g/d PO	Diarrhea, nausea, GI ulceration
Inhibitors of T-cell signaling			
Cyclosporine	Inhibits NF-AT (nuclear factor of activated T lymphocytes) activation	2.5–5.0 mg/kg/d PO	Nephrotoxicity, hypertension, gingival hyperplasia, GI upset, paresthesias
Tacrolimus	Inhibits NF-AT activation	0.1–0.2 mg/kg/d PO	Nephrotoxicity, hypertension, diabetes mellitus
Sirolimus*	Inhibits T-lymphocyte activation in G1 Blunts T- and B-lymphocyte responses to lymphokines	6 mg loading dose IV and then 4 mg/d IV increasing by 2-mg increments	Gastrointestinal, cutaneous at trough levels of >25 ng/mL
Alkylating agents			
Cyclophosphamide	Cross-links DNA	1–2 mg/d PO	Hemorrhagic cystitis, sterility, increased risk of malignancy
Chlorambucil	Cross-links DNA	2–12 mg/d PO	Sterility, increased risk of malignancy
Biologic response modifiers			
Infliximab	TNF-α inhibitor	3 mg/kg IV weeks 0, 2, 6 and then q 6–8 weeks	Infusion reactions, infections (TB reactivation—for all TNF-α inhibitors) Malignancy/ lymphoproliferative diseases Autoantibodies/ lupuslike syndrome Congestive heart failure
Adalimumab*	TNF-α inhibitor	40 mg q 1 week or q 2 weeks	Headache, nausea, rash, stomach upset
Daclizumab*	Binds the alpha subunit of IL-2 receptor	1.0 mg/kg IV q 2 weeks x 5 doses	Rare if any
Rituximab*	Binds CD20-positive lymphocytes (mainly B lymphocytes)	Two infusions 1.0 g IV given 2 weeks apart and repeated	Late-onset neutropenia; few case reports
Anakinra*	IL-1 receptor antagonist	100 mg subcutaneous injection daily	Few case reports; efficacy in posterior uveitis and JIA?

*Still under investigation.

similar to those who never took those medications. On the other hand, tumor necrosis factor inhibitors were associated with increased overall (twofold) and cancer (3.8-fold) risk of mortality. Trimethoprim-sulfamethoxazole prophylaxis against *Pneumocystis jiroveci* (previously known as *Pneumocystis carinii*) infection should be considered in patients receiving alkylating agents. The physician should obtain thorough informed consent prior to initiating IMT.

Although IMT may be associated with serious life-threatening complications, it can be extremely effective in the treatment of ocular inflammatory disease in patients unresponsive to, or intolerant of, systemic corticosteroids. All of these agents are potentially teratogenic, and patients should be advised to avoid becoming pregnant while taking them. Again, the physician should obtain informed consent prior to beginning therapy.

Jabs DA, Rosenbaum JT, Foster CS, et al. Guidelines for the use of immunosuppressive drugs in patients with ocular inflammatory disorders: recommendations of an expert panel. *Am J Ophthalmol.* 2000;130(4):492–513.

Kempen JH, Daniel E, Dunn JP, et al. Overall and cancer related mortality among patients with ocular inflammation treated with immunosuppressive drugs: retrospective cohort study. *BMJ.* 2009;339:b2480. doi:10.1136/bmj.b2480.

Smith JR, Rosenbaum JT. Management of uveitis: a rheumatologic perspective. *Arthritis Rheum.* 2002;46(2):309–318.

Antimetabolites

The antimetabolites include azathioprine, methotrexate, and mycophenolate mofetil. They have different clinical properties but all appear to have similar long-term efficacy. A recent study comparing antimetabolite drugs used to treat noninfectious uveitis found a slightly higher incidence of side effects among patients taking azathioprine and a significantly shorter time to treatment success for mycophenolate mofetil.

Azathioprine, a purine nucleoside analogue, interferes with DNA replication and RNA transcription. It is administered at a dose of 2 mg/kg/day. It is well absorbed orally and, in a randomized, placebo-controlled trial in patients with Behçet disease, it was shown to be effective in preventing ocular involvement among those without eye disease and in decreasing the occurrence of contralateral eye involvement among those with unilateral Behçet uveitis. It has also been found beneficial in patients with intermediate uveitis, VKH syndrome, sympathetic ophthalmia, and necrotizing scleritis. Overall, nearly 50% of patients treated with azathioprine achieve inflammatory control and are able to taper prednisone dosage to 10 mg/day or less. Many clinicians start administering azathioprine at 50 mg/day for 1 week to see if the patient develops any gastrointestinal side effects (nausea, upset stomach, and vomiting) before escalating the dose. These symptoms are common and may occur in up to 25% of patients, necessitating discontinuation. Bone marrow suppression is unusual at the doses of azathioprine used to treat uveitis. Reversible hepatic toxicity occurs in less than 2% of patients. Dose reduction may remedy mild hepatotoxicity. Complete blood counts and liver function tests must be obtained every 4–6 weeks. The variability of clinical response to azathioprine among patients is probably caused by genetic variability in the activity of thiopurine S-methyltransferase (TPMT), an enzyme responsible for the metabolism of 6-mercaptopurine (6-MP). A genotypic test is now becoming available that can help determine patient candidacy for azathioprine therapy before treatment and can help clinicians individualize patient doses. Evaluation of TPMT activity has revealed 3 groups of patients:

- low/no TPMT activity (0.3% of patients); azathioprine therapy not recommended
- intermediate TPMT activity (11% of patients); azathioprine therapy at reduced dosage
- normal/high TPMT activity (89% of patients); azathioprine therapy at higher doses than in patients with intermediate TPMT activity

Methotrexate is a folic acid analogue and inhibitor of dihydrofolate reductase; it inhibits DNA replication, but its anti-inflammatory effects result from extracellular release of adenosine. Numerous studies have shown methotrexate to be effective in treating various types of uveitis, including JIA-associated iridocyclitis, sarcoidosis, panuveitis, and scleritis. Treatment with this medication is unique in that it is given as a *weekly* dose, usually starting at 7.5–10.0 mg/week and gradually increasing to a maintenance dose of 15–25 mg/week. Methotrexate can be given orally, subcutaneously, intramuscularly, or intravenously and is usually well tolerated. It has greater bioavailability when given parenterally. Folate is given concurrently at a dose of 1 mg/day to reduce side effects. Methotrexate may take up to 6 months to produce its full effect in controlling intraocular inflammation. Gastrointestinal distress and anorexia may occur in 10% of patients. Reversible hepatotoxicity occurs in up to 15% of patients, and cirrhosis occurs in less than 0.1% of patients receiving long-term methotrexate. Methotrexate is teratogenic, and complete blood counts and liver function tests should be obtained every 4–6 weeks to monitor for side effects. The drug has a long record of success in the treatment of children with JIA. For that reason, it has been a first-line choice for IMT in children. Uncontrolled clinical trials have shown that it can enable corticosteroid sparing in two-thirds of patients with chronic ocular inflammatory disorders. Recently, a prospective study of intravitreal injections of methotrexate (400 μg) for the treatment of refractory uveitis and uveitic CME demonstrated reduction of inflammation and CME, and reduced need for other systemic IMT. This treatment is being actively investigated.

Mycophenolate mofetil inhibits both inosine monophosphate dehydrogenase and DNA replication. It has good oral bioavailability and is given at a dose of 1 g twice daily. It tends to work rapidly; median time to successful control of ocular inflammation (in combination with less than 10 mg/day of prednisone) is about 4 months. Reversible gastrointestinal distress and diarrhea are common side effects, although less than 20% of patients receiving mycophenolate mofetil have side effects; these can usually be managed by dose reduction. Very few patients find the drug intolerable. Complete blood counts should be performed every week for 1 month, then every 2 weeks for 2 months, and then monthly. Two large retrospective studies found mycophenolate mofetil to be an effective corticosteroid-sparing agent in up to 85% of patients with chronic uveitis. It has similar efficacy in children (88%) and can be a safe alternative to methotrexate in patients with pediatric uveitis. Its side effect profile makes it a reasonable first choice for IMT in adults.

Cutolo M, Sulli A, Pizzorni C, Seriolo B, Straub RH. Anti-inflammatory mechanisms of methotrexate in rheumatoid arthritis. *Ann Rheum Dis* 2001;60(8):729–735.

Doycheva D, Deuter C, Stuebiger N, Biester S, Zierhut M. Mycophenolate mofetil in the treatment of uveitis in children. *Br J Ophthalmol.* 2007;91(2):180–184.

Galor A, Jabs DA, Leder H, et al. Comparison of antimetabolite drugs as corticosteroid-sparing therapy for noninfectious ocular inflammation. *Ophthalmology.* 2008;115(10):1826–1832.

Malik AR, Pavesio C. The use of low dose methotrexate in children with chronic anterior and intermediate uveitis. *Br J Ophthalmol.* 2005;89(7):806–808.

Pasadhika S, Kempen JH, Newcomb CW, et al. Azathioprine for ocular inflammatory diseases. *Am J Ophthalmol* 2009;148(4):500–509.

Samson CM, Waheed N, Baltatzis S, Foster CS. Methotrexate therapy for chronic noninfectious uveitis: analysis of a case series of 160 patients. *Ophthalmology.* 2001;108(6):1134–1139.

Siepmann K, Huber M, Stubiger N, et al. Mycophenolate mofetil is a highly effective and safe immunosuppressive agent for the treatment of uveitis: a retrospective analysis of 106 patients. *Graefes Arch Clin Exp Ophthalmol.* 2006;244(7):788–794.

Taylor SR, Habot-Wilner Z, Pacheco P, Lightman SL. Intraocular methotrexate in the treatment of uveitis and uveitic cystoid macular edema. *Ophthalmology.* 2009;116(4):797–801.

Teoh SC, Hogan AC, Dick AD, Lee RWJ. Mycophenolate mofetil for the treatment of uveitis. *Am J Ophthalmol.* 2008;146(5):752–760.

Thorne JE, Jabs DA, Qazi FA, Nguyen QD, Kempen JH, Dunn JP. Mycophenolate mofetil therapy for inflammatory eye disease. *Ophthalmology.* 2005;112(8):1472–1477.

Inhibitors of T-cell signaling

Agents that inhibit T-cell signaling include cyclosporine, tacrolimus, and sirolimus. Cyclosporine, a macrolide product of the fungus *Beauveria nivea,* and tacrolimus, a product of *Streptomyces tsukubaensis,* are calcineurin inhibitors that eliminate T-cell receptor signal transduction and down-regulate interleukin-2 (IL-2) gene transcription and receptor expression of $CD4^+$ T-lymphocytes. Sirolimus, an antifungal product of *Streptomyces hygroscopicus,* is a noncalcineurin inhibitor of T-cell signaling that inhibits antibody production and B-lymphocytes.

Cyclosporine is available in 2 oral preparations. One is a microemulsion (Neoral, Novartis), which has better bioavailability than the other formulation (Sandimmune, Novartis). These 2 drugs are not bioequivalent. Neoral is begun at 2 mg/kg/day and Sandimmune at 2.5 mg/kg/day. The dose is adjusted based on toxicity and clinical response to 1–5 mg/kg/day. The most common side effects with cyclosporine are systemic hypertension and nephrotoxicity. Additional side effects include paresthesia, gastrointestinal upset, fatigue, hypertrichosis, and gingival hyperplasia. Blood pressure, serum creatinine levels, and complete blood counts must be assessed monthly. If serum creatinine rises by 30%, dose adjustment is required. Sustained elevation of serum creatinine levels will require a drug holiday until levels return to baseline. It is usually not necessary to check drug levels unless there is a concern about compliance or absorption. Patients with psoriasis treated with cyclosporine appear to be at greater risk of primary skin cancers. Cyclosporine was shown to be effective in a randomized, controlled clinical trial for the treatment of Behçet uveitis, with control of inflammation in 50% of patients. However, the dose used in this study was 10 mg/kg/day, substantially higher than what is used now (5 mg/kg/day), and led to substantial nephrotoxicity. Cyclosporine has also been shown to be effective in the treatment of intermediate uveitis and several types of posterior uveitis, including Behçet disease and VKH syndrome. Overall, cyclosporine combined with corticosteroids has been shown to be modestly effective in controlling ocular inflammation (in up to 33%) but toxicity necessitating cessation of therapy is more common in patients over the age of 55.

Tacrolimus is given orally at 0.10–0.15 mg/kg/day. Because of its lower dose and increased potency, its main side effect, nephrotoxicity, is less common than with cyclosporine. Serum creatinine level and complete blood count results are monitored monthly. A prospective trial of cyclosporine and tacrolimus suggested equal efficacy in controlling chronic posterior and intermediate uveitis, with tacrolimus demonstrating greater safety (less risk of hypertension and hyperlipidemia). Long-term tolerability and efficacy are excellent as well, with an 85% chance of reducing prednisone dosage to less than 10 mg/day.

In 1 open-label, prospective study, *sirolimus* was found to be effective in reducing or eliminating the need for systemic corticosteroids in patients with refractory noninfectious uveitis. Gastrointestinal and cutaneous side effects were common and dose-dependent, and most occurred at trough blood levels above 25 ng/mL. The drug is still under active investigation for the treatment of uveitis.

Hogan AC, McAvoy CE, Dick AD, Lee RWJ. Long-term efficacy and tolerance of tacrolimus for the treatment of uveitis. *Ophthalmology.* 2007;114(5):1000–1006.

Kaçmaz RO, Kempen JH, Newcomb C, et al. Cyclosporine for ocular inflammatory diseases. *Ophthalmology.* 2010;117(3):576–584.

Murphy CC, Greiner K, Plskova J, et al. Cyclosporine vs tacrolimus therapy for posterior and intermediate uveitis. *Arch Ophthalmol.* 2005;123(5):634–641.

Shanmuganathan VA, Casely EM, Raj D, et al. The efficacy of sirolimus in the treatment of patients with refractory uveitis. *Br J Ophthalmol.* 2005;89(6):666–669.

Alkylating agents

Alkylating agents include cyclophosphamide and chlorambucil. These drugs are at the top of the therapeutic stepladder and are used only if other immunomodulators fail to control uveitis; they are also used as first-line therapy for necrotizing scleritis associated with systemic vasculitides such as Wegener granulomatosis or relapsing polychondritis. They have been found beneficial as well in patients with intermediate uveitis, VKH syndrome, sympathetic ophthalmia, and Behçet disease. The most worrisome side effect of alkylating agents is an increased risk of malignancy. In the doses used for the treatment of uveitis, the risk is probably low, but this is controversial. Patients with polycythemia rubra vera treated with chlorambucil had a 13.5-fold greater risk of leukemia. Patients with Wegener granulomatosis treated with cyclophosphamide had a 2.4-fold increased risk of cancer and a 33-fold increased risk of bladder cancer. Therefore, these drugs should be used with great caution and only by clinicians experienced in the management of their dosing and potential toxicity. Patients may wish to consider sperm or embryo banking prior to beginning cyclophosphamide or chlorambucil therapy because of the high rate of sterility if the cumulative dose exceeds certain limits.

Cyclophosphamide is an alkylating agent whose active metabolites alkylate purines in DNA and RNA, resulting in impaired DNA replication and cell death. Cyclophosphamide is cytotoxic to resting and actively dividing lymphocytes. It is absorbed orally and metabolized in the liver into its active metabolites. It is probably more effective in controlling ocular inflammation when given orally at a dose of 2 mg/kg/day than when given as intermittent intravenous pulses. Most patients are treated for 1 year, and the dose is adjusted to maintain the leukocyte counts between 3000–4000 cells/µL after the patient has been tapered off corticosteroids. Inflammation control is achieved in three-quarters of patients within 12 months, disease remission occurs in two-thirds of patients within 2 years, and one-third discontinue therapy within 1 year because of reversible side effects. Patients receiving a cumulative dose of cyclophosphamide of up to 36 grams have no increased risk of secondary malignancy. After 1 year of disease quiescence, cyclophosphamide is tapered off. Myelosuppression and hemorrhagic cystitis are the most common side effects. Hemorrhagic cystitis is more common when cyclophosphamide is administered orally. Patients must be encouraged to drink more than 2 liters of fluid per day while on this regimen. Complete blood count and urinalysis are monitored weekly to monthly. Microscopic hematuria is a warning to increase hydration. Gross hematuria is an indication to discontinue therapy. If leukocyte counts fall below 2500 cells/µL, cyclophosphamide should be discontinued until cell counts recover. Other toxicities include teratogenicity, sterility, and reversible alopecia. Opportunistic infections such as *Pneumocystis* pneumonia occur more commonly in patients who are receiving cyclophosphamide; trimethoprim-sulfamethoxazole prophylaxis is recommended for these patients. Cyclophosphamide has been shown to be effective in treating necrotizing scleritis and retinal vasculitis and other uveitic conditions in uncontrolled case series.

Chlorambucil is a very long-acting alkylating agent that also interferes with DNA replication. It is absorbed well when administered orally. The drug is traditionally given as a single daily dose of 0.1–0.2 mg/kg. It may also be administered as short-term high-dose therapy; dosing starts at 2 mg/day for 1 week, then is increased by 2 mg/day each subsequent week until the inflammation is suppressed, the leukocyte count falls below 2800 cells/µL, or the platelet count drops below 100,000/µL. Short-term therapy is continued for 3–6 months. Concurrent oral corticosteroids may be tapered and discontinued once ocular inflammation becomes inactive. Because chlorambucil is myelosuppressive, complete blood counts should be obtained weekly. It is also teratogenic and causes sterility. Uncontrolled case series suggest that chlorambucil is effective, providing long-term, drug-free remissions in 66%–75% of patients with sympathetic ophthalmia, Behçet disease, and other sight-threatening uveitic syndromes.

Faurschou M, Sorensen IJ, Mellemkjaer L, et al. Malignancies in Wegener's granulomatosis: incidence and relation to cyclophosphamide therapy in a cohort of 293 patients. *J Rheumatol.* 2008;35(1):100–105.

Goldstein DA, Fontanilla FA, Kaul S, Sahin O, Tessler HH. Long-term follow-up of patients treated with short-term high-dose chlorambucil for sight-threatening ocular inflammation. *Ophthalmology.* 2002;109(2):370–377.

Miserocchi E, Baltatzis S, Ekong A, Roque M, Foster CS. Efficacy and safety of chlorambucil in intractable noninfectious uveitis: the Massachusetts Eye and Ear Infirmary experience. *Ophthalmology.* 2002;109(1):137–142.

Pujari SS, Kempen JH, Newcomb CW, et al. Cyclophosphamide for ocular inflammatory diseases. *Ophthalmology.* 2010; 117(2): 356–365.

Biologic response modifiers

Inflammation is driven by a complex series of cell–cell and cell–cytokine interactions. Inhibitors of various cytokines have been labeled *biologic response modifiers.* They already play an important role in the treatment of patients with uveitis, as these drugs result in targeted immunomodulation, thereby theoretically reducing the systemic side effects that are common with the previously discussed immunomodulatory agents. These drugs are considerably more expensive than traditional IMT and are reserved for specific conditions, such as Behçet disease, or situations in which traditional IMT has failed. Infliximab and adalimumab are biologics that inhibit the action of tumor necrosis factor α (TNF-α) and have changed the management of some uveitic entities. TNF-α is believed to play a major role in the pathogenesis of JIA, ankylosing spondylitis, and other spondyloarthropathies. Another biologic, daclizumab, is a humanized monoclonal antibody to the IL-2 receptor. It has also been used for treatment of recalcitrant uveitis. Adalimumab is given as subcutaneous injections, and infliximab and daclizumab are (usually) given as intravenous infusions. These drugs are generally prescribed and administered by uveitis specialists and rheumatologists experienced with their use, side effects, and toxicities.

Etanercept, a TNF receptor blocker, has been proven effective in controlling joint inflammation in polyarticular JIA and adult rheumatoid arthritis but showed no effect in controlling active intraocular inflammation or in allowing the taper of other immunomodulators in previously well-controlled patients. It is generally less effective than infliximab and is not a preferred biologic for uveitis treatment.

Infliximab, a chimeric, monoclonal IgG1κ antibody directed against TNF-α, is effective in controlling current inflammation and decreasing the likelihood of future attacks in Behçet uveitis, idiopathic uveitis, sarcoidosis, VKH syndrome, and many other entities in more than 75% of patients. It has a corticosteroid-sparing effect and appears to improve the visual prognosis of patients with recalcitrant Behçet uveitis. Similar favorable effects have been reported in patients with HLA-B27–associated anterior uveitis treated with infliximab. However, in 1 recent study, although 78% of patients achieved successful control of inflammation at 10 weeks, nearly one-half could not complete the 50 weeks of therapy because of drug-induced toxicity, which included lupus, systemic vascular thrombosis, congestive heart failure, new malignancy, demyelinating disease, and vitreous hemorrhage. As many as 75% of patients receiving more than 3 infusions developed antinuclear antibodies. Low-dose methotrexate (5–7.5 mg/week) may be administered concomitantly to reduce the risk of drug-induced lupus syndrome. Also, reports have clearly shown that some patients with unknown, inactive, postprimary tuberculosis treated with infliximab subsequently developed disseminated tuberculosis. Thus, a positive purified protein derivative (PPD) skin test is considered a contraindication for infliximab therapy. More recent reports suggest a lower frequency of side effects than that reported in earlier studies.

Adalimumab, a fully humanized monoclonal IgG1 antibody directed against TNF-α, has been shown to be as effective as infliximab in controlling inflammation, with success rates of up to 88% without relapse in pediatric patients with uveitis and 100% in adult patients with Behçet uveitis, posterior uveitis, and panuveitis. However, uveitis relapses requiring local corticosteroid injections occurred in 42% of adult patients while on adalimumab. Side effects, including development of antidrug antibodies, appear to be less common than with infliximab. Adalimumab is less expensive than infliximab and can be injected subcutaneously at home every 2 weeks, without the need for the intravenous infusions required by infliximab. Several other TNF-α inhibitors are currently under development.

Daclizumab, a humanized monoclonal antibody to the IL-2 receptor, has been shown in uncontrolled studies to be effective in controlling active chronic uveitis and in enabling discontinuation of other immunomodulators in 67%–80% of patients. It may be given intravenously or subcutaneously.

Rituximab, a chimeric monoclonal antibody directed against CD20-positive cells (mainly B lymphocytes) may also useful in treatment of Behçet retinal vasculitis and Wegener granulomatosis–associated necrotizing scleritis.

Anakinra is a recombinant IL-1 receptor antagonist that holds some promise as a biologic treatment alternative for JIA-associated uveitis. Only 1 human case report exists regarding its efficacy in posterior uveitis.

Several studies have shown interferon alfa-2a/2b (IFN-α2a/b) and intravenous immunoglobulin to be beneficial in some patients with uveitis. IFN-α2a seems to be an alternative to anti-TNF drugs. It has antiviral, immunomodulatory, and antiangiogenic effects. Recent reports in the European literature seem to indicate that IFN-α2a is efficacious and well-tolerated in patients with Behçet uveitis, controlling inflammation in almost 90%; it is somewhat less effective in non-Behçet uveitis, with inflammation control in 60%. Other immunosuppressive agents are discontinued prior to starting IFN-α2a therapy. A flulike syndrome has been observed, most frequently during the first weeks of therapy, but may be improved by prophylactic administration of acetaminophen. Despite the use of low interferon doses, leukopenia or thrombocytopenia may occur. Depression is another important side effect of interferon therapy.

Biester S, Deuter C, Michels H, et al. Adalimumab in the therapy of uveitis in childhood. *Br J Ophthalmol.* 2007;91(3):319–324.

Bodaghi B, Gendron G, Wechsler B, et al. Efficacy of interferon alpha in the treatment of refractory and sight threatening uveitis: a retrospective monocentric study of 45 patients. *Br J Ophthalmol.* 2007;91(3):335–339.

Braun J, Baraliakos X, Listing J, Sieper J. Decreased incidence of anterior uveitis in patients with ankylosing spondylitis treated with the anti-tumor necrosis factor agents infliximab and etanercept. *Arthritis Rheum.* 2005;52(8):2447–2451.

Foster CS, Tufail F, Waheed NK, et al. Efficacy of etanercept in preventing relapse of uveitis controlled by methotrexate. *Arch Ophthalmol.* 2003;121(4):437–440.

Gueudry J. Wechsler B, Terrada C, et al. Long-term efficacy and safety of low-dose interferon alpha2a therapy in severe uveitis associated with Behçet disease. *Am J Ophthalmol.* 2008;146(6):837–844.

Imrie FR, Dick AD. Biologics in the treatment of uveitis. *Curr Opin Ophthalmol.* 2007;18(6): 481–486.

Kötter I, Zierhut M, Eckstein AK, et al. Human recombinant interferon alfa-2a for the treatment of Behçet's disease with sight threatening posterior or panuveitis. *Br J Ophthalmol.* 2003;87(4):423–431.

Papaliodis GN, Chu D, Foster CS. Treatment of ocular inflammatory disorders with daclizumab. *Ophthalmology.* 2003;110(4):786–789.

Sfikakis PP, Markomichelakis N, Alpsoy E, et al. Anti-TNF therapy in the management of Behcet's disease—review and basis for recommendations. *Rheumatology (Oxford).* 2007;46(5):736–741.

Schmeling H, Horneff G. Etanercept and uveitis in patients with juvenile idiopathic arthritis. *Rheumatology (Oxford).* 2005;44(8):1008–1011.

Smith JR, Levinson RD, Holland GN, et al. Differential efficacy of tumor necrosis factor inhibition in the management of inflammatory eye disease and associated rheumatic disease. *Arthritis Rheum.* 2001;45(3):252–257.

Smith JA, Thompson DJ, Whitcup SM, et al. A randomized, placebo-controlled, double-masked clinical trial of etanercept for the treatment of uveitis associated with juvenile idiopathic arthritis. *Arthritis Rheum.* 2005;53(1):18–23.

Suhler EB, Smith JR, Wertheim MS, et al. A prospective trial of infliximab therapy for refractory uveitis. Preliminary safety and efficacy outcomes. *Arch Ophthalmol.* 2005;123(7):903–912.

Tugal-Tutkun I, Mudun A, Urgancioglu M, et al. Efficacy of infliximab in the treatment of uveitis that is resistant to treatment with the combination of azathioprine, cyclosporine, and corticosteroids in Behçet's disease: an open-label trial. *Arthritis Rheum.* 2005;52(8):2478–2484.

Surgical Management of Uveitis

Surgery is performed in patients with uveitis for diagnostic and/or therapeutic reasons. In fact, any time a surgical procedure is performed on a uveitic eye, intraocular fluid and/or tissue samples should be obtained, especially if the etiology of the inflammation is unknown. Therapeutic surgical procedures for uveitis and its complications are discussed in Chapter 10.

CHAPTER 6

Noninfectious (Autoimmune) Ocular Inflammatory Disease

Many different ocular inflammatory entities are triggered by environmental, genetic, and innate and adaptive immunologic stimuli. Often the trigger or inciting event or agent that causes the inflammation is unknown or undetectable. Once the common infectious pathogens have been ruled out and any systemic autoimmune diseases identified by appropriate diagnostic testing, these autoimmune, noninfectious entities can be treated with anti-inflammatory therapy. The noninfectious uveitic entities are discussed in this chapter.

Noninfectious Scleritis

Scleritis, inflammation of the sclera, is a typically painful, destructive condition with a potential risk of permanent structural damage to the eye and visual compromise. Scleritis may be classified similarly to uveitis, both anatomically and etiologically, the latter including infection, autoimmunity, and trauma. Scleritis not due to infection or trauma is the most common form of this disease. Approximately 40% of cases of scleritis are associated with a systemic disease, especially rheumatoid arthritis. See BCSC Section 8, *External Disease and Cornea* for a complete discussion of the epidemiology and classification of scleritis.

Treatment of Noninfectious Scleritis

Nonsteroidal anti-inflammatory drugs
Nonsteroidal anti-inflammatory drugs (NSAIDs) may be effective in the treatment of non-necrotizing scleritis. These agents serve to relieve pain and reduce inflammation, although they are primarily useful in milder cases. No one drug has been proven more effective than another, but indomethacin, flurbiprofen, and naproxen have all been used successfully. If the initial NSAID fails, a second can be tried before switching to corticosteroids.

Corticosteroids
Topical corticosteroids are potentially useful in very mild cases of scleritis, or as an adjunctive therapy. Subconjunctival injections of corticosteroid were recently shown to be effective in anterior nonnecrotizing scleritis. There remains some controversy surrounding this route of administration, because of the potential complication of localized necrotizing

disease following injection, although several case series suggest efficacy without significant risk. Extensive counseling of patients regarding these risks should be carried out. Systemic corticosteroids remain the mainstay of noninfectious scleritis therapy. These may be administered orally or as a high-dose intravenous pulse.

Immunomodulatory therapy

As with noninfectious uveitis, patients with scleritis that is nonresponsive to corticosteroids or that requires doses of corticosteroids too high for long-term use should be transitioned to steroid-sparing immunomodulatory therapy (IMT). No specific data exist that adequately guide the specific choice of agent, other than in a few situations. The antimetabolites such as methotrexate, azathioprine, and mycophenolate mofetil have all been successfully used. Calcineurin inhibitors are also an option. Cyclophosphamide is the drug of choice for Wegener granulomatosis and polyarteritis nodosa. Biologic agents such as tumor necrosis factor (TNF) inhibitors (infliximab and adalimumab) and rituximab have been reported to be useful in treatment of recalcitrant scleritis.

Pain management

Because scleritis can be an excruciatingly painful condition, attention to pain control is necessary. Oral NSAIDs may be of benefit, but their use in combination with oral corticosteroids or some of the antimetabolites should be monitored carefully. The judicious use of oral narcotics is entirely appropriate while anti-inflammatory therapy is instituted to achieve disease control. Topical cycloplegia may also be of benefit.

Surgery

Scleral reinforcement surgery may be needed to address scleral thinning and to avoid the complications of globe rupture, which can occur with minimal trauma in these patients. Materials used for grafting include cadaveric donor sclera, but the scleral graft may melt and some authors have recommended autogenous periosteum.

Doctor P, Sultan A, Syed S, Christen W, Bhat P, Quinones K, Foster S. Infliximab for the treatment of refractory scleritis. *Br J Ophthalmol.* 2010;94(5):579–583.

Raiji VR, Palestine AG, Parver DL. Scleritis and systemic disease association in a community-based referral practice. *Am J Ophthalmol.* 2009;148(6):946–950.

Anterior Uveitis

Anterior uveitis is the most common form of uveitis, accounting for the large majority of cases, with an annual incidence rate of 8 per 100,000 persons. The incidence increases with age to approximately 220 per 100,000 persons in patients aged 65 years and older.

Because uveitis may occur secondarily to inflammation of the cornea and sclera, the physician should evaluate these structures carefully to rule out a primary keratitis or scleritis. Inflammation of the sclera and the cornea is covered in depth in BCSC Section 8, *External Disease and Cornea;* see also the section on scleritis in this chapter.

Gritz DC, Wong IG. Incidence and prevalence of uveitis in Northern California. The Northern California Epidemiology of Uveitis Study. *Ophthalmology.* 2004;111(3):491–500.

Reeves SW, Sloan FA, Lee PP, Jaffe GJ. Uveitis in the elderly; epidemiological data from the National Long-term Care Survey Medicare Cohort. *Ophthalmology.* 2006;113(2):307–321.

Acute Nongranulomatous Iritis and Iridocyclitis

The classic presentation of acute anterior uveitis is the sudden onset of pain, redness, and photophobia that can be associated with decreased vision. Fine keratic precipitates (KPs) and fibrin dust the corneal endothelium in most cases. Endothelial dysfunction may cause the cornea to become acutely edematous. The anterior chamber shows an intense cellular response and variable flare. Severe cases may show a protein coagulum in the aqueous or, less commonly, a hypopyon (Fig 6-1). Occasionally, a fibrin net forms across the pupillary margin (Fig 6-2), potentially producing a seclusion membrane and iris bombé. Iris vessels may be dilated, and, on rare occasions, a spontaneous hyphema occurs. Cells may also be present in the anterior vitreous, and in rare cases patients develop severe, diffuse vitritis. Fundus lesions are not characteristic, although cystoid macular edema (CME), disc edema, pars plana exudates, or small areas of peripheral localized choroiditis may be noted. Occasionally, intraocular pressure (IOP) may be elevated because of blockage of the trabecular meshwork by debris and cells or by pupillary block.

The inflammation usually lasts several days to weeks, up to 3 months. Two patterns may occur. Typically, an attack is acute and unilateral, with a history of episodes alternating between the 2 eyes. Recurrences are common. Either eye may be affected, but recurrence is rarely bilateral. If damage to the vascular endothelium can be minimized, no silent, ongoing damage or low-grade inflammation should occur between attacks. The second pattern is acute and bilateral and occurs simultaneously with tubulointerstitial nephritis.

Corticosteroids are the mainstay of treatment to reduce inflammation, prevent cicatrization, and minimize damage to the uveal vasculature. Topical corticosteroids are the first line of treatment, and they often need to be given every 1–2 hours. If necessary,

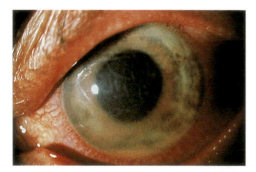

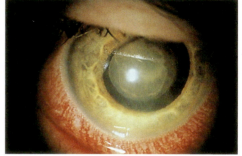

Figure 6-1 Acute HLA-B27–positive anterior uveitis with pain, photophobia, marked injection, fixed pupil, loss of iris detail from corneal edema, and hypopyon. *(Courtesy of David Meisler, MD.)*

Figure 6-2 Ankylosing spondylitis: acute unilateral iridocyclitis with severe anterior chamber reaction with central fibrinous exudate contracting anterior to the lens capsule, and posterior synechiae from 10 o'clock to 12 o'clock. *(Courtesy of David Meisler, MD.)*

periocular or oral corticosteroids may be used for severe episodes. Initial attacks may require all 3 routes, particularly in the severe cases found mostly in younger patients.

Severely damaged vessels may leak continuously, transforming the typical course from acute and intermittent to chronic and recalcitrant. This chronic course must be avoided at all costs by timely diagnosis, aggressive initial therapy, and patient compliance. Maintenance therapy is not indicated once the active inflammation has been controlled.

Anti-TNF therapy has been effective in decreasing recurrences of anterior uveitis in patients with HLA-B27–associated uveitis. Cycloplegic and mydriatic agents are used both to relieve pain and to break and prevent synechiae formation. They may be given topically or with conjunctival cotton pledgets soaked in tropicamide, cyclopentolate, and phenylephrine hydrochloride (Fig 6-3).

Braun J, Baraliakos X, Listing J, Sieper J. Decreased incidence of anterior uveitis in patients with ankylosing spondylitis treated with the anti-tumor necrosis factor agents infliximab and etanercept. *Arthritis Rheum.* 2005;53(8):2447–2451.

Cunningham ET Jr. Diagnosis and management of anterior uveitis. *Focal Points: Clinical Modules for Ophthalmologists.* San Francisco, CA: American Academy of Ophthalmology; 2002, module 1.

El-Shabrawi Y, Hermann J. Anti-tumor necrosis factor-alpha therapy with infliximab as an alternative to corticosteroids in the treatment of human leukocyte antigen B27-associated acute anterior uveitis. *Ophthalmology.* 2002;109(12):2342–2346.

HLA-B27–related diseases

HLA-B27 is a class I cell surface antigen that presents other antigens to T suppressor cells and is encoded by the B locus of the major histocompatibility complex (MHC); it is located on the short arm of chromosome 6. Although it is present in approximately 5% of the general population, about one-half of patients with acute iritis may be HLA-B27–positive. In nonwhite populations, HLA-B27 is seen less frequently. The precise trigger for acute iritis in genetically susceptible persons is not clear. Patients with recurrent anterior nongranulomatous uveitis should be tested for the presence of HLA-B27, but the test does not provide an absolute diagnosis.

Several autoimmune diseases known as the *seronegative spondyloarthropathies* are strongly associated with both acute anterior uveitis and HLA-B27. Patients with these

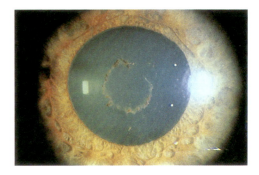

Figure 6-3 Acute iridocyclitis after intensive use of topical corticosteroids and perilimbal subconjunctival dilating agents, leaving an anterior capsular ring of pigment following posterior synechiolysis. *(Courtesy of John D. Sheppard, Jr, MD.)*

diseases, by definition, do not have a positive rheumatoid factor. The seronegative spondyloarthropathies include

- ankylosing spondylitis
- reactive arthritis syndrome
- inflammatory bowel disease
- psoriatic arthritis

These entities are sometimes clinically indistinguishable, and all may be associated with spondylitis and sacroiliitis. Women tend to experience more atypical spondyloarthropathies than do men.

Ankylosing spondylitis Ankylosing spondylitis varies from asymptomatic to severe and crippling. Symptoms of this disorder include lower back pain and stiffness after inactivity.

Up to 90% of patients with ankylosing spondylitis are positive for HLA-B27, although not all HLA-B27–positive patients (there is a prevalence of about 8% in the white population) develop the disease; in fact, most do not develop any form of autoimmune disease. The chance that an HLA-B27–positive patient will develop spondyloarthritis or eye disease is 1 in 4. Family members may also have ankylosing spondylitis or iritis. Often, symptoms of back disease are lacking in persons with iritis who test positive.

The ophthalmologist may be the first physician to suspect ankylosing spondylitis. Symptoms or family history of back problems together with HLA-B27 positivity suggest the diagnosis. Sacroiliac imaging studies should be obtained when indicated by a suggestive history of morning lower back stiffness that improves with exertion. Patients with ankylosing spondylitis should be informed of the risk of deformity and referred to a rheumatologist. Pulmonary apical fibrosis may develop; aortitis occurs in about 5% of cases and may be associated with aortic valvular insufficiency.

NSAIDs are the mainstay of treatment for ankylosing spondylitis. Sulfasalazine may be used in patients whose disease is not controlled with NSAIDs. Morning stiffness and the erythrocyte sedimentation rate (ESR) decrease in patients taking sulfasalazine, but it is not clear whether the drug improves pain, function, movement of the spine, or overall well-being. Sulfasalazine appears to reduce the frequency of recurrences of iritis. Side effects of sulfasalazine include skin rashes, stomach upset, and mouth ulcers.

Chang JH, McCluskey PJ, Wakefield D. Acute anterior uveitis and HLA-B27. *Surv Ophthalmol.* 2005;50(4):364–388.

Monnet D, Breban M, Hudry C, Dougados M, Brézin AP. Ophthalmic findings and frequency of extraocular manifestations in patients with HLA-B27 uveitis: a study of 175 cases. *Ophthalmology.* 2004;111(4):802–809.

Schmidt WA, Wierth S, Milleck D, Droste U, Gromnica-Ihle E. Sulfasalazine in ankylosing spondylitis: a prospective, randomized, double-blind placebo-controlled study and comparison with other controlled studies. *Z Rheumatol.* 2002;61(2):159–167.

Reactive arthritis syndrome Reactive arthritis syndrome consists of the classic diagnostic triad of nonspecific urethritis, polyarthritis, and conjunctival inflammation often accompanied by iritis. The HLA-B27 marker is found in up to 95% of patients. Prostatic fluid culture is negative. The condition occurs most frequently in young adult men, although 10% of patients are female.

Reactive arthritis syndrome may be triggered by episodes of diarrhea or dysentery without urethritis. *Ureaplasma urealyticum* as well as *Chlamydia, Shigella, Salmonella,* and *Yersinia* organisms have all been implicated as triggering infections. Arthritis begins within 30 days of infection in 80% of patients. The knees, ankles, feet, and wrists are affected asymmetrically and in an oligoarticular distribution. Sacroiliitis is present in as many as 70% of patients.

In addition to the classic triad, 2 other conditions are considered to be major diagnostic criteria:

- *keratoderma blennorrhagicum:* a scaly, erythematous, irritating disorder of the palms and soles of the feet (Figs 6-4, 6-5)
- *circinate balanitis:* a persistent, scaly, erythematous, circumferential rash of the distal penis

Numerous minor criteria are also useful in establishing a diagnosis of reactive arthritis syndrome, according to the American Rheumatologic Association guidelines. These include plantar fasciitis, Achilles tendinitis, sacroiliitis, nail bed pitting, palate ulcers, and tongue ulcers.

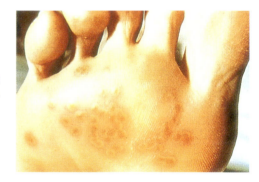

Figure 6-4 Reactive arthritis syndrome with keratoderma blennorrhagicum on the sole. *(Courtesy of John D. Sheppard, Jr, MD.)*

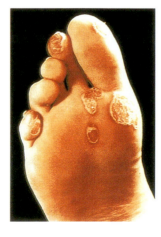

Figure 6-5 Reactive arthritis syndrome with pedal discoid keratoderma blennorrhagicum. *(Courtesy of John D. Sheppard, Jr, MD.)*

Conjunctivitis is the most common eye lesion associated with this disease, and it is usually mucopurulent and papillary. Punctate and subepithelial keratitis may also occur, occasionally leaving permanent corneal scars. Acute nongranulomatous iritis occurs in up to 10% of patients. In some cases, the iritis becomes bilateral and chronic because of a permanent breakdown of the blood–aqueous barrier.

Inflammatory bowel disease Ulcerative colitis and Crohn disease (granulomatous ileocolitis) are both associated with acute iritis. Up to 12% of patients with ulcerative colitis and 2.4% of patients with Crohn disease develop acute anterior uveitis. Occasionally, bowel disease is asymptomatic and follows the onset of iritis. Twenty percent of patients with inflammatory bowel disease have sacroiliitis; of these, 60% are HLA-B27–positive. Patients with both acute iritis and inflammatory bowel disease tend to exhibit HLA-B27 positivity as well as sacroiliitis. Patients with inflammatory bowel disease may also develop sclerouveitis. In contrast to patients who develop acute iritis, these individuals tend to be HLA-B27–negative, have symptoms resembling rheumatoid arthritis, and usually do not develop sacroiliitis.

Psoriatic arthritis Of patients with psoriatic arthritis, 20% may have sacroiliitis, and inflammatory bowel disease occurs more frequently than would be expected by chance. Diagnosis is based on the findings of typical cutaneous changes (Fig 6-6), terminal phalangeal joint inflammation (Fig 6-7), and ungual involvement. Up to 25% of patients with psoriatic arthritis develop acute iritis. Treatment consists of cycloplegic and mydriatic agents and corticosteroids, which are usually given topically. In severe cases, periocular or systemic corticosteroids may be required, and chronic cases may need IMT.

Iritis in patients with psoriasis without arthritis has distinct clinical features. The mean age of onset is older than in idiopathic or HLA-B27–associated uveitis (30–40 years vs 48 years). It tends to be bilateral and of longer duration and to require oral treatment with NSAIDs. Retinal vasculitis, CME, and papillitis are frequently seen.

Durrani K, Foster CS. Psoriatic uveitis: a distinct clinical entity? *Am J Ophthalmol.* 2005; 139(1):106–111.

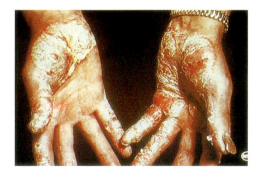

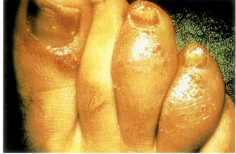

Figure 6-6 Psoriatic arthritis with classic erythematous, hyperkeratotic rash. *(Courtesy of John D. Sheppard, Jr, MD.)*

Figure 6-7 Psoriatic arthritis with sausage digits resulting from tissue swelling and distal interphalangeal joint inflammation. *(Courtesy of John D. Sheppard, Jr, MD.)*

Tubulointerstitial nephritis and uveitis syndrome

Tubulointerstitial nephritis and uveitis (TINU) syndrome occurs predominantly in adolescent girls and women up to their early 30s; the mean age of onset for TINU syndrome is 21 years. Patients present with redness and variable pain, blurred vision, and photophobia. Ocular symptoms and findings are more severe in patients with recurrent disease, with development of fibrin, posterior synechiae, larger KPs, and, rarely, hypopyon. Posterior segment findings may include diffuse vitreous opacities, optic nerve swelling, and retinal exudates.

Patients may present with ophthalmic findings before the development of systemic symptoms such as fever, arthralgias, rashes, and tubulointerstitial nephritis. More commonly, however, patients present with systemic symptoms before the development of iritis. The following criteria are required for a clinical diagnosis of TINU syndrome:

- abnormal serum creatinine level or decreased creatinine clearance
- abnormal urinalysis findings, with increased β_2-microglobulin, proteinuria, presence of eosinophils, pyuria or hematuria, urinary white cell casts, and normoglycemic glucosuria
- associated systemic illness consisting of fever, weight loss, anorexia, fatigue, arthralgias, and myalgias; patients may also have abnormal liver function, eosinophilia, and an elevated ESR

The etiology remains unclear. Seroreactivity against retinal and renal antigens has been demonstrated. The syndrome has a genetic susceptibility, as it has been reported to be associated with HLA-DQ in white North Americans and with HLA-DR14 in Spanish patients. The predominance of activated helper T lymphocytes in the kidney interstitium suggests a role for cellular immunity. Renal biopsies have shown severe interstitial fibrosis. TINU syndrome is very responsive to high-dose oral corticosteroids.

Abed L, Merouani A, Haddad E, Benoit G, Oligny LL, Sartelet H. Presence of autoantibodies against tubular and uveal cells in a patient with tubulointerstitial nephritis and uveitis (TINU) syndrome. *Nephrol Dial Transplant.* 2008;23(4):1452–1455.

Goda C, Kotake S, Ichiishi A, Namba K, Kitaichi N, Ohno S. Clinical features in tubulointerstitial nephritis and uveitis (TINU) syndrome. *Am J Ophthalmol.* 2005;140(4):637–641.

Mandeville JT, Levinson RD, Holland GN. The tubulointerstitial nephritis and uveitis syndrome. *Surv Ophthalmol.* 2001;49(3):195–208.

Shimazaki K, Jirawuthiworavong GV, Nguyen EV, Awazu M, Levinson RD, Gordon LK. Tubulointerstitial nephritis and uveitis syndrome: a case with an autoimmune reactivity against retinal and renal antigens. *Ocul Immunol Inflamm.* 2008;16(1):51–53.

Glaucomatocyclitic crisis

Glaucomatocyclitic crisis usually manifests as a recurrent unilateral mild acute iritis. Symptoms are vague: discomfort, blurred vision, halos. Signs include markedly elevated IOP, corneal edema, fine KPs, low-grade cell and flare, and a slightly dilated pupil. Episodes last from several hours to several days, and recurrences are common over many years. Treatment is with topical corticosteroids and antiglaucoma medication, including, if necessary, carbonic anhydrase inhibitors. Pilocarpine probably should be avoided because it may exacerbate ciliary spasm.

Glaucomatocyclitic crisis, like Vogt-Koyanagi-Harada (VKH) syndrome, which is discussed later in this chapter, may be associated with the HLA-B54 gene locus. Because it is rare, it should be a diagnosis of exclusion, established only after other, more common syndromes such as herpetic uveitis have been ruled out. Recent studies link cytomegalovirus (CMV) infection with glaucomatocyclitic crisis.

Chee SP, Jap A. Presumed Fuchs heterochromic iridocyclitis and Posner-Schlossman syndrome: comparison of cytomegalovirus-positive and negative eyes. *Am J Ophthalmol.* 2008;146(6): 883–889.

Lens-associated uveitis

Uveitis may result from an immune reaction to lens material. This can occur following disruption of the lens capsule (traumatic or surgical) or from leakage of lens protein through the lens capsule in mature or hypermature cataracts (Figs 6-8, 6-9).

This type of uveitis was once divided into several categories, including phacoanaphylactic endophthalmitis, phacotoxic uveitis, and phacolytic glaucoma. Some of these terms are misleading and do not accurately describe the disease process. For example, the term *phacoanaphylactic* is not appropriate because anaphylaxis involves immunoglobulin E (IgE), mast cells, and basophils, none of which are present in phacogenic uveitis. Also, the term *phacotoxic* is misleading because there is no evidence that lens proteins are directly toxic to ocular tissues.

The exact mechanism of lens-induced uveitis, although unknown, is thought to represent an immune reaction to lens protein. Experimental animal studies suggest that altered tolerance to lens protein leads to the inflammation, which usually has an abrupt onset but may occasionally occur insidiously. Patients previously sensitized to lens protein (eg, after cataract extraction in the fellow eye) can experience inflammation within 24 hours after capsular rupture.

Clinically, patients show an anterior uveitis that may be granulomatous or nongranulomatous. KPs are usually present and may be small or large. Anterior chamber reaction varies from mild (eg, postoperative inflammation where there is a small amount of

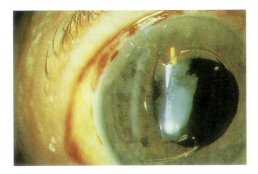

Figure 6-8 Low-grade postoperative uveitis in this patient could be secondary to retained lens cortex or to the anterior chamber intraocular lens (IOL). *(Courtesy of John D. Sheppard, Jr, MD.)*

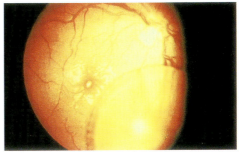

Figure 6-9 Traumatically dislocated nucleus atop the optic nerve produced progressively severe phacoantigenic uveitis and glaucoma, necessitating pars plana lensectomy and vitrectomy. *(Courtesy of John D. Sheppard, Jr, MD.)*

retained cortex) to severe (eg, traumatic lens capsule disruption); hypopyon may be present. Posterior synechiae are common, and IOP is often elevated. Inflammation in the anterior vitreous cavity is common, but fundus lesions do not occur.

Histologically, a zonal granulomatous inflammation is centered at the site of lens injury. Neutrophils are present about the lens material with surrounding lymphocytes, plasma cells, epithelioid cells, and occasional giant cells.

Treatment consists of topical and, in severe cases, systemic corticosteroids, as well as cycloplegic and mydriatic agents. Surgical removal of all lens material is usually curative. When small amounts of lens material remain, corticosteroid therapy alone may be sufficient to allow resorption of the inciting material.

Phacolytic glaucoma Phacolytic glaucoma involves an acute increase in IOP caused by clogging of the trabecular meshwork by lens protein and engorged macrophages. This form occurs with hypermature cataracts. The diagnosis is suggested by elevated IOP, lack of KPs, refractile bodies in the aqueous (representing lipid-laden macrophages), and lack of synechiae. Therapy includes pressure reduction, often with osmotic agents and topical medications, and prompt cataract extraction. An aqueous tap may reveal swollen macrophages.

Kalogeropoulos CD, Malamou-Mitsi VD, Asproudis I, Psilas K. The contribution of aqueous humor cytology in the differential diagnosis of anterior uvea inflammations. *Ocul Immunol Inflamm.* 2004;12(3):215–225.

Postoperative inflammation: infectious

Infectious endophthalmitis must be included in the differential diagnosis of postoperative inflammation and hypopyon. *Propionibacterium acnes, Staphylococcus epidermidis,* and *Candida* species can cause delayed or late-onset endophthalmitis following cataract surgery. Infectious endophthalmitis is discussed in more detail in Chapter 8.

Postoperative inflammation: IOL-associated

Intraocular lens (IOL)–associated uveitis may range from mild inflammation to the uveitis-glaucoma-hyphema (UGH) syndrome. Surgical manipulation results in breakdown of the blood–aqueous barrier, leading to vulnerability in the early postoperative period. IOL implantation can activate complement cascades and promote neutrophil chemotaxis, leading to cellular deposits on the IOL, synechiae formation, capsular opacification, and anterior capsule phimosis. Retained lens material from extracapsular cataract extraction may exacerbate the usual transient postoperative inflammation. Iris chafing caused by the edges or loops of IOLs on either the anterior or the posterior surface of the iris can result in mechanical irritation and inflammation. In particular, metal-loop lenses and poorly polished lenses can cause this reaction. The incidence of this type of complication with modern lenses is 1% or less. The motion of an iris-supported or anterior chamber IOL may cause intermittent corneal touch and lead to corneal endothelial damage or decompensation, low-grade iritis, peripheral anterior synechiae, recalcitrant glaucoma, and CME (Figs 6-10, 6-11). These lenses should be removed and exchanged when penetrating keratoplasty is performed.

UGH syndrome still occurs today, although it has become much less common. The syndrome may be caused by irritation of the iris root by the warped footplates of poorly

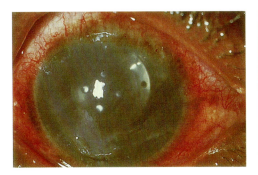

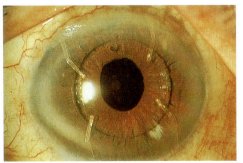

Figure 6-10 Pseudophakic bullous keratopathy and chronic iridocyclitis caused by an iris-fixated anterior chamber IOL, with corneal touch, iris stromal erosion, and chronic recalcitrant cystoid macular edema. *(Courtesy of John D. Sheppard, Jr, MD.)*

Figure 6-11 Fixed-haptic anterior chamber IOL associated with peripheral and superior corneal edema, chronic low-grade iridocyclitis, peripheral anterior synechiae, globe tenderness, and intermittent microhyphema. *(Courtesy of John D. Sheppard, Jr, MD.)*

made rigid anterior chamber IOLs or other implanted devices such as cosmetic iris implants. Flexible anterior chamber IOLs are less likely to cause UGH syndrome. Various polymers used in the manufacture of IOLs may activate complement and cause neutrophil chemotaxis and resultant inflammation.

As a general rule, the more biocompatible the IOL material, the less likely it is to incite an inflammatory response. Irregular or damaged IOL surfaces as well as polypropylene haptics have been associated with enhanced bacterial and leukocyte binding and probably should be avoided in patients with uveitis. Several attempts have been made to modify the IOL surface to increase its biocompatibility. These modifications have had little clinical impact on postoperative inflammation and have been abandoned with the advent of acrylic IOLs.

Foldable implant materials have also been found to be well tolerated in many patients with uveitis. Some studies have shown increased cellular deposition on silicone optics compared with acrylic or hydrogel optics, but others have shown no difference between the lens materials. In general, acrylic IOLs appear to have excellent biocompatibility, with low rates of cellular deposits and capsular opacification.

One of the most important factors in the success of cataract surgery in patients with uveitis is aggressive control of the intraocular inflammation in both the preoperative and postoperative periods. For further discussion and illustrations, see Chapter 10 in this book and BCSC Section 11, *Lens and Cataract.*

Arthur SN, Wright MM, Kramarevsky N, Kaufman SC, Grajewski AL. Uveitis-glaucoma-hyphema syndrome and corneal decompensation in association with cosmetic iris implants. *Am J Ophthalmol.* 2009;148(5):790–793.

Rauz S, Stavrou P, Murray PI. Evaluation of foldable intraocular lenses in patients with uveitis. *Ophthalmology.* 2000;107(5):909–919.

Ravalico G, Baccara F, Lovisato A, Tognetto D. Postoperative cellular reaction on various intraocular lens materials. *Ophthalmology.* 1997;104(7):1084–1091.

Drug-induced uveitis

Treatment with certain medications has been associated with the development of intra-ocular inflammation. Systemic medications reported to cause uveitis include rifabutin (a semisynthetic derivative of rifamycin and rifampin effective in the treatment of *Myco-bacterium avium-intracellulare* infection), bisphosphonates (inhibitors of bone resorption that are used in the prevention of osteoporosis and in the treatment of hypercalcemia, bone metastasis, and Paget disease), sulfonamides (commonly used in the treatment of urinary tract infections), diethylcarbamazine (an antifilarial agent), and oral contraceptives.

Numerous topical antiglaucoma medications have been associated with uveitis: metipranolol (a nonselective adrenergic blocking agent used in the treatment of glau-coma), anticholinesterase inhibitors, and prostaglandin $F_{2\alpha}$ analogues (travoprost, latano-prost, bimatoprost). Drugs that are injected directly into the eye have also been associated with uveitis. These include antibiotics, urokinase (a plasminogen activator), cidofovir (a cytosine analogue effective against CMV) and agents directed against vascular endothelial growth factor (VEGF). Treatment generally involves topical corticosteroids and cyclople-gic agents, if necessary. Recalcitrant cases may require cessation or tapering of the offend-ing systemic medication.

Bacille Calmette-Guérin (BCG) and influenza vaccines, as well as the purified protein derivative (PPD) used in the tuberculin skin test, have also been implicated in the devel-opment of uveitis.

Faulkner WJ, Burk SE. Acute anterior uveitis and corneal edema associated with travoprost. *Arch Ophthalmol.* 2003;121(7):1054–1055.

Kourlas H, Abrams P. Ranibizumab for the treatment of neovascular age-related macular de-generation: a review. *Clin Ther.* 2007;29(9):1850–1861.

Moorthy RS, Valluri S, Jampol LM. Drug-induced uveitis. *Surv Ophthalmol.* 1998;42(6): 557–570.

Wu L, Martínez-Castellanos MA, Quiroz-Mercado H, et al, and the Pan American Collab-orative Retina Group (PACORES). Twelve-month safety of intravitreal injections of be-vacizumab (Avastin): results of the Pan-American Collaborative Retina Study Group (PACORES). *Graefes Arch Clin Exp Ophthalmol.* 2008;246(1):81–87.

Chronic Anterior Uveitis (Iridocyclitis)

Inflammation of the anterior segment that is persistent and relapses less than 3 months after discontinuation of therapy is termed *chronic iridocyclitis;* it may persist for years. This type of inflammation usually starts insidiously, with variable amounts of redness, discomfort, and photophobia. Some patients have no symptoms. The disease can be uni-lateral or bilateral, and the amount of inflammatory activity is variable. CME is common.

Juvenile idiopathic arthritis

The classification of juvenile arthritis has been complicated by the differences between the European classification developed by the European League Against Rheumatism (EULAR) and the classification used by the American College of Rheumatology (ACR) and the American Rheumatism Association (ARA). In 1997, the International League of Associations of Rheumatologists (ILAR) adopted the term *juvenile idiopathic arthritis*

(JIA) to replace the previously used terms *juvenile chronic arthritis* and *juvenile rheumatoid arthritis*. JIA is the most common systemic disorder associated with iridocyclitis in the pediatric age group; it is characterized by arthritis beginning before age 16 and lasting for at least 6 weeks.

Ocular involvement in JIA JIA can be classified into 3 types based on medical history and other presenting factors.

- *Systemic onset (Still disease)*. This type, usually seen in children under age 5, is characterized by fever, rash, lymphadenopathy, and hepatosplenomegaly. Joint involvement may be minimal or absent initially. This type accounts for approximately 20% of all cases of JIA, but ocular involvement is rare; fewer than 6% of patients with systemic onset JIA have uveitis.
- *Polyarticular onset*. Patients with this type show involvement of more than 4 joints in the first 6 months of the disease; it represents 40% of JIA cases overall but only about 10% of cases of JIA-associated iridocyclitis. Patients with a positive rheumatoid factor may not develop uveitis.
- *Pauciarticular onset*. This type includes the vast majority (80%–90%) of patients with JIA who have uveitis. Four or fewer joints may be involved during the first 6 months of disease, and patients may have no joint symptoms. Pauciarticular onset JIA is further subdivided: type 1 disease is seen in girls under age 5 who typically have positive test results for antinuclear antibody (ANA); chronic iridocyclitis occurs in up to 25% of these patients. Type 2 disease is seen in older boys, many of whom go on to develop evidence of seronegative spondyloarthropathy (75% are HLA-B27–positive). The uveitis in these patients tends to be acute and recurrent rather than chronic, as in those with systemic onset JIA.

The average age of onset of uveitis in patients with JIA is 6 years. Uveitis generally develops within 5–7 years of the onset of joint disease but may occur as long as 28 years after the development of arthritis. There is usually little or no correlation between ocular and joint inflammation. Risk factors for the development of chronic iridocyclitis in patients with JIA include female gender, pauciarticular onset, and the presence of circulating ANA. Most patients have negative test results for rheumatoid factor.

The eye is often white and uninflamed. Symptoms include mild to moderate pain, photophobia, and blurring, although some patients do not have pain. Often, the eye disease is found incidentally during a routine school physical examination. The signs of inflammation include fine KPs, band keratopathy, flare and cells, posterior synechiae, and cataract (Figs 6-12, 6-13). Patients in whom JIA is suspected should undergo ANA testing and should be evaluated by a pediatric rheumatologist, because the joint disease may be minimal or absent at the time the uveitis is diagnosed. The differential diagnosis in these patients includes Fuchs heterochromic iridocyclitis, sarcoidosis, Behçet disease, the seronegative spondyloarthropathies, herpetic uveitis, and Lyme disease.

Prognosis Because of the frequently asymptomatic nature of the uveitis in these patients, profound silent ocular damage can occur, and the long-term prognosis often depends on the extent of damage at the time of first diagnosis. Complications are frequent and often

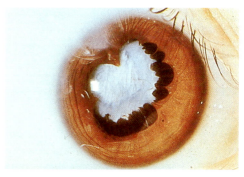

Figure 6-12 Juvenile idiopathic arthritis, with chronic iridocyclitis and cataract.

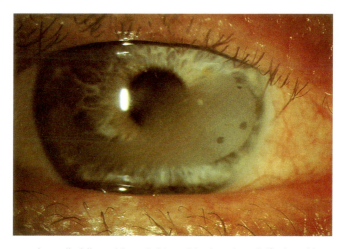

Figure 6-13 Juvenile idiopathic arthritis, with chronic calcific band keratopathy.

severe and include band keratopathy, cataract, glaucoma, vitreous debris, macular edema, chronic hypotony, and phthisis. Children with JIA, especially those who are ANA-positive or have pauciarticular disease, should undergo regular slit-lamp examinations. Table 6-1 outlines the recommended schedule for screening patients with JIA for uveitis, as developed by the American Academy of Pediatrics.

Treatment The initial treatment for patients with JIA who have uveitis consists of topical corticosteroids. More severe cases may require use of systemic or periocular corticosteroids. Corticosteroid therapy is not indicated in patients with chronic aqueous flare in the absence of active cellular reaction. Short-acting mydriatic agents are useful in patients with chronic flare to keep the pupil mobile and to prevent posterior synechiae formation. Use of systemic NSAIDs may permit a lower dose of corticosteroids.

Because of the chronic nature of the inflammation, corticosteroid-induced complications are common. The long-term use of systemic corticosteroids in children presents numerous problems, including growth retardation from premature closure of the epiphyses. In addition, there is evidence that even low-grade inflammation, if present for a prolonged period, can result in unacceptable ocular morbidity and visual loss. For these reasons, many of these children are now treated with weekly low-dose methotrexate. Numerous

Table 6-1 Frequency of Ophthalmologic Examination in Patients With JIA

Type	ANA	Age at Onset, y	Duration of Disease, y	Risk Category	Eye Examination Frequency, mo
Oligoarthritis or polyarthritis	+	≤6	≤4	High	3
	+	≤6	>4	Moderate	6
	+	≤6	>7	Low	12
	+	>6	≤4	Moderate	6
	+	>6	>4	Low	12
	–	≤6	≤4	Moderate	6
	–	≤6	>4	Low	12
	–	>6	NA	Low	12
Systemic disease (fever, rash)	NA	NA	NA	Low	12

JIA = juvenile idiopathic arthritis; ANA = antinuclear antibodies; NA = not applicable.
Recommendations for follow-up continue through childhood and adolescence.

Reprinted with permission from Cassidy J, Kivlin J, Lindsley C, Nocton J; Section on Rheumatology; Section on Ophthalmology. Ophthalmologic examinations in children with juvenile rheumatoid arthritis. *Pediatrics.* 2006;117(5):1844.

studies have shown that this treatment regimen can effectively control the uveitis, is generally well tolerated, and can spare patients the complications of long-term corticosteroid use. In addition, newer studies have revealed benefit from TNF inhibitors and other biologic agents in the treatment of JIA, with a reduction in ocular inflammation, a decrease in topical and systemic corticosteroid use, and fewer recurrences.

Treatment of cataracts in patients with JIA remains a challenge, and the use of IOLs remains controversial. Children who are left aphakic may develop amblyopia. There is a high complication rate following cataract surgery in patients with JIA-associated iridocyclitis, due to the difficulty in controlling the more aggressive inflammatory response seen in these children. Lensectomy and vitrectomy via the pars plana have been advocated.

However, there have been reports of more successful cataract surgery with IOL implants in patients with JIA. BenEzra and Cohen studied 5 children with JIA who received IOL implants. Although the vision initially improved in 4 of 5 eyes, it later decreased due to the development of retrolental membranes. Lam and colleagues reported good results following cataract extraction and IOL implants in 5 children with JIA. The major difference between the 2 studies was the more aggressive, long-term preoperative and postoperative use of IMT in the latter.

The following guidelines must be followed when selecting patients with JIA for cataract surgery with IOL implants:

- The patient's intraocular inflammation must be well controlled for at least 3 months before surgery with systemic IMT and must not require frequent instillation of topical corticosteroids.
- Only acrylic lenses should be implanted.
- Patients must be followed up very frequently after cataract surgery to detect any inflammation, and inflammation that occurs must be aggressively treated.
- IMT must be used preoperatively and postoperatively, not just perioperatively.

- Because long-term results are not available, patients must be strongly advised about the need for careful, regular, lifelong follow-up to detect late complications that may lead to loss of the eye.
- The ophthalmologist must have a low threshold for IOL explantation in patients who have persistent postoperative inflammation and recurrent cyclitic membranes.

Patients with band keratopathy should be treated (eg, scraping or chelation with sodium ethylenediaminetetraacetic acid [EDTA]) and allowed to heal well before cataract surgery is attempted. See also Chapter 10 and BCSC Section 6, *Pediatric Ophthalmology and Strabismus,* Chapter 21.

Glaucoma should be treated with medical therapy initially, although surgical intervention is often necessary in severe cases. Standard filtering procedures are usually unsuccessful, and the use of antifibrotic agents or aqueous drainage devices is usually required for successful control of the glaucoma.

BenEzra D, Cohen E. Cataract surgery in children with chronic uveitis. *Ophthalmology.* 2000; 107(7):1255–1260.

Cunningham ET Jr. Uveitis in children. *Ocul Immunol Inflamm.* 2000;8(4):251–261.

Ducos de Lahitte G, Terrada C, Tran TH, et al. Maculopathy in uveitis of juvenile idiopathic arthritis: an optical coherence tomography study. *Br J Ophthalmol.* 2008;92(1):64–69.

Holland GN, Denove CS, Yu F. Chronic anterior uveitis in children: clinical characteristics and complications. *Am J Ophthalmol.* 2009;147(4):667–678.

Kanski JJ. Juvenile arthritis and uveitis. *Surv Ophthalmol.* 1990;34(4):253–267.

Lam L, Lowder CY, Baerveldt G, Smith SD, Traboulsi EI. Surgical management of cataracts in children with juvenile rheumatoid arthritis-associated uveitis. *Am J Ophthalmol.* 2003;135(6):772–778.

Paroli MP, Spinucci G, Fabiani C, Pivetti-Pezzi P. Retinal complications of juvenile idiopathic arthritis-related uveitis: a microperimetry and optical coherence tomography study. *Ocul Immunol Inflamm.* 2010;18(1):54–59.

Probst LE, Holland EJ. Intraocular lens implantation in patients with juvenile rheumatoid arthritis. *Am J Ophthalmol.* 1996;122(2):161–170.

Rajaraman RT, Kimura Y, Li S, Haines K, Chu DS. Retrospective case review of pediatric patients with uveitis treated with infliximab. *Ophthalmology.* 2006;113(2):308–314.

Sen HN, Levy-Clarke G, Faia LJ, et al. High-dose daclizumab for the treatment of juvenile idiopathic arthritis-associated active anterior uveitis. *Am J Ophthalmol.* 2009;148(5):696–703.

Tynjälä P, Kotaniemi K, Lindahl P, et al. Adalimumab in juvenile idiopathic arthritis-associated chronic anterior uveitis. *Rheumatology (Oxford).* 2008;47(3):339–344.

Fuchs heterochromic iridocyclitis

Fuchs heterochromic iridocyclitis, or Fuchs uveitis syndrome, is an entity that is frequently overlooked. Between 2% and 3% of patients referred to uveitis clinics have Fuchs heterochromic iridocyclitis. This condition is usually unilateral, and its symptoms vary from none to mild blurring and discomfort. Signs include

- diffuse iris stromal atrophy with variable pigment epithelial layer atrophy (Fig 6-14)
- small white stellate KPs scattered *diffusely* over the entire endothelium (Fig 6-15); diffusely distributed KPs also occur with herpetic keratouveitis
- cells presenting in the anterior chamber as well as the anterior vitreous

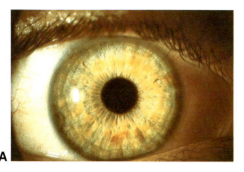
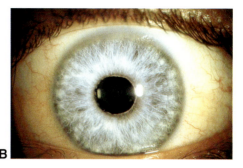

A **B**

Figure 6-14 Heterochromia in Fuchs heterochromic iridocyclitis. **A,** Right eye. **B,** Left eye. Note the lighter iris color and stromal atrophy ("moth-eaten appearance") in the left eye, which was the affected eye. *(Courtesy of David Forster, MD.)*

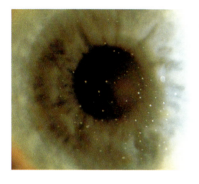

Figure 6-15 Diffusely distributed keratic precipitates in a patient with Fuchs heterochromic iridocyclitis. *(Courtesy of David Forster, MD.)*

Synechiae almost never form, but glaucoma and cataracts occur frequently. Generally, fundus lesions are absent, but fundus scars and retinal periphlebitis have been reported on rare occasions. Macular edema seldom occurs.

The diagnosis is based on the distribution of KPs, lack of synechiae, lack of symptoms, and heterochromia. Heterochromia may be subtle in a brown-eyed patient and one must look carefully for signs of iris stromal atrophy. Often, the inflammation is discovered on a routine examination, such as when a unilateral cataract develops. Usually, but not invariably, a lighter-colored iris indicates the involved eye (Fig 6-16). In blue-eyed persons, however, the affected eye may become darker as the stromal atrophy progresses and the darker iris pigment epithelium shows through.

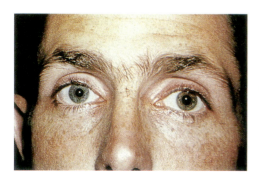

Figure 6-16 Heterochromia in Fuchs heterochromic iridocyclitis in a brown-eyed patient.

The etiology of Fuchs heterochromic iridocyclitis remains unclear. Associations with ocular toxoplasmosis, herpes simplex virus, and CMV infection have been suggested. de Groot-Mijnes and colleagues recently reported the association of rubella virus in patients with Fuchs heterochromic iridocyclitis; 13 of 14 patients with the disease demonstrated intraocular immunoglobulin G (IgG) production against rubella virus, whereas none had antibodies against herpes simplex virus, herpes zoster virus, or *Toxoplasma gondii.*

Patients generally do well with cataract surgery, and IOLs can usually be implanted successfully. However, some patients may suffer significant visual disability as a result of extensive vitreous opacification, even after uncomplicated cataract surgery with IOL implantation in the capsular bag. Pars plana vitrectomy should be carefully considered in such patients. Glaucoma control can be difficult. Abnormal vessels may bridge the angle on gonioscopy. These vessels may bleed during surgery, resulting in postoperative hyphema.

Few cases of Fuchs heterochromic iridocyclitis require therapy. The prognosis is good in most cases even though the inflammation persists for decades. Because topical corticosteroids can lessen the inflammation but typically do not resolve it, aggressive treatment to eradicate the cellular reaction is not indicated. Cycloplegia is seldom necessary. Histological examination shows plasma cells in the ciliary body, indicating that true inflammation occurs.

Birnbaum AD, Tessler HH, Schultz KL, et al. Epidemiologic relationship between Fuchs heterochromic iridocyclitis and the United States rubella vaccination program. *Am J Ophthalmol.* 2007;144(3):424–428.

de Groot-Mijnes JD, de Visser L, Rothova A, Schuller M, van Loon AM, Weersink AJ. Rubella virus is associated with Fuchs heterochromic iridocyclitis. *Am J Ophthalmol.* 2006;141(1): 212–214.

Idiopathic iridocyclitis

In many patients with chronic iridocyclitis, the cause is unknown. Therapy, including cycloplegia, may be necessary before a specific diagnosis is possible. In some cases initially labeled as idiopathic, repeat diagnostic testing at a later date may reveal an underlying systemic condition.

Intermediate Uveitis

The Standardization of Uveitis Nomenclature (SUN) Working Group defines *intermediate uveitis* as the subset in which the major site of inflammation is in the vitreous; it accounts for up to 15% of all cases of uveitis. It is characterized by ocular inflammation concentrated in the anterior vitreous and the vitreous base overlying the ciliary body and peripheral retina–pars plana complex. Inflammatory cells may aggregate in the vitreous ("snowballs"), where some coalesce. In some patients, inflammatory exudative accumulation on the inferior pars plana ("snowbanking") seems to correlate with a more severe disease process. There may be associated retinal phlebitis. Anterior chamber reaction may occur, but in adults it is usually mild and attributed to spillover from the vitreous.

Intermediate uveitis is associated with various conditions, including sarcoidosis, multiple sclerosis (MS), Lyme disease, peripheral toxocariasis, syphilis, tuberculosis, primary Sjögren syndrome, and infection with human T-cell lymphotropic virus type 1 (HTLV-1).

Pars Planitis

The term *pars planitis* refers to the subset of intermediate uveitis where there is snowbank or snowball formation in the absence of an associated infection or systemic disease. It is the most common form of intermediate uveitis, constituting approximately 85%–90% of cases. Previously also known as *chronic cyclitis* and *peripheral uveitis,* the condition most commonly affects persons aged 5–40 years. It has a bimodal distribution, concentrating in younger (5–15 years) and older (20–40 years) groups. No overall gender predilection is apparent. The pathogenesis of pars planitis is not well understood but is thought to involve autoimmune reactions against the vitreous, peripheral retina, and ciliary body. An association with the HLA-DR15 and HLA-DR51 alleles has been found. HLA-DR15 is also associated with MS, suggesting a common immunogenetic predisposition to both diseases.

Clinical characteristics

Approximately 80% of cases of pars planitis are bilateral but can often be asymmetric in severity. In children, the initial presentation may consist of significant anterior chamber inflammation accompanied by redness, photophobia, and discomfort. The onset in teenagers and young adults may be more insidious, with the presenting complaint generally being floaters. Ocular manifestations include variable numbers of spillover anterior chamber cells, vitreous cells, snowballs (Fig 6-17), and pars plana exudates. Inferior peripheral retinal phlebitis with retinal venous sheathing is common. With long-standing inflammation, CME often develops; this becomes chronic and refractory in approximately 10% of patients and is the major cause of visual loss. Ischemia from retinal phlebitis, combined with angiogenic stimuli from intraocular inflammation, can lead to neovascularization along the inferior snowbank in up to 10% of cases. These neovascular complexes can

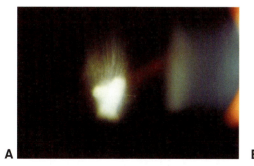
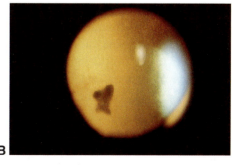

A   **B**

Figure 6-17 **A,** Vitreous snowball opacity in the anterior, inferior retrolental vitreous of a patient with pars planitis. **B,** Same vitreous snowball opacity in retroillumination, showing its location with respect to the lens. Note also the vitreous cellularity as evidenced by retroillumination. *(Courtesy of Ramana S. Moorthy, MD.)*

bleed, resulting in vitreous hemorrhages, and contract, leading to peripheral tractional and rhegmatogenous retinal detachments; in rare cases, the complexes evolve into peripheral retinal angiomas. Retinal detachments occur in 10% of patients with pars planitis. With chronicity, posterior synechiae and band keratopathy may also develop. Other possible causes of visual loss associated with chronic inflammation include posterior subcapsular cataracts, epiretinal membrane, and vitreous cellular opacification.

Differential diagnosis

The differential diagnosis of pars planitis includes syphilis, Lyme uveitis, sarcoidosis, intermediate uveitis associated with MS, and toxocariasis. Lyme and syphilitic uveitis may simulate any anatomical subtype of uveitis. Measurement of Lyme antibody titers may be particularly useful in areas where the disease is endemic, especially in the presence of cutaneous and articular disease. Iridocyclitis and intermediate uveitis may occur in up to 20% of patients with MS. Sarcoid uveitis presents as an intermediate disease in 7% of cases. Periphlebitis and retinal neovascularization frequently occur in sarcoidosis; however, anterior uveitis is much more common. Elevated levels of serum angiotensin-converting enzyme (ACE) and chest computed tomography (CT) findings can help differentiate sarcoidosis from idiopathic pars planitis. A peripheral *Toxocara* granuloma can mimic the unilateral pars plana snowbank in a child and should be ruled out. Serologic testing can be helpful in these cases.

Vitritis without other ocular findings can be suggestive of primary central nervous system (CNS) lymphoma. These patients are generally much older at presentation than those with pars planitis, usually in their sixth decade of life or older. Fuchs heterochromic iridocyclitis can produce mild to dense vitritis but has characteristic KPs and iris heterochromia.

Ancillary tests and histology

Diagnosis of pars planitis is based on classic clinical findings. Laboratory workup to exclude other causes of intermediate uveitis, including sarcoidosis, Lyme disease, and syphilis, is essential. Measurement of serum ACE and Lyme antibody titers, chest CT scanning, and syphilis serologic investigations should be considered. Fluorescein angiography (FA) may show diffuse peripheral venular leakage, disc leakage, and CME. Ultrasound biomicroscopy may be used in the case of a small pupil or dense cataract to demonstrate peripheral exudates or membranes over the pars plana.

Histologic examination of eyes with pars planitis shows vitreous condensation and cellular infiltration in the vitreous base. The inflammatory cells consist mostly of macrophages, lymphocytes, and a few plasma cells. Pars planitis is also characterized by peripheral lymphocytic cuffing of venules and a loose fibrovascular membrane over the pars plana.

Prognosis

The clinical course of pars planitis may be divided into 3 types. Approximately 10% of cases have a self-limiting, benign course; 30% have a smoldering course with remissions and exacerbations; and 60% have a prolonged course without exacerbations. Pars planitis may remain active for many years and has occasionally been documented to last more than 30 years. In most cases, the disease "burns out" after a few years. If CME is treated until resolution and kept from returning by adequate control of inflammation, the long-term visual prognosis can be good, with nearly 75% of patients maintaining visual acuity of 20/50 or better.

Treatment

Therapy should be directed toward treating the underlying cause of the inflammation, if possible. For example, infectious causes such as Lyme disease, tuberculosis, and syphilis should be treated with appropriate antimicrobial agents. If an underlying condition is not identified, as in pars planitis, or if therapy of an associated condition consists of nonspecific control of inflammation, as with sarcoidosis, anti-inflammatory therapy should be implemented. Treatment is begun if visual acuity is affected and the patient is symptomatic or if CME and retinal vasculitis are present. Mild cases without CME may not require treatment. A classic 4-step approach has been described.

Step 1 Periocular corticosteroids usually constitute the first line of therapy. These may be administered by local injection of depot corticosteroids, using the posterior sub-Tenon route (see Chapter 5, Fig 5-8). Triamcinolone or methylprednisolone may be used. Injections are usually repeated every 4 weeks until 4 injections have been administered. Generally, the inflammation responds and the CME improves. These injections may be repeated as necessary. Patients, especially those with a history of glaucoma, must be carefully monitored for corticosteroid-induced IOP elevation. Other complications of periocular corticosteroids include aponeurotic ptosis, enophthalmos, and, in rare instances, globe perforation. Cataract formation can occur with any form of corticosteroid therapy.

Intravitreal triamcinolone injections may be an alternative to periocular injections in severe refractory cases. These injections carry a risk of retinal detachment, vitreous hemorrhage, endophthalmitis, and sustained IOP elevation and glaucoma. Meticulous attention must be directed to the location of the intravitreal injection, with care to avoid areas of snowbanking and areas with peripheral retinal pathology.

Systemic corticosteroid therapy may be started if local therapy is not effective; it is generally reserved for more severe or bilateral cases. Patients may be treated with an initial dosage of 1–1.5 mg/kg/day, with a gradual tapering every week to dosages of less than 10 mg/day.

Step 2 If corticosteroid therapy fails, peripheral ablation of the pars plana snowbank with cryotherapy and/or indirect laser photocoagulation to the peripheral retina can be performed. Re-treatment is sometimes necessary. How peripheral laser photocoagulation and cryotherapy decrease inflammation is unknown. In their initial report, Aaberg and colleagues showed that following treatment with cryotherapy, 13 of 23 eyes (57%) had a decrease in vitritis and improvement in visual acuity. Cryotherapy is performed by applying a double row of transconjunctival cryopexy to an area 1 clock-hour beyond all evidence of disease activity, using a freeze–thaw technique.

Other authors have subsequently reported on cryotherapy treatment of the retina posterior to the snowbank. Peripheral FA revealed marked peripheral fluorescein leakage before peripheral retinal cryotherapy; after treatment, these areas of leakage were no longer noted. Peripheral retinal cryoablation has been associated with retinal detachments. Cryotherapy probably should not be performed in the presence of a tractional retinal detachment with peripheral neovascularization because of the increased risk of progressive traction and development of rhegmatogenous retinal detachment.

Peripheral scatter laser photocoagulation seems to be as effective as cryotherapy in treating inflammation and peripheral neovascularization and does not seem to increase the risk of rhegmatogenous retinal detachment. Photocoagulation burns may be placed confluently in 3 or 4 rows just posterior to the snowbank. Treatment may be extended to the equator posterior to the snowbank on each side.

Because peripheral laser photocoagulation appears to decrease inflammation in a manner similar to that of peripheral retinal cryoablation, direct treatment of the snowbank is unnecessary and is, in fact, contraindicated. Direct treatment may cause contraction of the vitreous base and lead to secondary retinal tears. Treatment of the peripheral retina may be a safer approach to this disease. In 1 series, no retinal detachments occurred following peripheral laser photocoagulation.

Step 3 If cryotherapy fails and systemic IMT is contraindicated or not desired because of the risk of systemic side effects, pars plana vitrectomy with induction of posterior hyaloidal separation and peripheral laser photocoagulation of the pars plana snowbank may be performed. Vitrectomy may be necessary to treat severe visual loss caused by dense vitreous cellular accumulation and veils, vitreal hemorrhage or traction, retinal detachment, and CME. Vitrectomy may reduce the need for high doses of maintenance oral corticosteroids in some patients. Separation of the posterior hyaloid membrane during vitrectomy may have a beneficial effect in reducing CME. Potential complications include retinal detachment, endophthalmitis, and cataract formation.

Step 4 Systemic immunomodulatory agents such as methotrexate, cyclosporine, azathioprine, mycophenolate mofetil, and cyclophosphamide may also be tried, and are indicated for treatment of bilateral disease. It should be noted that a rigid adherence to this stepwise approach to pars planitis treatment may prevent the benefits of combined therapy. For example, steroid-sparing therapies may be used to wean patients from long-term or high-dose systemic steroids. Additionally, IMT may be used to achieve disease quiescence prior to vitrectomy for those patients who suffer the neovascular or tractional complications of pars planitis.

Complications

Complications of pars planitis include cataract, glaucoma, CME, retinal neovascularization, vitreous hemorrhage, and tractional or rhegmatogenous retinal detachment. Cataracts occur in up to 60% of cases. Cataract surgery with IOL implantation may be complicated by smoldering low-grade inflammation; repeated opacification of the posterior capsule despite capsulotomy; recurrent retrolental membranes; and chronic CME, even in burned-out cases. Combining pars plana vitrectomy with cataract extraction and IOL implantation may reduce the risk of these complications. Glaucoma—both angle-closure and open-angle—occurs in approximately 10% of patients with pars planitis. CME may occur in 50% of patients with intermediate uveitis and is a hallmark of pars planitis. Retinal neovascularization occurs in up to 15% of patients with pars planitis.

Neovascularization of the disc as well as a peripheral snowbank have been reported. Occasionally, vitreous hemorrhage is the presenting sign of pars planitis, especially in children. Less than 5% of patients with pars planitis develop vitreous hemorrhage, which can be effectively treated with pars plana vitrectomy. Tractional and rhegmatogenous retinal detachments occur in up to 15% of patients and require scleral buckling, sometimes combined with vitrectomy. Risk factors for rhegmatogenous retinal detachment include severe inflammation, use of cryotherapy at the time of a vitrectomy, and neovascularization of the pars plana snowbank.

Donaldson MJ, Pulido JS, Herman DC, Diehl N, Hodge D. Pars planitis: a 20-year study of incidence, clinical features, and outcomes. *Am J Ophthalmol.* 2007;144(6):812–817.

Kaplan HJ. Intermediate uveitis (pars planitis, chronic cyclitis)—a four step approach to treatment. In: Saari KM, ed. *Uveitis Update.* Amsterdam: Excerpta Medica; 1984:169–172.

Potter MJ, Myckatyn SO, Maberley AL, Lee AS. Vitrectomy for pars planitis complicated by vitreous hemorrhage: visual outcome and long-term follow-up. *Am J Ophthalmol.* 2001;131(4):514–515.

Pulido JS, Mieler WF, Walton D, et al. Results of peripheral laser photocoagulation in pars planitis. *Trans Am Ophthalmol Soc.* 1998;96:127–137.

Sobrin L, D'Amico DJ. Controversies in intravitreal triamcinolone acetonide use. *Int Ophthalmol Clin.* 2005;45(4):133–141.

Standardization of Uveitis Nomenclature (SUN) Working Group. Standardization of uveitis nomenclature for reporting of clinical data. Results of the First International Workshop. *Am J Ophthalmol.* 2005;140(3):509–516.

Multiple Sclerosis

Patients with MS may develop variants of intermediate uveitis. The reported frequency of uveitis in patients with MS is as high as 30%, and uveitis is 10 times more common in this group than in the general population. MS usually affects white women 20–50 years of age. The onset of uveitis may precede the diagnosis of MS in up to 25% of patients, and by 5–10 years. Up to 15% of patients with pars planitis may eventually develop MS. Intermediate uveitis and panuveitis are the most common categories of MS-associated uveitis, and up to 95% of cases are bilateral. Periphlebitis in MS is not clearly related to optic neuritis, systemic exacerbations, or disease severity.

The immunopathogenesis of MS is not well understood but appears to involve humoral, cellular, and immunogenetic components directed against myelin. HLA-DR15 appears to be associated with the combination of MS and uveitis. Immunocytologic studies have shown some cross-reactivity between myelin-associated glycoprotein and Müller cells.

The severity of intermediate uveitis in MS appears to be milder than in idiopathic cases. Macular edema is less common. Most patients develop mild vitritis with periphlebitis. It is unclear whether treatment of MS with interferon has any effect on intermediate uveitis.

As biologic therapies for uveitis become more common, it is particularly important to consider the possibility of MS in any patient who presents with intermediate uveitis or pars planitis, as these agents are detrimental to patients with MS.

Chen L, Gordon LK. Ocular manifestations of multiple sclerosis. *Curr Opin Ophthalmol.* 2005;16(5):315–320.

Zein G, Berta A, Foster CS. Multiple sclerosis-associated uveitis. *Ocul Immunol Inflamm.* 2004;12(2):137–142.

Zierhut M, Foster CS. Multiple sclerosis, sarcoidosis and other diseases in patients with pars planitis. *Dev Ophthalmol.* 1992;23:41–47.

Posterior Uveitis

Posterior uveitis is defined by the SUN classification system as intraocular inflammation primarily involving the retina and/or choroid. Inflammatory cells may be observed diffusely throughout the vitreous cavity, overlying foci of active inflammation, or on the posterior vitreous face. Macular edema, retina vasculitis, and retinal or choroidal neovascularization (CNV), although not infrequent structural complications of certain uveitic entities, are not considered essential to the anatomical classification of posterior uveitis. Noninfectious syndromes with primarily posterior segment involvement are included in this section; diagnoses routinely producing both anterior and posterior segment involvement are addressed in the Panuveitis section later in the chapter.

Collagen Vascular Diseases

Systemic lupus erythematosus

Systemic lupus erythematosus (SLE) is a connective tissue disorder with multisystem involvement that primarily affects women of childbearing age, with higher incidence rates among African Americans and Hispanic persons in the United States. The pathogenesis of SLE is incompletely understood. Several major histocompatibility complex genes, including HLA-A1, HLA-B8, and HLA-DR3, as well as null alleles producing a deficiency of certain complement components may confer a susceptibility to the disease. It is thought to be an autoimmune disorder characterized by B-lymphocyte hyperactivity, polyclonal B-lymphocyte activation, hypergammaglobulinemia, autoantibody formation, and T-lymphocyte autoreactivity with immune complex deposition, leading to end-organ damage. Autoantibodies arising in SLE include ANA, antibodies to both single- and double-stranded DNA (anti-ssDNA and anti-dsDNA), antibodies to cytoplasmic components (anti-Sm, anti-Ro, and anti-La), and antiphospholipid antibodies. Cytokine patterns and abnormalities in signal transduction pathways may also be important in disease pathogenesis. The systemic manifestations of SLE are protean and include acute cutaneous diseases in approximately 70%–80% of patients (malar rash, discoid lupus, photosensitivity, mucosal lesions); arthritis in 80%–85%; renal disease in approximately 50%–75%; Raynaud phenomenon in 30%–50%; neurologic involvement in 35%; cardiac, pulmonary, and hepatic disease; and hematologic abnormalities. The diagnosis is essentially clinical, based on the identification of 4 of 11 criteria enumerated by the American College of Rheumatology (Table 6-2).

Ocular manifestations occur in 50% of patients with SLE and include cutaneous lesions on the eyelids (discoid lupus erythematosus), secondary Sjögren syndrome (occurring in approximately 20% of patients), all subtypes of scleral inflammatory disease, neuro-ophthalmic lesions (cranial nerve palsies, optic neuropathy, and retrochiasmal and cerebral visual disorders), retinal vasculopathy, and, in rare cases, uveitis.

Table 6-2 Revised Criteria for the Diagnosis of Systemic Lupus Erythematosus*

1. Malar rash
2. Discoid rash
3. Photosensitivity
4. Mucosal ulcers
5. Arthritis
6. Serositis (pleuritis, pericarditis)
7. Renal disorder (proteinuria, nephritis)
8. Neurologic disorder (seizures, psychosis)
9. Hematologic disorder (hemolytic anemia, or leukopenia, lymphopenia, or thrombocytopenia)
10. Immunologic disorder (anti-dsDNA, anti-Sm, antiphospholipid, or anticardiolipin antibodies; positive lupus anticoagulant test result; false-positive test result for syphilis)
11. Antinuclear antibody

*Diagnosis of systemic lupus erythematosus if 4 or more of the 11 criteria are met.

Adapted from Tan EM, Cohen AS, Fries JF, et al. The 1982 revised criteria for the classification of systemic lupus erythematosus. *Arthritis Rheum*. 1982;25(11):1271–1277; and Hochberg MC. Updating the American College of Rheumatology revised criteria for the classification of systemic lupus erythematosus [letter]. *Arthritis Rheum*. 1997;40(9):1725.

Lupus retinopathy, the most well-recognized posterior segment manifestation, is considered an important marker of systemic disease activity, with a prevalence ranging from 3% among outpatients with mild disease to 29% among those with more active disease. Its clinical spectrum varies from mild to severe and is characterized by the following:

- *Cotton-wool spots with or without intraretinal hemorrhages.* These occur independently of hypertension, and are thought to be due to the underlying microangiopathy of the disease (Fig 6-18).
- *Severe retinal vascular occlusive disease (arterial and venous thrombosis).* Retinal vaso-occlusion results in retinal nonperfusion and ischemia, secondary retinal neovascularization, and vitreous hemorrhage (Fig 6-19). More severe retinal vascular occlusive disease in SLE appears to be associated with CNS lupus and the presence

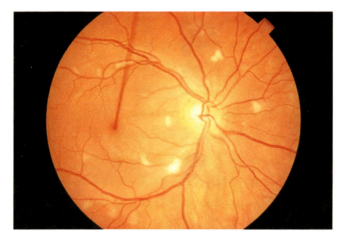

Figure 6-18 Systemic lupus erythematosus: multiple cotton-wool spots. *(Courtesy of E. Mitchel Opremcak, MD.)*

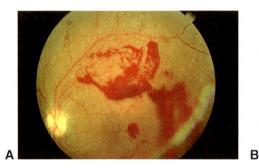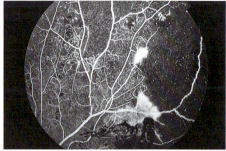

A   B

Figure 6-19 **A,** Ischemic retinal vasculitis and neovascularization in a patient with systemic lupus erythematosus. **B,** Fluorescein angiogram of the same patient as in **A** showing capillary nonperfusion. *(Courtesy of E. Mitchel Opremcak, MD.)*

of antiphospholipid antibodies, including lupus anticoagulant and anticardiolipin antibodies, found in 34% and 44% of these patients, respectively. Antiphospholipid antibodies may also arise primarily, unassociated with other autoimmune diseases, and produce a similar clinical picture; these are frequently associated with spontaneous abortion. Retinal vascular thrombosis is thought to be related to these autoantibodies and to the induction of a hypercoagulable state rather than to an inflammatory retinal vasculitis.

- *Lupus choroidopathy.* This entity is characterized by serous elevations of the retina, retinal pigment epithelium (RPE), or both; choroidal infarction; and CNV. It may be observed with severe systemic vascular disease, due to either hypertension from lupus nephritis or systemic vasculitis (Fig 6-20). SLE-induced hypertension and nephritis may also result in arteriolar narrowing, retinal hemorrhage, and disc edema.

Treatment is directed toward control of the underlying disease, using NSAIDs, corticosteroids, IMT, plasmapheresis, and systemic antihypertensive medications. Patients with severe vaso-occlusive disease or antiphospholipid antibodies may benefit from antiplatelet

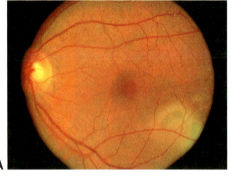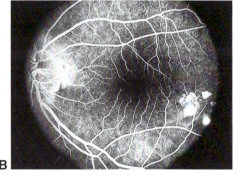

A   B

Figure 6-20 **A,** Multifocal choroiditis in a patient with systemic lupus erythematosus. **B,** Fluorescein angiogram showing multifocal areas of hyperfluorescence. *(Courtesy of E. Mitchel Opremcak, MD.)*

therapy or systemic anticoagulation. Ischemic complications, including proliferative reti-nopathy and vitreous hemorrhage, are managed with panretinal photocoagulation and vitrectomy surgery.

Davies JB, Rao PK. Ocular manifestation of systemic lupus erythematosus. *Curr Opin Ophthal-mol.* 2008;19(6):512–518.

D'Cruz DP, Khamashta MA, Hughes GR. Systemic lupus erythematosus. *Lancet.* 2007; 369(9561):587–596.

Jabs DA, Fine SL, Hochberg MC, Newman SA, Heiner GG, Stevens MB. Severe retinal vaso-occlusive disease in systemic lupus erythematosus. *Arch Ophthalmol.* 1986;104(4):558–563.

Nguyen QD, Uy HS, Akpek EK, Harper SL, Zacks DN, Foster CS. Choroidopathy of systemic lupus erythematosus. *Lupus.* 2000;9(4):288–298.

Polyarteritis nodosa and microscopic polyangiitis

Polyarteritis nodosa (PAN) is an uncommon systemic vasculitis characterized by sub-acute or chronic, focal, episodic necrotizing inflammation of medium-sized and small muscular arteries. Classic PAN and microscopic polyangiitis (microscopic polyarteritis) are differentiated by the presence or absence of small vessel involvement. The disease presents in patients between the ages of 40 and 60 years and affects men 3 times more frequently than women, with an annual incidence rate of approximately 0.7 per 100,000 individuals. Although there are no racial or geographic predisposing factors, 10% of the patients are positive for hepatitis B surface antigen, implicating hepatitis B as an etiologic agent. Indeed, the demonstration of circulating immune complexes composed of hepatitis B antigen and antibodies to hepatitis B in vessel walls during the early stages of the disease strongly implicate immune-complex–mediated mechanisms in the pathogenesis of PAN.

Constitutional symptoms, including fatigue, fever, weight loss, and arthralgia, are seen in up to 75% of patients, with mononeuritis multiplex being the most common symptom, if not the initial presenting sign. Renal involvement, related to vasculitis, is common, as is secondary hypertension, which affects approximately one-third of patients. Gastrointesti-nal disease with small bowel ischemia and infarction occurs less frequently but may lead to serious complications. Other systemic manifestations include cutaneous involvement (eg, subcutaneous nodules), purpura or Raynaud phenomenon, coronary arteritis, peri-carditis, and hematologic abnormalities. CNS disease associated with PAN is rare.

Ocular involvement is present in up to 20% of patients with PAN, arising as a con-sequence of the underlying vascular disease. In the posterior pole, this may manifest as hypertensive retinopathy replete with macular star formation, cotton-wool spots, and in-traretinal hemorrhage in patients with renal disease; retinal arteriolar occlusive disease; or choroidal infarcts with exudative retinal detachment secondary to vasculitis involving the posterior ciliary arteries and choroidal vessels (Fig 6-21). Elschnig spots may be observed in the posterior pole as a result of choroidal ischemia. Neuro-ophthalmic manifestations include cranial nerve palsies, amaurosis fugax, homonymous hemianopia, Horner syn-drome, and optic atrophy. Scleral inflammatory disease of all types, including necrotizing and posterior scleritis, has been reported. Peripheral ulcerative keratitis (PUK), typically accompanied by scleritis, may be the presenting manifestation of PAN.

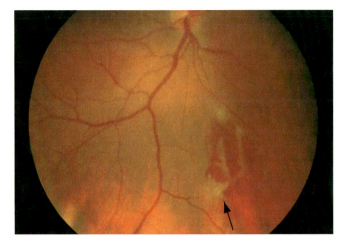

Figure 6-21 Polyarteritis nodosa with retinal vasculitis associated with vascular sheathing *(arrow)* and intraretinal hemorrhage. *(Courtesy of E. Mitchel Opremcak, MD.)*

The diagnosis of PAN is made by fulfilling 3 of the 10 classification criteria:

- weight loss of more than 4 kg
- livedo reticularis
- testicular pain or tenderness
- myalgia, weakness, or leg tenderness
- mononeuropathy or polyneuropathy
- elevated diastolic blood pressure (≥90 mm Hg)
- elevated blood urea nitrogen
- positive hepatitis B serology
- abnormal arteriographic findings
- demonstration of neutrophils on biopsy specimens of small or medium-sized arteries

The presence of antineutrophil cytoplasmic antibody (ANCA) further suggests the diagnosis (see the discussion of Wegener granulomatosis in the following section). The 5-year mortality rate of untreated PAN is 90%. Although systemic corticosteroid use may reduce this rate to 50%, appropriate treatment mandates combination therapy with immunomodulatory medications such as cyclophosphamide, which improves 5-year survival to 80% and may induce long-term remission of the disease. It is therefore important to consider PAN in the differential diagnosis of retinal vasculitis presenting in patients with multiple systemic complaints in whom an underlying necrotizing vasculitis is suspected; appropriate diagnosis and management can be life-saving. Tissue biopsy confirms the diagnosis.

Akova YA, Jabbur NS, Foster CS. Ocular presentation of polyarteritis nodosa. Clinical course and management with steroid and cytotoxic therapy. *Ophthalmology.* 1993;100(12):1775–1781.

Gayraud M, Guillevin L, Cohen P, et al, and the French Cooperative Study Group for Vasculitides. Treatment of good-prognosis polyarteritis nodosa and Churg-Strauss syndrome: comparison of steroids and oral or pulse cyclophosphamide in 25 patients. *Br J Rheumatol.* 1997;36(12):1290–1297.

Perez VL, Chavala SH, Ahmed M, et al. Ocular manifestations and concepts of systemic vasculitides. *Surv Ophthalmol.* 2004;49(4):399–418.

Wegener granulomatosis

Wegener granulomatosis is a multisystem autoimmune disorder characterized by the classic triad of necrotizing granulomatous vasculitis of the upper and lower respiratory tract, focal segmental glomerulonephritis, and necrotizing vasculitis of small arteries and veins. Involvement of the paranasal sinuses is the most characteristic clinical feature of this disorder, followed by pulmonary and renal disease. Renal involvement may or may not be evident at presentation, but its early detection is important, as up to 85% of patients develop glomerulonephritis during the course of the disease, which, if left untreated, carries significant mortality. A limited form of this disease has also been described, consisting of granulomatous inflammation involving the respiratory tract without overt involvement of the kidneys; however, subclinical renal disease may be present on tissue biopsy.

Patients may present with constitutional symptoms, sinusitis associated with bloody nasal discharge, pulmonary symptomatology, and arthritis. Dermatologic involvement is seen in approximately one-half of patients, with purpura involving the lower extremities occurring most frequently; less common are ulcers and subcutaneous nodules. Nervous system involvement may be seen in approximately one-third of patients with peripheral neuropathies, the most common being mononeuritis multiplex; less frequently observed are cranial neuropathies, seizures, stroke syndromes, and cerebral vasculitis.

Ocular or orbital involvement is seen in 15% of patients at presentation and in up to 50% of patients during the course of the disease. Orbital involvement, one of the most frequently reported ocular findings, is usually secondary to contiguous extension of the granulomatous inflammatory process from the paranasal sinuses into the orbit. Orbital pseudotumor, distinct from the sinus inflammation; orbital cellulitis; and dacryocystitis may arise from the involved and secondarily infected nasal mucosa. Scleritis of any type, particularly diffuse anterior or necrotizing disease, with or without peripheral ulcerative keratitis, affects up to 40% of patients. Posterior scleritis has also been reported.

Approximately 10% of patients with Wegener granulomatosis and ocular involvement have been reported to have an associated nonspecific unilateral or bilateral anterior, intermediate, or posterior uveitis, with varying degrees of vitritis. Retinal involvement is relatively uncommon, occurring in up to 10% of patients. Retinal vascular manifestations range from relatively benign cotton-wool spots, with or without associated intraretinal hemorrhages, to more severe vaso-occlusive disease, including branch or central retinal artery or vein occlusion. Retinitis has been reported in up to 20% of patients; those with accompanying retinal vasculitis may develop retinal neovascularization, vitreous hemorrhage, and neovascular glaucoma (Fig 6-22). Optic nerve involvement, especially ischemic optic neuropathy, is not uncommon. Vision loss in Wegener granulomatosis may occur in up to 40% of patients, especially among those with long-standing or inadequately treated disease.

Tissue biopsy establishes the histologic diagnosis; chest x-ray may disclose nodular, diffuse, or cavitary lesions; and laboratory evaluation may note proteinuria or hematuria, elevated ESR, and the presence of C-reactive protein and ANCAs.

ANCAs are antibodies directed against cytoplasmic azurophilic granules of neutrophils and monocytes, which are specific markers for a group of related systemic vasculitides

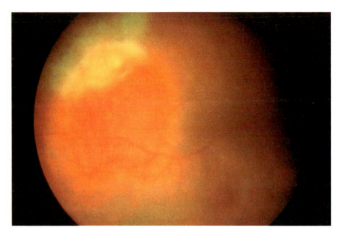

Figure 6-22 Wegener granulomatosis: retinitis. *(Courtesy of E. Mitchel Opremcak, MD.)*

that include Wegener granulomatosis, PAN, microscopic polyarteritis nodosa, Churg-Strauss syndrome, and pauci-immunoglomerulonephritis. Two main classes of ANCA have been described based on the immunofluorescence staining pattern on ethanol-fixed neutrophils and the main target antigen. The cytoplasmic pattern, or c-ANCA, is both sensitive and specific for Wegener granulomatosis and is present in up to 95% of patients; proteinase 3 is the most common target antigen. The perinuclear pattern, or p-ANCA, is associated with PAN, microscopic polyarteritis nodosa, relapsing polychondritis, and renal vasculitis. Myeloperoxidase is the most common antigenic target. In contrast to the results found in Wegener granulomatosis, the diagnostic sensitivities of c-ANCA and p-ANCA for PAN are only 5% and 15%, respectively; in patients with microscopic polyarteritis nodosa, p-ANCA (myeloperoxidase) positivity is more common (50%–80%), with a smaller percentage (40%) having the c-ANCA (proteinase 3) marker.

As with PAN, appropriate treatment mandates combination therapy with oral corticosteroids and IMT, specifically cyclophosphamide. Without therapy, the 1-year mortality rate is 80%. However, 93% of patients treated with cyclophosphamide and corticosteroids successfully achieve remission with resolution of ocular manifestations. As with PAN, ophthalmologists must be intimately familiar with Wegener granulomatosis, as ocular inflammatory manifestations are frequently present, and timely diagnosis and treatment are essential in reducing not only ocular morbidity but overall patient mortality.

Hoffman GS, Kerr GS, Leavitt RY, et al. Wegener's granulomatosis: an analysis of 158 patients. *Ann Intern Med.* 1992;116(6):488–498.

Pakrou N, Selva D, Leibovitch I. Wegener's granulomatosis: ophthalmic manifestations and management. *Semin Arthritis Rheum.* 2006;35(5):284–292.

Susac Syndrome

Susac syndrome (also known as *SICRET syndrome,* for small infarctions of cochlear, retinal, and encephalic tissue) is a rare entity, initially reported in 1979 by Susac et al and consisting of the clinically observed triad of encephalopathy, hearing loss, and retinal artery branch occlusions. It occurs mostly in young women but has been noted in patients aged

16 to 58 years. Differential diagnosis at presentation includes MS, herpetic encephalitis, acute disseminated encephalomyelitis, and Behçet disease. However, ocular findings are highly specific and allow prompt diagnostic confirmation with subsequent therapeutic adjustments. Ophthalmoscopy shows diffuse or localized narrowing of retinal arteries with a "boxcar" segmentation of the blood column at the level of peripheral retinal arteries. Vitreous haze or cells are absent. Retinal FA discloses focal nonperfused retinal arterioles with hyperfluorescent walls (Fig 6-23). There is usually no evidence of embolic material or inflammatory reactions around the vessels. Magnetic resonance imaging (MRI) is another useful diagnostic tool and shows multifocal supratentorial white matter lesions; the corpus callosum may be involved. Treatment remains controversial and includes high-dose intravenous corticosteroids, anticoagulants, and IMT. The course of Susac syndrome is not always self-limiting and isolated retinal arteriolar involvement may occur as a very late manifestation.

Aubart-Cohen F, Klein I, Alexandra JF, et al. Long-term outcome in Susac syndrome. *Medicine (Baltimore).* 2007;86(2):93–102.

Susac JO, Hardman JM, Selhorst lB. Microangiopathy of the brain and retina. *Neurology.* 1979;29(3):313–316.

Inflammatory Chorioretinopathies of Unknown Etiology

The inflammatory chorioretinopathies, or white dot syndromes, are a heterogeneous group of inflammatory disorders with overlapping clinical features that share in common the presence of discrete, multiple, well-circumscribed, yellow-white lesions at the level of the retina, outer retina, RPE, choriocapillaris, and choroid during some phase of their course. The white dot syndromes consist of the predominantly noninfectious ocular syndromes listed in Table 6-3. Their differential diagnosis includes systemic and ocular infectious entities such as syphilis, diffuse unilateral subacute neuroretinitis (DUSN), and ocular histoplasmosis syndrome (OHS), as well as noninfectious entities such as sarcoidosis, sympathetic ophthalmia, VKH syndrome, and intraocular lymphoma (Table 6-4). Common presenting symptoms include photopsias, blurred vision, nyctalopia, floaters,

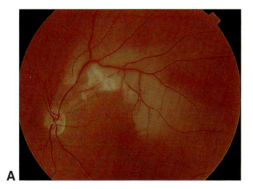
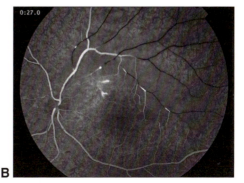

Figure 6-23 Susac syndrome. **A,** Color fundus photograph disclosing an area of intraretinal whitening corresponding to a supratemporal branch artery occlusion in the left eye. **B,** Fluorescein angiogram showing a supratemporal branch artery occlusion with multiple areas of segmental staining well away from sites of bifurcation. *(Courtesy of Albert T. Vitale, MD.)*

Table 6-3 Inflammatory Chorioretinopathies

	Birdshot	APMPPE	Serpiginous Choroiditis	MCP	PIC	SFU	MEWDS	ARPE	AZOOR
Age	Older (30–70)	Young (20–50)	Young, middle-age (20–60)	Young (9–69)	Young (18–40)	Young (14–34)	Young (10–47)	Young (16–40)	Young (13–63)
Sex	F>M	M=F	M=F	F (3:1)	F (90%)	F (100%)	F (3:1)	M=F	F (3:1)
Laterality	Bilateral	Bilateral	Bilateral, asymmetric	Bilateral	Bilateral	Asymmetric	Unilateral	Unilateral (75%)	Unilateral (24%), bilateral (76%)
Systemic associations	80%–98% HLA-A29+, lymphocyte proliferation to retinal S-antigen	Viral prodrome, cerebrovasculitis, CSF abnormalities	HLA-B7	None	None	None	Viral prodrome (50%)	None	Systemic autoimmune disease (28%)
Pathogenesis	Autoimmune?	Viral?	Autoimmune? Infectious (herpes)?	Viral?	Variant of MCP? Limited myopic degeneration?	Autoimmune	Viral? Common non–disease-specific genetics?	Viral?	Viral vs autoimmune
Onset	Insidious	Acute	Variable	Insidious	Acute	Insidious	Acute	Acute	Insidious
Course	Chronic, recurrent	Self-limited	Chronic, recurrent	Chronic, recurrent	Self-limited	Chronic, recurrent	Self-limited	Self-limited	Chronic, recurrent (31%)
Symptoms	Blurred vision, floaters, photopsias, disturbed night and color vision	Blurred vision, scotomata, photopsias	Blurred vision, scotomata	Blurred vision, floaters, photopsias, metamorphopsia, scotomata	Paracentral scotomata, photopsias, metamorphopsia	Blurred vision, decreased vision	Blurred or decreased vision, scotomata, photopsias	Central metamorphopsia, scotomata	Photopsias

Examination	Vitritis; ovoid, creamy, white-yellow, postequatorial lesions (50–1500 μm), do not pigment	Multifocal, flat, gray-white lesions, 1–2 disc areas, outer retina/RPE with evolving pigmentation	Geographic, yellow-gray, peripapillary, macular chorioretinal lesions with centripedal extension; activity at leading, peripheral edge with RPE/choriocapillaris atrophy in its wake	Myopia, iridocyclitis (50%), vitritis (100%), active white-yellow chorioretinal lesions (50–200 μm) evolving to punched-out scars	Myopia, vitritis absent, white-yellow chorioretinal lesions	Moderate vitritis, 50–500 μm yellow-white lesions posterior pole to midperiphery, RPE, hypertrophy, atrophy, large stellate zones of subretinal fibrosis	Myopia; mild iridocyclitis; vitritis; small white-orange, evanescent, perifoveal dots (100–200 μm) outer retina/RPE; macular granularity	Small, hyperpigmented lesions with yellow halo (100–200 μm), unassociated vitritis	Initially normal to subtle RPE changes, late pigment migration, focal perivenous sheathing
Structural complications	Retinal vasculitis, disc edema, CME, CNVM (6%)	Disc edema	CNVM (25%), RPE mottling, scarring, loss of choriocapillaris	Optic disc edema, peripapillary pigment changes, CME (14%–44%), CNVM (33%)	CNVM (17%–40%), serous detachment over confluent lesions	Neurosensory retinal detachment, CME, CNVM	Disc edema, venous sheathing	None	RPE mottling, occasional CME
Fluorescein angiography (FA)	Early hypofluorescence vs silence, subtle late stain; leakage from disc, vessels, CME; delayed retinal circulation time	Acute lesions: early blockage, late staining; late window defects	Early hypofluorescence, late staining/leakage of active border, leakage in presence of CNVM	Early blockage, late staining of lesions, leakage from CME, CNVM	Early hyperfluorescence, variable late leakage/staining acute lesions, leakage in presence of CME, CNVM	Multiple areas of alternating hypo- and hyperfluorescence; early, late staining	Early punctate hyperfluorescence, wreathlike configuration, late staining of lesions, optic nerve	Early hyperfluorescence with surrounding halo of hyperfluorescence and late staining	In acute stage, normal with increased retinal circulation time; in late stage, diffuse hyperfluorescence, RPE atrophy

(Continued)

Table 6-3 *(continued)*

	Birdshot	APMPPE	Serpiginous Choroiditis	MCP	PIC	SFU	MEWDS	ARPE	AZOOR
Indocyanine green angiography (ICG)	Corresponding hypofluorescent lesions more numerous than on exam, FA	Hypofluorescent spots corresponding to those seen on exam, FA	Early hypofluorescence, late staining, more widespread extent than seen on exam, FA	Multiple hypofluorescent lesions, confluence around optic nerve, more numerous than on exam, FA	Multiple hypofluorescent, peripapillary, posterior pole lesions, corresponding to those seen on exam, FA		Multiple hypofluorescent spots, more numerous than on exam, FA		
Electrophysiology, visual fields (VF)	ERG: abnormal rod and cone responses	EOG: variably abnormal	ERG: normal	ERG: abnormal, extinguished responses	ERG: normal VF: enlargement of blind spot (41%)	VF, ERG, and EOG markedly attenuated	ERG: diminished a wave, early receptor potentials (reversible); VF: enlarged blind spot, paracentral scotomata	ERG: normal EOG: abnormal	ERG, mfERG: abnormal; VF: temporal, superior defects, enlarged blind spot
Visual prognosis	Guarded without treatment	Good	Guarded	Guarded	Good in absence of CNVM	Guarded	Excellent	Excellent	Guarded
Treatment	Systemic corticosteroids, IMT	Observation; systemic corticosteroids with CNS involvement	Systemic corticosteroids, IMT, laser for CNVM	Systemic corticosteroids, IMT, laser for CNVM	Observation; systemic/periocular corticosteroids, laser for CNVM	Corticosteroids for CME, IMT of equivocal efficacy long term	Observation	None	Corticosteroids, IMT, antivirals of equivocal efficacy

APMPPE = acute posterior multifocal placoid pigment epitheliopathy, ARPE = acute retinal pigment epitheliitis, AZOOR = acute zonal occult outer retinopathy, CNVM = choroidal neovascular membrane, IMT = immunomodulatory therapy, MCP = multifocal choroiditis and panuveitis syndrome, MEWDS = multiple evanescent white dot syndrome, PIC = punctate inner choroiditis, SFU = subretinal fibrosis and uveitis syndrome.

Table 6-4 Differential Diagnosis for Chorioretinopathies

Syphilis
Diffuse unilateral subacute neuroretinitis (DUSN)
Ocular histoplasmosis syndrome (OHS)
Tuberculosis
Toxoplasmosis
Pneumocystis choroidopathy
Candidiasis
Acute retinal necrosis (ARN)
Ophthalmomyasis
Sarcoidosis
Sympathetic ophthalmia
Vogt-Koyanagi-Harada (VKH) syndrome
Intraocular lymphoma

and visual field loss contiguous with a blind spot. In many cases, a prodromal viral syndrome can be identified. Bilateral involvement, albeit asymmetrically (with the exception of multiple evanescent white dot syndrome [MEWDS]), is the rule. Other than patients with birdshot retinochoroidopathy or serpiginous choroiditis, the majority of individuals are younger than age 50. A female predominance is observed in patients with MEWDS, birdshot retinochoroidopathy, multifocal choroiditis and panuveitis, punctate inner choroiditis (PIC), and acute zonal occult outer retinopathy.

The etiology of the white dot syndromes is unknown. Some investigators have postulated an infectious cause; others have suggested an autoimmune/inflammatory pathogenesis arising in individuals with common non–disease-specific genetics, triggered by some exogenous agent. An increased prevalence of systemic autoimmunity in both patients with white dot syndromes and their first- and second-degree relatives suggests that inflammatory chorioretinopathies may occur in families with inherited immune dysregulation that predisposes to autoimmunity. Whether the white dot syndromes represent a clinical spectrum of a single disease entity or are each discrete diseases awaits identification of the underlying mechanisms. Although they have similarities, the white dot syndromes can be differentiated clinically based on their variable lesion morphology and evolution, distinct natural histories, and angiographic behavior. This has important implications with respect to disease-specific treatments and predictions of the ultimate visual prognosis.

Gass JD. Are acute zonal occult outer retinopathy and the white dot syndromes (AZOOR complex) specific autoimmune diseases? *Am J Ophthalmol.* 2003;135(3):380–381.

Jampol LM, Becker KG. White spot syndromes of the retina: a hypothesis based on the common genetic hypothesis of autoimmune/inflammatory disease. *Am J Ophthalmol.* 2003;135(3): 376–379.

Quillen DA, Davis JB, Gottlieb JL, et al. The white dot syndromes. *Am J Ophthalmol.* 2004; 137(3):538–550.

Pearlman RB, Golchet PR, Feldmann MG, et al. Increased prevalence of autoimmunity in patients with white spot syndromes and their family members. *Arch Ophthalmol.* 2009;127(7): 869–874.

Birdshot retinochoroidopathy

Birdshot retinochoroidopathy (vitiliginous chorioretinitis) is an uncommon disease presenting predominantly in white women of northern European descent past the fourth decade of life. While no consistent systemic disease association has been identified, birdshot retinochoroidopathy is highly correlated with the HLA-A29 gene, with a sensitivity of 96% and a specificity of 93%. The presence of the haplotype confers considerable increased relative risk (224-fold) for the development of this disease. HLA-A29 is confirmatory rather than diagnostic, as 7% of the general population carries this haplotype, and in the absence of characteristic clinical features, an alternative diagnosis should be considered. Retinal autoimmunity is thought to play an important role in the pathogenesis of birdshot retinochoroidopathy, as is suggested by the similarities between it and experimental autoimmune uveitis and by the demonstration of lymphocyte proliferation to retinal S-antigen. Alternatively, it has been hypothesized that an infectious agent may enhance the expression, by the HLA-A29 molecule, of self-peptides to T lymphocytes. Both T and B lymphocytes, but no organisms, have been seen on histologic examination of the chorioretinal lesions from autopsy eyes with birdshot retinochoroidopathy.

Presenting symptoms include blurred vision, floaters, nyctalopia, and disturbance of color vision. Anterior segment inflammation may be minimal or lacking; however, varying degrees of vitritis are commonly noted. Funduscopy reveals characteristic multifocal, hypopigmented, ovoid, cream-colored lesions (50–1500 µm) at the level of the choroid and RPE in the postequatorial fundus; typically these show a nasal and radial distribution, emanating from the optic nerve, and frequently they follow the underlying choroidal vessels (Fig 6-24). They do not become pigmented over time and are best appreciated by indirect ophthalmoscopy. Retinal vasculitis, CME, and optic nerve head inflammation are important components of active disease. Late complications include optic atrophy, epiretinal membrane (ERM) formation, and, rarely, CNV.

FA reveals inconsistent findings depending on age, lesions, and phase of study. Although early birdshot lesions may show initial hypofluorescence with subtle late staining, in general, FA does not typically highlight the birdshot lesions themselves but rather is

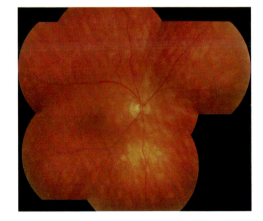

Figure 6-24 Birdshot retinochoroidopathy with multiple postequatorial, cream-colored ovoid lesions. *(Courtesy of Ramana S. Moorthy, MD.)*

useful in identifying more subtle indices of active inflammation such as retinal vasculitis, CME, and optic nerve head leakage (Figs 6-25, 6-26). Late hypopigmented lesions typically do not show transmission defects, implying loss of pigment concurrent with loss of choriocapillaris. Indocyanine green (ICG) angiography discloses multiple hypofluorescent spots, which are typically more numerous than those seen on clinical examination or on FA (Fig 6-27). Fundus autofluorescence (FAF) imaging reveals hypoautofluorescence in areas of RPE atrophy that are more numerous and not uniformly correspondent with the birdshot lesions, suggesting that the choroid and RPE may be affected independently. Placoid macular hypoautofluorescence may be an important predictor of central vision loss (Fig 6-28).

Important differential diagnostic considerations include pars planitis, VKH syndrome, sympathetic ophthalmia, OHS, and especially sarcoidosis, which may present with chorioretinal lesions of similar morphology and distribution as those seen in birdshot retinochoroidopathy.

Progressive visual field loss and abnormal electroretinogram (ERG) results are commonly seen with extended follow-up, suggesting that a more diffuse retinal dysfunction not fully explained by the presence of CME or other structural abnormalities contributes to visual loss. For this reason full-field ERGs (with attention to the 30-Hz flicker implicit time and scotopic-b wave amplitudes) and both Goldmann and automated visual fields (30-2 with attention to the mean deviation) are more useful parameters in following disease course and response to therapy than changes in funduscopic examination results or visual acuity.

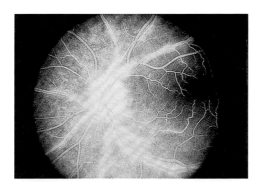

Figure 6-25 Fluorescein angiogram showing diffuse retinal phlebitis in a patient with birdshot retinochoroidopathy. *(Courtesy of E. Mitchel Opremcak, MD.)*

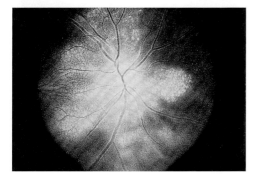

Figure 6-26 Fluorescein angiogram showing cystoid retinal edema in a patient with birdshot retinochoroidopathy. *(Courtesy of E. Mitchel Opremcak, MD.)*

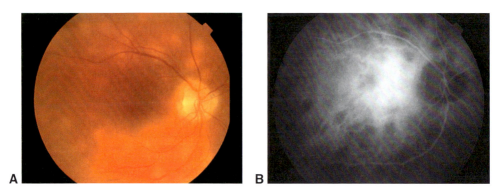

Figure 6-27 Birdshot retinochoroidopathy. Fundus photograph **(A)** and indocyanine green angiogram **(B)** showing numerous midphase hypofluorescent spots corresponding to fundus lesions. *(Courtesy of Albert T. Vitale, MD.)*

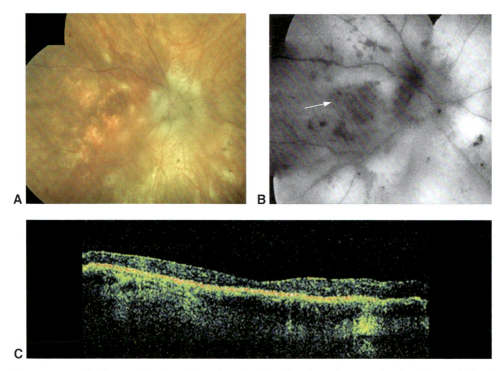

Figure 6-28 Birdshot retinochoroidopathy. **A,** Color fundus photograph showing multifocal hypopigmented spots within the macula and outside the arcades. **B,** Autofluorescence photograph showing placoid hypoautofluorescence in the central macula *(arrow).* **C,** Optical coherence tomography image showing foveal thinning. *(Reprinted with permission from Koizumi H, Pozzoni MC, Spaide RF. Fundus autofluorescence in birdshot chorioretinopathy. Ophthalmology. 2008:115(5):e17. Epub Apr 18.)*

Although it has been reported that 20% of patients may have self-limiting disease, the course is generally marked by multiple exacerbations and remissions, with few patients maintaining good vision without treatment. It was recently reported that among patients with disease duration longer than 30 months, more than two-thirds had visual acuity worse than 20/50 and one-third worse than 20/200. The overall 5-year cumulative incidence of visual acuity of 20/200 or worse was 20%.

Treatment consists of the initial administration of systemic corticosteroids, with early introduction of corticosteroid-sparing IMT, because birdshot retinochoroidopathy is typically incompletely responsive to corticosteroids alone and extended treatment is anticipated in most patients. Corticosteroid-sparing immunomodulators include low-dose cyclosporine (2–5 mg/kg/day), mycophenolate mofetil, azathioprine, methotrexate, daclizumab, and intravenous polyclonal immunoglobulin. Periocular corticosteroid injections are useful as adjunctive therapy in managing CME and inflammatory recurrences. This approach is effective in reducing intraocular inflammation, inflammatory recurrences, and the risk of developing CME, as well as preserving visual acuity. The intravitreal fluocinolone acetonide implant is an option for patients who cannot tolerate systemic therapy.

Gordon LK, Monnet D, Holland GN, Brézin AP, Yu F, Levinson RD. Longitudinal cohort study of patients with birdshot chorioretinopathy. IV. Visual field results at baseline. *Am J Ophthalmol.* 2007;144(6):829–837.

Holder GE, Robson AG, Pavesio C, Graham EM. Electrophysiological characterisation and monitoring in the management of birdshot chorioretinopathy. *Br J Ophthalmol.* 2005;89(6):709–718.

Kiss S, Ahmed M, Letko E, Foster CS. Long-term follow-up of patients with birdshot retinochoroidopathy treated with corticosteroid-sparing systemic immunomodulatory therapy. *Ophthalmology.* 2005;112(6):1066–1071.

Koizumi H, Pozzoni MC, Spaide RF. Fundus autofluorescence in birdshot chorioretinopathy. *Ophthalmology.* 2008;115(5):e15–e20. Epub Apr 18.

Levinson RD, Gonzales CR. Birdshot retinochoroidopathy: immunopathogenesis, evaluation, and treatment. *Ophthalmol Clin North Am.* 2002;15(3):343–350.

Oh KT, Christmas NJ, Folk JC. Birdshot retinochoroiditis: long term follow-up of a chronically progressive disease. *Am J Ophthalmol.* 2002;133(5):622–629.

Thorne JE, Jabs DA, Peters GB, Hair D, Dunn JP, Kempen JH. Birdshot retinochoroidopathy: ocular complications and visual impairment. *Am J Ophthalmol.* 2005;140(1):45–51.

Acute posterior multifocal placoid pigment epitheliopathy

Acute posterior multifocal placoid pigment epitheliopathy (APMPPE), an uncommon condition presenting in otherwise healthy young adults, typically occurs with an influenza-like illness (50%) and affects men and women equally. A genetic predisposition may be present given the association of HLA-B7 and HLA-DR2 with the development of this entity. A number of noninfectious systemic conditions have been reported in connection with APMPPE, including erythema nodosum, Wegener granulomatosis, PAN, cerebral vasculitis, scleritis and episcleritis, sarcoidosis, and ulcerative colitis. Infectious conditions including group A streptococcal and adenovirus type 5 infections, tuberculosis, Lyme disease, and mumps have also been associated with APMPPE, as has hepatitis B vaccination. These diverse disease associations reinforce the concept that APMPPE is an immune-driven vascular alteration.

Patients typically present with a sudden onset of bilateral, asymmetric visual loss associated with central and paracentral scotomata, with the fellow eye becoming involved within days to weeks. Photopsias may precede visual loss. There is minimal anterior segment inflammation, but vitritis of a mild to moderate degree is present in 50% of patients.

Funduscopic findings include multiple, large, flat, yellow-white placoid lesions at the level of the RPE, varying in size from 1 to 2 disc areas, located throughout the posterior pole to the equator (Fig 6-29). New peripheral lesions may appear in a linear or radial array over the next 3 weeks. Papillitis may be observed, but CME is uncommon. Atypical findings include retinal vasculitis, retinal vascular occlusive disease, retinal neovascularization, and exudative retinal detachment. The lesions resolve over a period of 2 to 6 weeks, leaving a permanent, well-defined alteration in the RPE consisting of alternating areas of depigmentation and pigment clumping.

The diagnosis of APMPPE is based on the characteristic clinical presentation and FA findings during the acute phase of the disease: early hypofluorescence (blockage) lesions corresponding to but typically more numerous than those seen on funduscopy and late hyperfluorescent staining (Fig 6-30). Subacute lesions may show increased central hyperfluorescence with late staining; with resolution, transmission defects are typically observed. ICG angiography reveals choroidal hypofluorescence with hypervisualization of the underlying choroidal vessels in both the acute and inactive stages of the disease, with these lesions becoming smaller in the inactive stages (Fig 6-31). Whether the lesions of APMPPE themselves are due primarily to involvement of the RPE or represent choroidal/choriocapillary perfusion abnormalities with secondary involvement of the RPE and

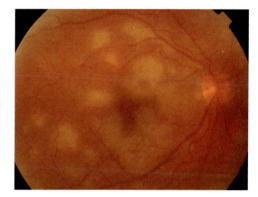

Figure 6-29 Acute posterior multifocal placoid pigment epitheliopathy (APMPPE). Multifocal, placoid lesions in the macula. *(Courtesy of Albert T. Vitale, MD.)*

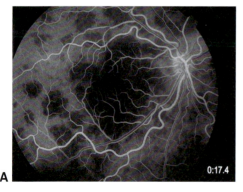
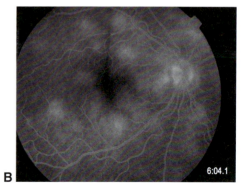

Figure 6-30 Fluorescein angiogram in a patient with APMPPE. **A,** Early blockage of choroidal circulation. **B,** Late-phase staining. *(Courtesy of Albert T. Vitale, MD.)*

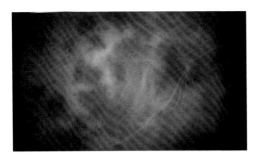

Figure 6-31 Indocyanine green angiogram in a patient with APMPPE showing multiple midphase hypofluorescent spots. *(Courtesy of Albert T. Vitale, MD.)*

photoreceptors remains controversial; however, taken together, the FA, ICG, and FAF imaging findings suggest the latter. Choroidal perfusion abnormalities seen early on FA and ICG angiography are more numerous than the overlying placoid lesions; abnormalities noted on FAF imaging lag the appearance of these lesions, are fewer in number, and lack the perfusion changes seen during angiography; and RPE alterations seen during recovery appear well after the choroid is affected. All of these implicate a primary choroidal process.

In addition to choroidal metastasis, viral retinitis, toxoplasmic retinochoroiditis, and pneumocystis choroiditis, an important differential diagnostic consideration is serpiginous choroiditis. APMPPE is an acute, usually nonrecurring disease, whereas serpiginous choroiditis is insidious and relentlessly progressive.

An uncommon variant termed *relentless placoid chorioretinitis* that has features of both serpiginous choroiditis and APMPPE has been reported. Men or women between the second and sixth decade of life present with floaters, photopsia, paracentral scotomata, and decreased vision with a variable degree of both anterior segment inflammation and vitritis. The acute retinal lesions are similar to those of APMPPE or serpiginous choroiditis both clinically and angiographically, but the clinical course is atypical for both entities. Patients have numerous posterior and peripheral lesions predating or occurring simultaneously with macular involvement. Acute lesions heal over a period of weeks with resultant chorioretinal atrophy. Older pigmented areas are observed together with new active white placoid lesions that are not necessarily extensions of previous areas of activity. Prolonged periods of disease activity with the appearance of numerous (>50) multifocal lesions scattered throughout the fundus are seen. Relapses are common, with the appearance of new lesions and the growth of subacute lesions for up to 2 years after the initial presentation. FA demonstrates early hypofluorescence and late staining of these lesions. Although macular involvement can result in vision loss, metamorphopsia, or scotomata, visual acuity is preserved in most patients upon healing of the lesions (Fig 6-32).

Although visual acuity returns to 20/40 or better within 6 months in the majority of patients with APMPPE, 20% are left with residual visual dysfunction. Risk factors for visual loss include foveal involvement at presentation, older age at presentation, unilateral disease, a longer interval between initial and fellow eye involvement, and recurrence. There are no convincing data to suggest that treatment with systemic corticosteroids is beneficial in altering the visual outcome, although some authorities advocate their use in patients presenting with extensive macular involvement, in an effort to limit subsequent RPE derangement of the foveal center, and in individuals with an associated

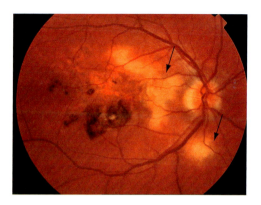

Figure 6-32 Relentless placoid chorioretinitis. Retinal pigment epithelial hyperpigmentation and atrophy in the central macula in areas of previous inflammation, with new, yellow-white foci of active disease temporal and inferior to the optic nerve *(arrows)*. *(Courtesy of Albert T. Vitale, MD.)*

CNS vasculitis. Similarly, the precise role of systemic steroids, antiviral agents, and IMT for the treatment of relentless placoid chorioretinitis is incompletely understood. Systemic steroids are commonly employed, but the disease may recur despite their use.

Fiore T, Iaccheri B, Androudi S, et al. Acute posterior multifocal placoid pigment epitheliopathy. Outcome and visual prognosis. *Retina*. 2009;29(7):994–1001.

Jones BE, Jampol LM, Yannuzzi LA, et al. Relentless placoid chorioretinitis: a new entity or an unusual variant of serpiginous chorioretinitis? *Arch Ophthalmol*. 2000;118(7):931–938.

Pagliarini S, Piguet B, Ffytche TJ, Bird AC. Foveal involvement and lack of visual recovery in APMPPE associated with uncommon features. *Eye*. 1995;9(pt 1):42–47.

Spaide RF. Autofluorescence imaging of acute posterior multifocal placoid pigment epitheliopathy. *Retina*. 2006;26(4):479–482.

Stanga PE, Lim JI, Hamilton P. Indocyanine green angiography in chorioretinal diseases: indications and interpretation: an evidence-based update. *Ophthalmology*. 2003;110(1):15–21.

Wolf MD, Folk JC, Panknen CA, Goeken NE. HLA-B7 and HLA-DR2 antigens and acute posterior multifocal placoid pigment epitheliopathy. *Arch Ophthalmol*. 1990;108(5):698–700.

Serpiginous choroiditis

Serpiginous choroiditis, also known as *geographic* or *helicoid choroidopathy,* is an uncommon, chronic, progressive inflammatory condition affecting adult men and women equally in the second to seventh decades of life. Its etiology is unknown, but it is thought to represent an immune-mediated occlusive vasculitis, as suggested by the finding of lymphocytes in the choroidal infiltrates of patients with this disease as well as by the increased frequency of HLA-B7 and retinal S-antigen associations. An infectious etiology is suggested by the demonstration of elevated antibacterial antibodies, such as antistreptolysin O antibodies, and the association of viral meningitis in patients with this disease. A possible association with herpesviruses has also been postulated but not conclusively demonstrated. Serpiginous choroiditis has been reported to occur in patients with Crohn disease, sarcoidosis, and PAN, but no consistent systemic disease associations have been identified. Although serpiginous choroiditis may occur more frequently in individuals with positive PPD skin test results and tuberculous choroiditis may be indistinguishable from serpiginous choroiditis, treatment with antituberculous agents does not ameliorate the course of the latter.

Patients present with painless, unilateral, paracentral scotomata and decreased vision with minimal vitreous involvement and a quiet anterior chamber. Classically, funduscopy reveals asymmetric bilateral disease with characteristic gray-white lesions at the level of the RPE projecting in a pseudopodial or geographic manner from the optic nerve in the posterior fundus (Fig 6-33). Far less commonly, macular or peripheral lesions may present without peripapillary involvement. Disease activity is typically confined to the leading edge of the advancing lesion and may be associated with shallow subretinal fluid. Occasionally, vascular sheathing has been reported along with RPE detachment and neovascularization of the disc. Late findings include atrophy of the choriocapillaris, RPE, and retina, with extensive RPE hyperpigmentation and subretinal fibrosis, and CNV occurring at the border of the old scar in up to 25% of patients.

The disease course is marked by progressive centrifugal extension, with marked asymmetry between the 2 eyes. New lesions and recurrent attacks are typical, with up to 38% of patients reaching a final visual acuity of between 20/200 and counting fingers in the affected eye. FA shows blockage of the choroidal flush in the early phase of the study and staining of the active edge of the lesion in the later stage of the angiogram (Fig 6-34). In contrast, early hyperfluorescence with late leakage is indicative of the presence of CNV.

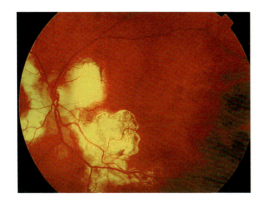

Figure 6-33 Serpiginous choroiditis. *(Courtesy of Albert T. Vitale, MD.)*

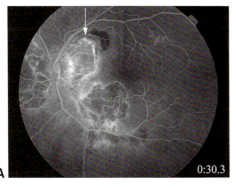 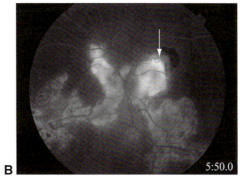

A 0:30.3 B 5:50.0

Figure 6-34 Fluorescein angiogram in a patient with serpiginous choroiditis. **A,** Early blocked fluorescence *(arrow)*. **B,** Late staining and leakage at the active margin of the lesion *(arrow)*. *(Courtesy of Albert T. Vitale, MD.)*

ICG angiography reveals hypofluorescence throughout all phases of the study for both acute and old lesions; it may reveal more extensive involvement than FA or clinical examination and may be useful in distinguishing active new serpiginous lesions, which are hypofluorescent, from CNV, which may appear as localized areas of hyperfluorescence during the middle to late phases of the study. FAF imaging may be an exquisitely sensitive modality in detecting damage to the RPE and in monitoring the clinical course of patients with serpiginous choroiditis, with characteristic hypoautofluorescence corresponding closely to areas of regressed disease activity and hyperfluorescence highlighting areas of active disease (Fig 6-35).

Given the small number of patients with serpiginous choroiditis, there is no consensus regarding the optimal treatment regimen or its efficacy. Systemic, periocular, and even intravitreal corticosteroids may be used in the treatment of active lesions, particularly

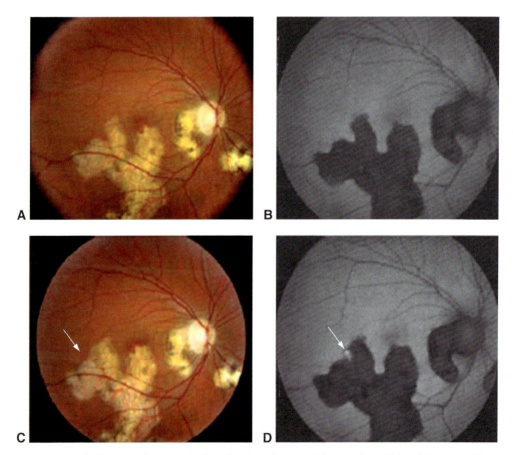

Figure 6-35 **A,** Fundus photograph showing inactive serpiginous choroiditis with peripapillary chorioretinal atrophy extending into the macula beneath fovea. **B,** Corresponding fundus autofluorescence (FAF) image showing hypoautofluorescence corresponding to the chorioretinal atrophy. **C,** Fundus photograph showing discoloration of retinal pigment epithelium during exacerbation of disease activity *(arrow).* **D,** Corresponding hyperautofluorescent signal on FAF *(arrow). (Reprinted with permission from Yeh S, Forooghian F, Wong W, et al. Fundus autofluorescence imaging of the white dot syndromes. Arch Ophthalmol. 2010;128(1):51.)*

those threatening the fovea. The addition of systemic IMT at the outset has been suggested as corticosteroids alone are ineffective and patients require prolonged anti-inflammatory therapy. Cyclosporine monotherapy has been effectively used in small numbers of patients, as has triple therapy with prednisone, cyclosporine, and azathioprine. Although this approach may induce rapid remission of acute disease, prolonged therapy is required and disease recurrence is frequently observed as these agents are tapered. Cytotoxic therapy with cyclophosphamide or chlorambucil has been shown to induce long drug-free remissions. The intravitreal fluocinolone acetonide implant may be used in patients intolerant of systemic therapy. Intravitreal anti-VEGF agents, focal laser photocoagulation, and photodynamic therapy are important therapeutic modalities for the treatment of associated CNV.

Akpek EK, Jabs DA, Tessler HH, Joondeph BC, Foster CS. Successful treatment of serpiginous choroiditis with alkylating agents. *Ophthalmology*. 2002;109(8):1506–1513.

Christmas NJ, Oh KT, Oh DM, Folk JC. Long-term follow-up of patients with serpiginous choroiditis. *Retina*. 2002;22(5):550–556.

Gupta V, Gupta A, Arora S, Bambery P, Dogra AR, Agarwal A. Presumed tubercular serpiginous like choroiditis: clinical presentations and management. *Ophthalmology*. 2003;110(9): 1744–1749.

Hooper PL, Kaplan HJ. Triple agent immunosuppression in serpiginous choroiditis. *Ophthalmology*. 1991;98(6):944–951.

Lim WK, Buggage RR, Nussenblatt RB. Serpiginous choroiditis. *Surv Ophthalmol*. 2005;50(3): 231–244.

Piccolino F, Grosso A, Savini E. Fundus autofluorescence in serpiginous choroiditis. *Graefes Arch Clin Exp Ophthalmol*. 2009;247(2):179–185.

Priya K, Madhavan HN, Reiser BJ, et al. Association of herpesviruses in the aqueous humor of patients with serpiginous choroiditis: a polymerase chain reaction-based study. *Ocul Immunol Inflamm*. 2002;10(4):253–261.

Multifocal choroiditis and panuveitis

Multifocal choroiditis and panuveitis (MCP), PIC, and the subretinal fibrosis and uveitis syndrome represent a subset of the white dot syndromes; some authorities regard them as discrete entities while others view them as a single disease with a variable severity continuum. MCP, although classified as a panuveitis, is presented here among the white dot syndromes, given its characteristic funduscopic appearance and the predominance of posterior pole involvement.

MCP is an idiopathic inflammatory disorder of unknown etiology affecting the choroid, retina, and vitreous that presents asymmetrically, most often in young myopic women with photopsias, enlargement of the physiologic blind spot, and decreased vision. In contrast to patients with OHS, those with MCP and CNV are less likely to have the HLA-DR2, HLA-B7, or HLA-DR1 haplotypes. The ophthalmoscopic hallmarks include the presence of punched-out white-yellow dots (50–200 μm) in a peripapillary, midperipheral, and anterior equatorial distribution (Fig 6-36). Varying degrees of anterior segment inflammation and an associated vitritis are uniformly present, effectively excluding a diagnosis of OHS or PIC. The lesions are smaller than those seen in birdshot retinochoroidopathy or APMPPE and evolve into atrophic scars with varying degrees of hyperpigmentation. They are larger and more pigmented than those seen in patients with PIC.

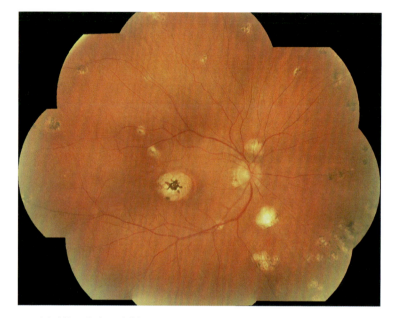

Figure 6-36 Multifocal choroiditis and panuveitis (MCP). *(Courtesy of Ramana S. Moorthy, MD.)*

New lesions may appear, and peripheral chorioretinal streaks and peripapillary pigment changes similar to those seen in OHS have been observed. Subretinal fibrosis with RPE clumping is much more common in MCP than OHS. Structural complications noted at presentation, including cataract (32%), CME (14%), ERM (5%), and CNV (28%), as well as those that develop over the chronic course of this disease, are frequent causes of visual impairment.

FA shows early hypofluorescence with late staining of acute active lesions, whereas atrophic lesions behave as transmission defects (early hyperfluorescence that fades in the late phases of the angiogram). Early hyperfluorescence and late leakage are observed in the presence of macular edema and CNV (Fig 6-37). As with birdshot retinochoroidopathy,

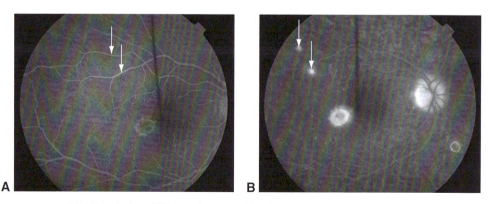

A   B

Figure 6-37 Multifocal choroiditis and panuveitis: fluorescein angiogram. **A,** Early blocked fluorescence *(arrows)*. **B,** Late staining of lesions *(arrows)*. *(Courtesy of Ramana S. Moorthy, MD.)*

ICG angiography shows multiple midphase hypofluorescent lesions compatible with active choroiditis that are more numerous than those seen on clinical examination or FA, frequently clustered around the optic nerve. This finding may correlate with the enlarged blind spot revealed by visual field testing. The hypofluorescent spots may fade with treatment and resolution of the intraocular inflammation. The most common finding on FAF imaging is punctate hypoautofluorescent spots (≥125 μm) corresponding to multiple areas of chorioretinal atrophy; however, smaller (<125 μm) spots numbering in the hundreds may be seen in the macular and peripapillary regions not visible on fundus photography, some of which will later develop into clinically evident chorioretinal scars (Fig 6-38). Active MCP lesions display hyperautofluorescence that disappears with minimal RPE disruption following anti-inflammatory treatment. FAF imaging suggests that patients with MCP have more widespread involvement of the RPE than indicated by other imaging modalities, and it therefore may be useful in monitoring response to treatment.

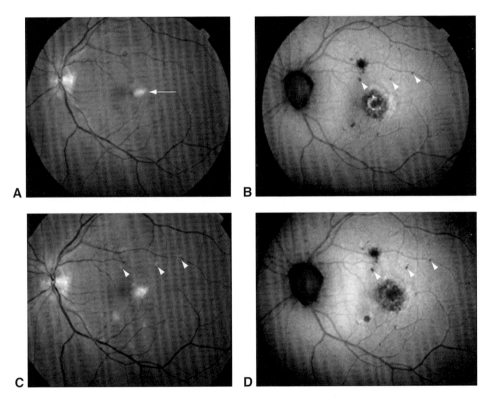

Figure 6-38 A 36-year-old woman with MCP. **A,** Area of choroidal neovascularization (CNV) *(arrow)* treated with photodynamic therapy 3 years earlier. **B,** Fundus autofluorescence (FAF) photograph shows multiple hypoautofluorescent spots *(arrowheads)* that did not correspond to ophthalmoscopically visible lesions. **C,** Three years later, fundus photograph shows multiple visible spots *(arrowheads)* corresponding to previously visualized hypoautofluorescent spots. **D,** FAF photograph taken at the same time as **C** shows corresponding hypoautofluorescent spots *(arrowheads)*, which are slightly enlarged from the previous study. *(Reprinted with permission from Haen S, Spaide RF. Fundus autofluorescence in multifocal choroiditis and panuveitis. Am J Ophthalmol. 2008;145(5):850.)*

A viral etiology involving herpes simplex and Epstein-Barr virus has been postulated, but neither has been conclusively demonstrated. Pathologic specimens obtained from eyes with MCP have shown variable findings, ranging from large numbers of B lymphocytes in the choroid to a predominance of T lymphocytes, suggesting that different immune mechanisms may produce a similar clinical picture and that an initial viral infection may trigger an autoimmune process. Recently, histologic examination of CNV samples excised from eyes with active MCP showed infiltration of B lymphocytes, suggesting that the presence of inflammatory cells in the anterior chamber and vitreous noted on clinical examination is a marker for active inflammatory CNV. No differences in histologic findings between eyes with MCP without intraocular inflammation and those with PIC were observed.

The diagnosis is one of exclusion as many other conditions, such as sarcoidosis, syphilis, and tuberculosis, may produce lesions similar in appearance to those of MCP. The visual prognosis is guarded, with permanent visual loss in at least 1 eye occurring in up to 75% of patients as a result of the complications associated with chronic, recurrent inflammation. In 1 study, the incidence rates of visual loss to 20/50 or worse and to 20/200 or worse were 19%/eye-year and 12%/eye-year in the affected eyes and 7%/person-year and 4%/person-year in the better-seeing eyes, respectively.

Systemic and periocular corticosteroids may be effective for the treatment of macular edema and have been shown to induce regression of CNV in some patients. Corticosteroid-sparing strategies with IMT are frequently required due to the chronic, recurrent nature of the inflammation; these have been successful in achieving not only inflammatory quiescence, but also an 83% reduction in the risk of posterior pole complications (CME, ERM, and CNV) and a 92% reduction in the risk of vision loss to 20/200 or worse in affected eyes. Intravitreal anti-VEGF agents and laser modalities (thermal photocoagulation and photodynamic therapy) are important adjuncts to the treatment of CNV. The intravitreal fluocinolone acetonide implant is a possible treatment option for patients unable to tolerate systemic therapy.

Dreyer RF, Gass JD. Multifocal choroiditis and panuveitis. A syndrome that mimics ocular histoplasmosis. *Arch Ophthalmol.* 1984(12);102:1776–1784.

Haen S, Spaide RF. Fundus autofluorescence in multifocal choroiditis and panuveitis. *Am J Ophthalmol.* 2008;145(5):847–853.

Michel SS, Ekong A, Baltatzis S, Foster CS. Multifocal choroiditis and panuveitis: immunomodulatory therapy. *Ophthalmology.* 2002;109(2):378–383.

Shimada H, Yuzawa M, Hirose T, Nakashizuka H, Hattori T, Kazato Y. Pathological findings of multifocal choroiditis with panuveitis and punctate inner choroidopathy. *Jpn J Ophthalmol.* 2008;52(4):282–288.

Thorne JE, Wittenberg S, Jabs DA, et al. Multifocal choroiditis with panuveitis. incidence of ocular complications and loss of visual acuity. *Ophthalmology.* 2006;113(12):2310–2315.

Yeh S, Forooghian F, Wong W, et al. Fundus autofluorescence imaging of the white dot syndromes. *Arch Ophthalmol.* 2010;128(1):46–56.

Punctate inner choroiditis

PIC is an idiopathic inflammatory disorder that, like MCP, occurs in otherwise healthy myopic white women, but it presents at a younger median age (29 vs 45 years, respectively). Patients with PIC complain of metamorphopsia, paracentral scotomata, photopsias, and asymmetric loss of central acuity. In contrast to the lesions of MCP, those of PIC (100–200 µm) rarely extend to the midperiphery and are never associated with vitritis (Fig 6-39). They progress to atrophic scars, typically leaving a halo of pigmentation, and are deeper and more punched out than those of MCP. New lesions and CME are rarely seen, whereas serous retinal detachment may be found over confluent PIC lesions. With the exception of CNV, patients with PIC have few structural complications (cataract, CME, or ERM) at presentation in comparison to those with MCP, undoubtedly related to the presence of chronic intraocular inflammation in the latter. CNV, a common vision-threatening complication in both entities, may be more frequent at presentation in patients with PIC (79%) than MCP (28%), but those with MCP are more likely to have bilateral visual impairment of 20/50 or worse (Fig 6-40).

In contrast to MCP, FA in patients with PIC shows early hyperfluorescence with late staining of the lesions (Figs 6-41, 6-42). ICG angiography displays midphase hypofluorescence throughout the posterior pole in a peripapillary distribution that corresponds to the lesions seen on FA and on clinical examination, which may be useful in delineating disease extent and monitoring its activity (Fig 6-43).

The visual prognosis is favorable in eyes without CNV involving the foveal center. Treatment options include observation or periocular and/or systemic corticosteroids for

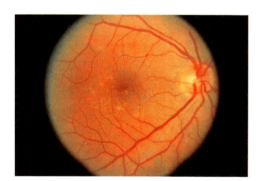

Figure 6-39 Punctate inner choroiditis (PIC). *(Courtesy of E. Mitchel Opremcak, MD.)*

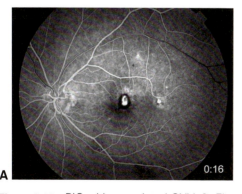

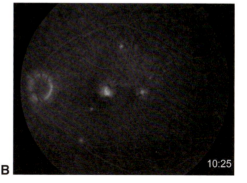

A   0:16   B   10:25

Figure 6-40 PIC with associated CNV. **A,** Fluorescein angiogram showing early hyperfluorescence of the PIC lesions, with lacey hyperfluorescence of CNV. **B,** Late hyperfluorescence and staining of PIC lesions and leakage due to CNV. *(Courtesy of Albert T. Vitale, MD.)*

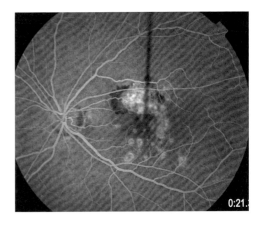

Figure 6-41 Early hyperfluorescence of PIC lesions and CNV. *(Courtesy of Albert T. Vitale, MD.)*

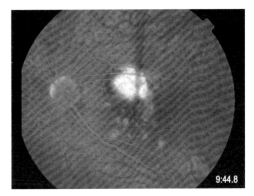

Figure 6-42 Late staining of PIC lesions with leakage from CNV. *(Courtesy of Albert T. Vitale, MD.)*

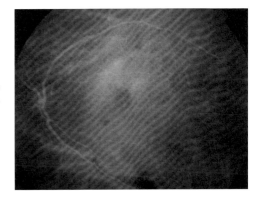

Figure 6-43 PIC: indocyanine green angiogram showing multiple midphase hypofluorescent spots. *(Courtesy of Albert T. Vitale, MD.)*

eyes presenting with poor initial visual acuity or multiple acute PIC lesions proximate to the fovea. Intravitreal anti-VEGF agents, laser photocoagulation, photodynamic therapy with or without intravitreal corticosteroids, and submacular surgery may be considered in eyes with CNV, as previously described.

Brown J Jr, Folk JC, Reddy CV, Kimura AE. Visual prognosis of multifocal choroiditis, punctate inner choroidopathy, and the diffuse subretinal fibrosis syndrome. *Ophthalmology.* 1996;103(2):1100–1105.

Kedhar SR, Thorne JE, Wittenberg S, Dunn JP, Jabs DA. Multifocal choroiditis with panuveitis and punctate inner choroidopathy: comparison of clinical characteristics at presentation. *Retina*. 2007;27(9):1174–1179.

Spaide RF, Freund KB, Slakter J, Sorenson J, Yannuzzi LA, Fisher Y. Treatment of subfoveal choroidal neovascularization associated with multifocal choroiditis and panuveitis with photodynamic therapy. *Retina*. 2002;22(5):545–549.

Subretinal fibrosis and uveitis syndrome

Subretinal fibrosis and uveitis syndrome is an extremely uncommon panuveitis of unknown etiology affecting otherwise healthy myopic women between the ages of 14 and 34 years. Significant anterior segment inflammation and mild to moderate vitritis are typically present bilaterally, with white-yellow lesions (50–500 μm) located in the posterior pole to midperiphery at the level of the RPE. These lesions may fade without RPE alterations, become atrophic, or enlarge and coalesce into large, white, stellate zones of subretinal fibrosis (Figs 6-44, 6-45). Serous neurosensory retinal detachment, CME, and CNV may also be observed.

Immune mechanisms have been implicated in the pathogenesis of subretinal fibrosis and uveitis syndrome, as suggested by the presence of local antibodies directed against the RPE, granulomatous infiltration of the choroid, enhanced expression of the Fas-Fas ligand in the retina, choroidal scars, and choroidal granulomas. A predominance of B lymphocytes, plasma cells, and subretinal fibrotic tissue with islands of RPE and Müller cells is observed histologically. The disease course is marked by chronic recurrent inflammation and the visual prognosis is guarded. Treatment with systemic corticosteroids and IMT is of equivocal efficacy.

FA shows multiple areas of blocked choroidal fluorescence and hyperfluorescence in the early stages of the study; in the late phase, staining of the lesions without leakage is observed. Again, the differential diagnosis includes ocular inflammatory conditions producing panuveitis and those in the differential diagnosis of the white dot syndromes, including sarcoidosis, OHS, APMPPE, syphilis, tuberculosis, birdshot retinochoroidopathy, pathologic myopia, sympathetic ophthalmia, and toxoplasmosis.

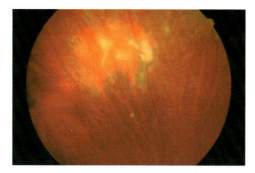

Figure 6-44 Subretinal fibrosis and uveitis syndrome: fundus photograph showing multifocal white subretinal lesions. *(Courtesy of E. Mitchel Opremcak, MD.)*

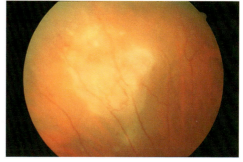

Figure 6-45 Subretinal fibrosis and uveitis syndrome: fundus photograph from the same patient as in Figure 6-44, showing progressive subretinal fibrosis. *(Courtesy of E. Mitchel Opremcak, MD.)*

Brown J Jr, Folk JC. Current controversies in the white dot syndromes. Multifocal choroiditis, punctate inner choroidopathy, and the diffuse subretinal fibrosis syndrome. *Ocul Immunol Inflamm.* 1998;6(6):125–127.

Chan CC, Matteson DM, Li Q, Whitcup SM, Nussenblatt RB. Apoptosis in patients with posterior uveitis. *Arch Ophthalmol.* 1997;115(12):1559–1567.

Kim MK, Chan CC, Belfort R Jr, et al. Histopathologic and immunohistopathologic features of subretinal fibrosis and uveitis syndrome. *Am J Ophthalmol.* 1987;104(1):15–23.

Multiple evanescent white dot syndrome

MEWDS is an uncommon idiopathic inflammatory condition of the retina that typically affects otherwise healthy, young, moderately myopic females in the second to fourth decades of life. Patients present with acute unilateral (80%) blurred or decreased vision, photopsias, and central or paracentral scotomata corresponding to an enlarged physiologic blind spot. An antecedent viral prodrome occurs in approximately one-third of cases. Funduscopy during the acute phase of the disease reveals multiple, discrete, white to orange spots (100–200 µm) at the level of the RPE or deep retina, typically in a perifoveal location (Fig 6-46). These spots are transitory and are frequently missed; they leave instead a granular macular pigmentary change, a pathognomonic finding. Bilateral cases have been reported and a small minority of patients with chronic MEWDS may develop choroidal scarring. There may be variable vitreous inflammation, mild blurring of the optic disc, and, in rare instances, isolated vascular sheathing.

FA reveals characteristic punctate hyperfluorescent lesions in a wreathlike configuration surrounding the fovea that stain late (Fig 6-47). ICG angiography shows multiple hypofluorescent lesions that are more numerous than those seen on clinical examination or FA and that typically fade with resolution of the disease (Fig 6-48). Visual field abnormalities are variable and include generalized depression, paracentral or peripheral scotomata, and enlargement of the blind spot. The ERG reveals diminished a-wave and early receptor potential (ERP) amplitudes, both of which are reversible. The multifocal ERG (mfERG) and electro-oculogram (EOG) localize the disease process to the RPE–photoreceptor complex rather than to the choroid. The recent demonstration of abnormal photoreceptor inner/outer segment junction reflectivity on spectral-domain optical coherence tomography (SD-OCT) and its correspondence with hypofluorescent spots visualized on ICG angiography and changes in microperimetry sensitivity further supports the localization of

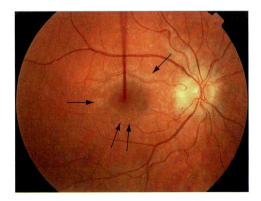

Figure 6-46 Multiple evanescent white dot syndrome (MEWDS). Multiple, discrete, punctate yellowish perifoveal dots *(arrows)*. *(Courtesy of Albert T. Vitale, MD.)*

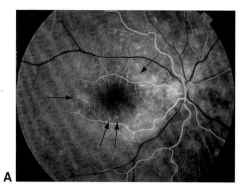
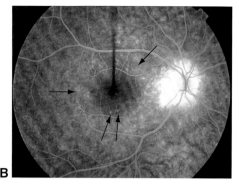

A **B**

Figure 6-47 MEWDS: fluorescein angiogram. **A,** Early phase with multiple punctate hyper-fluorescent lesions surrounding the fovea *(arrows)*. **B,** The lesions stain late in a wreathlike configuration *(arrows)*. *(Courtesy of Albert T. Vitale, MD.)*

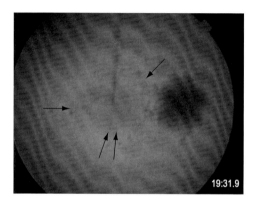

Figure 6-48 MEWDS: indocyanine green an-giogram of the same patient as in Figure 6-47, showing multiple, midphase, hypofluores-cent spots, more numerous than appreciated on fluorescein angiography or clinical exami-nation *(arrows)*. *(Courtesy of Albert T. Vitale, MD.)*

the disease process to the RPE–photoreceptor complex, as these abnormalities completely resolve during the course of the disease.

The prognosis is excellent with visual recovery within 2–10 weeks without treatment; however, residual symptoms including photopsias and enlargement of the blind spot may persist for months. Recurrences are uncommon (10%–15% of patients) and have a simi-larly good prognosis.

MEWDS has been reported in association with MCP, acute zonal occult outer reti-nopathy, and acute macular neuroretinopathy, suggesting a common genetic susceptibil-ity and/or pathogenetic factor. The latter is a rare condition, occurring among otherwise healthy young women, and is characterized by the acute onset of visual impairment and multifocal scotomata that correspond precisely to reddish, flat, wedge-shaped lesions in the macula. Although most patients experience a minimal decrease in visual acuity, symp-toms frequently persist despite resolution of the fundus lesions. No treatment is required, given the condition's favorable natural history.

Fine HF, Spaide RF, Ryan EH Jr, Matsumoto Y, Yannuzzi LA. Acute zonal occult outer reti-nopathy in patients with multiple evanescent white dot syndrome. *Arch Ophthalmol.* 2009;127(1):66–70.

Hangai M, Fujimoto M, Yoshimura N. Features and function of multiple evanescent white dot syndrome. *Arch Ophthalmol.* 2009; 127(10):1307–1313.

Jampol LM, Sieving PA, Pugh D, Fishman GA, Gilbert H. Multiple evanescent white dot syndrome. I. Clinical findings. *Arch Ophthalmol.* 1984;102(5):671–674.

Schaal S, Schiff WM, Kaplan HJ, Tezel TH. Simultaneous appearance of multiple evanescent white dot syndrome and multifocal choroiditis indicate a common causal relationship. *Ocul Immunol Inflamm.* 2009;17(5):325–327.

Sieving PA, Fishman GA, Jampol LM, Pugh D. Multiple evanescent white dot syndrome. II. Electrophysiology of the photoreceptors during retinal pigment epithelial disease. *Arch Ophthalmol.* 1984;102(5):675–679.

Acute retinal pigment epitheliitis

Acute retinal pigment epitheliitis, or Krill disease, is a benign self-limited inflammatory disorder of the RPE of unknown etiology. It typically presents in otherwise healthy young adults between the ages of 16 and 40 years with acute unilateral visual loss, central metamorphopsia, and scotomata. Ophthalmoscopic findings include clusters of small, discrete, hyperpigmented lesions, typically with a yellow halo in the posterior pole unassociated with vitritis or other abnormalities noted on funduscopy (Fig 6-49). FA shows early hyperfluorescence of the pinpoint dots with a surrounding halo of hyperfluorescence and late staining. Visual field testing shows central scotomata. Normal results on ERG with abnormal results on EOG serve to localize the disease process to the RPE. No treatment is required, as the lesions resolve without sequelae with excellent visual acuity over 6–12 weeks.

Deutman AF. Acute retinal pigment epitheliitis. *Am J Ophthalmol.* 1974;78(4):571–578.

Luttrull JK, Chittum EM. Acute retinal pigment epitheliitis. *Am J Ophthalmol.* 1995;120(3): 389–391.

Acute zonal occult outer retinopathy

Acute zonal occult outer retinopathy (AZOOR) is typified by acute loss of 1 or more zones of outer retinal function associated with photopsia, minimal funduscopic changes, and abnormal ERG findings; unilateral disease is more common at first, but 1 or both eyes

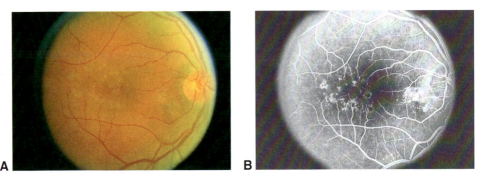

Figure 6-49 **A,** Acute retinal pigment epitheliitis. **B,** Fluorescein angiogram in patient with acute retinal pigment epitheliitis showing honeycomb lesions at the level of the RPE. *(Courtesy of E. Mitchel Opremcak, MD.)*

may be affected. Patients are typically young, myopic women who present with acute unilateral visual disturbances not infrequently associated with a mild vitritis (50%), apparently normal results on funduscopic examination, and visual acuity in the 20/40 range. Electrophysiological studies may demonstrate a consistent pattern of dysfunction, not only at the photoreceptor–RPE complex but also at the inner retinal level. Essentially, this consists of a delayed 30-Hz–flicker ERG and a reduction in the EOG light rise, which when present with classic symptomatology may be helpful diagnostically, obviating extensive neurologic evaluation. Visual field defects include enlargement of the blind spot and paracentral inferior, superior, and temporal defects with no corresponding retinal defect. Results of mfERG show decreased response from the blind spots and other visual field defects with corresponding loss or irregularity of the inner/outer segment line on OCT, suggesting that photoreceptor outer segment dysfunction and/or degeneration are the primary lesions in AZOOR. During the early stages of the disease, FA findings may be entirely normal, showing only a prolonged retinal circulation time. However, with disease progression, diffuse areas of hyperfluorescence and hypofluorescence and window defects corresponding to zones of RPE derangement become common. FAF imaging may be particularly useful in observing patients with AZOOR as it reveals conspicuous areas of central hypoautofluorescence corresponding to RPE and choriocapillary atrophy; peripheral hyperautofluorescence is seen at the border of the expanding lesion due to the presence of lipofuscin-laden cells that presage RPE cell death (Fig 6-50).

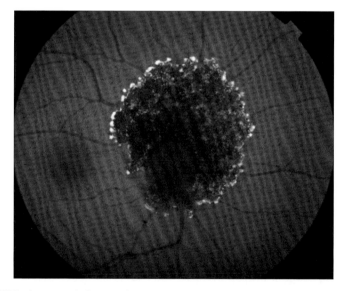

Figure 6-50 FAF photograph in a patient with acute zonal occult outer retinopathy (AZOOR) showing peripapillary hypoautofluorescence corresponding to atrophy of the RPE–choriocapillaris with intense hyperautofluorescence at the outer border of the lesion corresponding to the yellowish drusen-like material thought to represent the accumulation of large amounts of lipofuscin. *(Reprinted with permission from Spaide RF. Collateral damage in acute zonal occult outer retinopathy. Am J Ophthalmol. 2004;138(5):889.)*

With extended follow-up, the majority of patients develop bilateral disease, with recurrences in approximately one-third. Similarly, the funduscopic appearance varies with the stage of the disease, ranging from initial subtle RPE changes with depigmentation in areas of visual loss to vessel attenuation, late pigment migration, and focal perivenous sheathing. Visual field abnormalities typically stabilize in approximately three-quarters of patients and partially improve in about 25%. Visual acuity remains in the 20/40 range in 68% of patients; however, legal blindness has been reported in as many as 18% with long-term follow-up.

Cancer-associated retinopathy and retinitis pigmentosa should be considered in the differential diagnosis of AZOOR. It is unclear whether treatment with systemic corticosteroids or IMT alters the disease course or visual outcome.

The considerable similarities between AZOOR and other white dot syndromes—namely, MEWDS, MCP, OHS, PIC, acute macular neuroretinopathy, and acute idiopathic blind spot enlargement syndrome—have led some investigators to group these entities together in the so-called *AZOOR complex* of diseases. Although an infectious etiology has been postulated, systemic autoimmune disease has been observed in 28% of patients, supporting the notion that these diseases are of an inflammatory etiology and arise in patients with a common non–disease-specific genetic background, possibly triggered by some exogenous agent.

Francis PJ, Marinescu A, Fitzke FW, Bird AC, Holder GE. Acute zonal occult outer retinopathy: towards a set of diagnostic criteria. *Br J Ophthalmol.* 2005;89(1):70–73.

Gass JD, Agarwal A, Scott IU. Acute zonal occult outer retinopathy: a long-term follow-up study. *Am J Ophthalmol.* 2002;134(3):329–339.

Li D, Kishi S. Loss of photoreceptor outer segment in acute zonal occult outer retinopathy. *Arch Ophthalmol.* 2007;125(9):1194–1200.

Spaide RF. Collateral damage in acute zonal occult outer retinopathy. *Am J Ophthalmol.* 2004;138(5):887–889.

Panuveitis

Although intraocular inflammation can originate as an iritis, retinitis, or choroiditis, the designation "panuveitis" (or "diffuse uveitis") by definition requires involvement of all anatomical compartments of the eye—namely, the anterior chamber, vitreous, and retina or choroid—with no single predominant site of inflammation. As with posterior uveitis, structural complications such as macular edema, retinal or choroidal neovascularization, and vasculitis, although not infrequent accompaniments, are not considered essential in the anatomical classification of panuveitis. Generally, panuveitis is bilateral, although 1 eye may affected be first and the severity is not necessarily symmetric. The discussion of panuveitis in this chapter is limited to the noninfectious entities.

Sarcoidosis

Sarcoidosis is a multisystem granulomatous disorder of unknown etiology with protean systemic and ocular manifestations. Although intrathoracic manifestations are most common (90%), other organs frequently involved include the lymph nodes, skin, eyes, CNS, bones and joints, liver, and heart. Ocular involvement may be seen in up to 50% of patients with systemic disease, with uveitis being the most frequent manifestation. In most large series, sarcoidosis accounts for up to 10% of all cases of uveitis.

Sarcoidosis has a worldwide distribution, affecting all ethnic groups, with the highest prevalence seen in the northern European countries (40 cases per 100,000 people). In the United States the disease is up to 20 times more prevalent among African Americans than whites. Both sexes are affected, albeit with a slight female predominance; onset usually occurs usually between the ages of 20 and 50 years. Pediatric involvement is uncommon, and the clinical course is atypical. Children with early-onset sarcoidosis (younger than 5 years) are less likely than adults to manifest pulmonary disease and far more likely to have cutaneous and articular involvement; the disease course in older children (8–15 years) approximates that in adults.

The recently completed ACCESS (A Case Control Etiologic Study of Sarcoidosis) project suggests that specific occupations (in agricultural and pesticide-using industries) and workplace exposures (mold or mildew, musty odors, and insecticides) associated with microbe-rich environments may modestly increase the risk of developing sarcoidosis; however, no dominant factor could be identified. Similarly, molecular studies of tissue specimens of patients with sarcoidosis provide evidence that suggests that mycobacterial and, less convincingly, propionibacterial organisms may be important etiologic factors. A genetic predisposition for the development of the disease is suggested by the increased expression of class I and II HLA molecules, especially HLA-DRB1, in patients with biopsy-confirmed sarcoidosis. Familial clustering is observed, with siblings of patients having a fivefold increased risk of developing the disease. Patients with systemic sarcoidosis characteristically exhibit peripheral anergy on skin testing due to depression in delayed-type hypersensitivity, but at the target organ site, an active macrophage- and helper T lymphocyte (CD4$^+$)–driven immunologic response is present, leading to granuloma formation.

The basic pathologic lesion of sarcoidosis is a noncaseating granuloma without histologic evidence of infection (Fig 6-51). The epithelioid cell is a polyhedral mononuclear histiocyte that is derived from monocytes of the peripheral blood or macrophages of the tissue. The tubercle of sarcoidosis is composed of the following:

- epithelioid cells
- multinucleate giant cells of the Langhans type, with nuclei at the periphery of the cell arranged in an arc or incomplete circle
- a thin rim of lymphocytes

Central areas of the tubercle seldom undergo fibrinoid degeneration or, in skin lesions (lupus pernio), micronecrosis. Various types of inclusion bodies may occur in the cytoplasm of giant cells, including

- *Schaumann, or lamellar bodies:* ovoid, basophilic, calcific bodies measuring up to 100 μm in diameter and also containing iron
- *asteroid bodies:* star-shaped acidophilic bodies measuring up to 25 μm in diameter

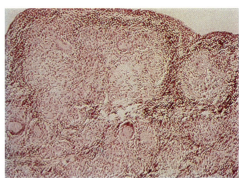

Figure 6-51 Sarcoidosis: histologic view of conjunctival biopsy. Note the giant cells and granulomatous inflammation.

Systemic sarcoidosis may present acutely, frequently with associated iridocyclitis in young patients, and spontaneously remit within 2 years of onset. One form of acute sarcoidosis is called *Löfgren syndrome* and consists of erythema nodosum, febrile arthropathy, bilateral hilar adenopathy, and acute iritis and is quite responsive to systemic corticosteroids; it has a good long-term prognosis. Another, termed *Heerfordt syndrome* (uveoparotid fever), is characterized by uveitis, parotitis, fever, and facial nerve palsy. Chronic sarcoidosis presents insidiously and is characterized by persistent disease of more than 2 years' duration, frequently with interpulmonary involvement and chronic uveitis. Extended corticosteroid therapy may be required. Pulmonary disease is the major cause of morbidity; overall mortality from sarcoidosis approaches 5% but may be as high as 10% with neurosarcoidosis.

Sarcoidosis can affect any ocular tissue, including the orbit and adnexa. Cutaneous involvement is frequent, and orbital and eyelid granulomas are common (Fig 6-52). Palpebral and bulbar conjunctival nodules may also be observed and provide a readily accessible site for tissue biopsy (Fig 6-53). Lacrimal gland infiltration may cause keratoconjunctivitis sicca.

Anterior uveitis, presenting either acutely or as a chronic granulomatous iridocyclitis, is the most common ocular lesion, occurring in approximately two-thirds of patients with ocular sarcoidosis. Symptoms of uveal involvement are variable and frequently include

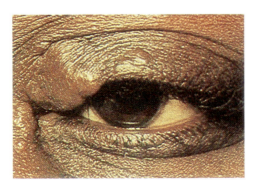

Figure 6-52 Sarcoidosis: skin lesions.

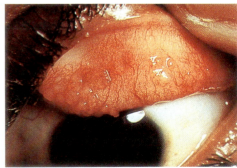

Figure 6-53 Sarcoidosis: conjunctival nodules.

mild to moderate blurring of vision and aching around the eyes. Typical biomicroscopic findings include

- mutton-fat KPs (Fig 6-54), including those involving the anterior chamber angle
- Koeppe and Busacca iris nodules (Fig 6-55)
- white clumps of cells ("snowballs") in the inferior anterior vitreous

Although the cornea is infrequently involved, nummular corneal infiltrates and inferior corneal endothelial opacification may be seen; band keratopathy may develop due to either chronic uveitis or hypercalcemia. Large iris granulomas, together with extensive posterior synechiae, may lead to iris bombé and angle-closure glaucoma. Peripheral anterior synechiae may also be extensive, encompassing the entire angle for 360° in advanced cases. Secondary glaucoma, together with sarcoid uveitis, may be severe and portends a poor prognosis with associated severe visual loss.

Posterior segment lesions occur in up to 20% of patients with ocular sarcoidosis. Vitreous infiltration is common and may be diffuse or appear more classically as yellowish white aggregates (snowballs), or linearly as a "string of pearls." Nodular granulomas measuring ¼ to 1 disc diameter may be observed on the optic nerve, in both the retina and the choroid, either posteriorly or peripherally (Fig 6-56). Perivascular sheathing is also common, appearing most often as either a linear or segmental periphlebitis (Fig 6-57). Irregular nodular granulomas along venules have been termed *candle-wax drippings,* or *taches de bougie.* Occlusive retinal vascular disease, especially branch retinal vein occlusion and, less commonly, central retinal vein occlusion, together with peripheral retinal capillary nonperfusion, may lead to retinal neovascularization and vitreous hemorrhage. CME is frequently present, and optic disc edema without granulomatous invasion of the optic nerve may be observed in patients with papilledema and neurosarcoidosis.

Diagnosis and treatment

Given its heterogeneous presentation, sarcoidosis should be considered in the differential diagnosis of any patient presenting with intraocular inflammation. Early-onset sarcoidosis in children (5 years of age or younger) must be differentiated from JIA-associated

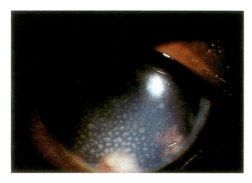

Figure 6-54 Sarcoidosis with keratic precipitates and iridocyclitis.

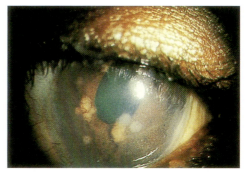

Figure 6-55 Sarcoidosis: iris nodules.

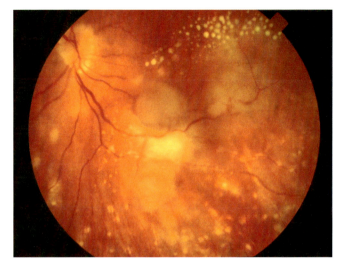

Figure 6-56 Multiple retinal and choroidal nodular granulomas, perivasculitis, and vitritis in a patient with sarcoidosis-associated posterior segment involvement. *(Courtesy of Albert T. Vitale, MD.)*

Figure 6-57 Sarcoidosis: retinal vascular sheathing.

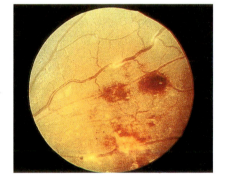

iridocyclitis and from familial juvenile systemic granulomatosis (Blau syndrome), given the overlap of ocular and articular involvement. Familial juvenile systemic granulomatosis, an autosomal dominantly inherited syndrome with 100% phenotypic correspondence to mutations in the *NOD2* gene (also known as *CARD15*), may produce ocular disease that is virtually identical to sarcoidosis and should be suspected in patients with a family history of granulomatous disease.

A chest radiograph is the single best screening test for the diagnosis of sarcoidosis, because it is reveals abnormalities in approximately 90% of patients with this disease. Thin-cut, spiral CT imaging is a more sensitive imaging modality and may be particularly valuable in patients who have normal chest radiograph results but in whom a high clinical index of suspicion remains. In such cases, parenchymal, mediastinal, and hilar structures with distinctive CT patterns highly suggestive for sarcoidosis may lead to the diagnosis. Although the serum ACE and lysozyme levels may be abnormally elevated, neither is diagnostic or specific; rather, they are reflective of total-body granuloma content and, as such, may be useful in tracking patients with active disease. Similarly, positive gallium scanning results in combination with an elevated ACE level appear to be highly specific for sarcoidosis in patients with active disease in whom clinical suspicion is high; however, routine screening of patients with uveitis with both modalities may be inappropriate given the low positive predictive value in this clinical setting. Ultimately, the diagnosis of sarcoidosis is made histologically, from tissue obtained from the lungs, mediastinal lymph nodes, skin, peripheral lymph nodes, liver, conjunctiva, minor salivary glands, or lacrimal glands. Readily accessible and clinically evident lesions (such as those on the skin, palpable lymph nodes, and nodules on the conjunctiva) should be sought for biopsy, because they are associated with a high yield and low morbidity and may obviate the need for more invasive transbronchial biopsy. Diagnostic criteria for ocular sarcoidosis were recently proposed by an international workshop of ophthalmologists but have yet to be validated. These consist of diagnostic grades ranging from "definitive" (based on tissue biopsy), to "presumed" (based on typical ocular findings with bilateral hilar adenopathy), to "probable" or "possible" disease (with supporting ancillary evidence).

Topical, periocular, and systemic corticosteroids are the mainstays of therapy for ocular sarcoidosis. Cycloplegia is useful for comfort and for prevention of synechiae. Vision-threatening posterior segment lesions generally require, and are responsive to, systemic corticosteroids (prednisone, 40–80 mg/day). Intravitreal corticosteroids, including the fluocinolone acetonide implant, are potential treatment options for patients intolerant of systemic therapy, but they leave the systemic disease untreated. Systemic IMT with methotrexate, azathioprine, mycophenolate mofetil, or cyclosporine may be required in patients who either are intolerant of or fail to respond to corticosteroids. Recently, the TNF-α inhibitor infliximab was shown to be effective in the treatment of sarcoidosis-associated uveitis. Prognostic factors associated with visual loss in patients with ocular sarcoidosis include the presence of chronic posterior uveitis, glaucoma, a delay in presentation to a uveitis specialist of more than 1 year, and the presence of intermediate or posterior uveitis. The likelihood of significant visual improvement is substantially increased with systemic therapy.

Chen ES, Moller DR. Etiology of sarcoidosis. *Clin Chest Med.* 2008;29(3):365–377.

Dana MR, Merayo-Lloves J, Schaumberg DA, Foster CS. Prognosticators for visual outcome in sarcoid uveitis. *Ophthalmology.* 1996;103(11):1846–1853.

Dev S, McCallum RM, Jaffe GJ. Methotrexate treatment for sarcoid-associated panuveitis. *Ophthalmology.* 1999;106(1):111–118.

Herbort CP, Rao NA, Mochizuki M, and the members of the Scientific Committee of the First International Workshop on Ocular Sarcoidosis. International criteria for the diagnosis of ocular sarcoidosis: results of the first International Workshop on Ocular Sarcoidosis (IWOS). *Ocul Immunol Inflamm.* 2009;17(3):160–169.

Kaiser PK, Lowder CY, Sullivan P, et al. Chest computerized tomography in the evaluation of uveitis in elderly women. *Am J Ophthalmol.* 2002;133(4):499–505.

Power WJ, Neves RA, Rodriguez A, Pedroza-Seres M, Foster CS. The value of combined serum angiotensin-converting enzyme and gallium scan in diagnosing ocular sarcoidosis. *Ophthalmology.* 1995;102(2):2007–2011.

Sympathetic Ophthalmia

Sympathetic ophthalmia (SO) is a rare, bilateral, diffuse granulomatous, nonnecrotizing panuveitis that may develop after either surgical or accidental trauma to 1 eye (the exciting eye), followed by a latent period and the appearance of uveitis in the uninjured fellow eye (the sympathizing eye). SO accounts for up to 2% of all uveitis cases. Although the precise incidence of SO is difficult to ascertain due to its rarity, significant improvements in the management of ocular trauma, together with the more widespread use of IMT, have led to an overall decrease. Earlier estimates of the incidence of SO ranged from up to 0.5% in eyes with nonsurgical trauma and 10/100,000 cases after intraocular surgery. Although the most recent minimum incidence estimate is low (0.03/100,000), SO remains a disease with a persistent and potentially devastating presence.

Until recently, accidental penetrating ocular trauma was the classic, most common precipitating event for SO. Ocular surgery—particularly vitreoretinal surgery—has now emerged as the main risk for the development of SO. In the early 1980s, the prevalence of SO in patients who had undergone pars plana vitrectomy was reported to be 0.01%, increasing to 0.06% when the procedure was performed in the context of other penetrating ocular injuries. More recent studies suggest that the risk of developing SO following pars plana vitrectomy is more than twice this figure and may be significantly greater than the risk of infectious endophthalmitis after vitrectomy. Improved access to emergency surgical care following penetrating ocular trauma and improved microsurgical technique have undoubtedly influenced this etiologic shift from penetrating injury to surgical trauma. Similarly, the demographic of SO has changed from earlier reports, in which there was higher prevalence among men, children, and the elderly (due to their presumed increased risk of accidental trauma), to more recent studies, which show no sex predominance and a lower risk in children (due in part to a reduced incidence of pediatric ocular injuries) and an increased risk in the elderly (likely due to an increased frequency of ocular surgery and retinal detachment in this population). Finally, although SO has been traditionally reported to develop in 80% of patients within 3 months of injury and in 90% within 1 year, the time interval may be longer than previously assumed; in recent series, only one-third of patients developed SO within 3 months and fewer than one-half did so within 1 year of injury.

Patients with SO typically present with asymmetric bilateral panuveitis, with more severe inflammation in the exciting eye than in the sympathizing eye, at least initially. Signs and symptoms in the sympathizing eye vary in their severity and onset, ranging from minimal problems in near vision, mild photophobia, and slight redness to severe granulomatous anterior uveitis. Both eyes may show mutton-fat KPs, thickening of the iris from lymphocytic infiltration, posterior synechiae formation, and elevated IOP due either to trabeculitis or to hypotony as a result of ciliary body shutdown (Fig 6-58).

Posterior segment findings include moderate to severe vitritis with characteristic yellowish white, midequatorial choroidal lesions (so-called *Dalen-Fuchs nodules*) that may become confluent. Peripapillary choroidal lesions and exudative retinal detachment may also develop (Fig 6-59). Structural complications of SO include cataract, chronic CME, peripapillary and macular CNV, and optic atrophy. In a recent study, complications in the

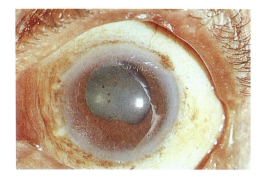

Figure 6-58 Sympathetic ophthalmia. Photo-graph shows sympathizing eye with synechiae.

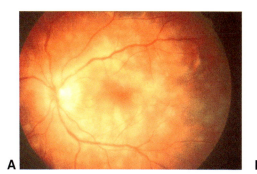

A

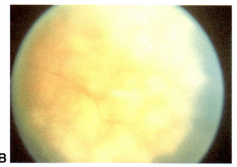

B

Figure 6-59 Sympathetic ophthalmia. **A,** Peripapillary and multifocal choroiditis (yellowish sub-retinal inflammatory infiltrates) with exudative retinal detachment in the macula. **B,** Peripheral multifocal choroiditis and hazy view due to vitritis. *(Courtesy of Ramana S. Moorthy, MD.)*

sympathizing eye at presentation were frequent (up to 47%), with cataract and optic nerve abnormalities most often associated with decreased vision and the further development of new complications, which occurred at a rate of 40% per person-year. Furthermore, traumatic etiology, the presence of active intraocular inflammation, and exudative retinal detachment correlated with poorer vision in the sympathizing eye. Extraocular findings similar to those observed with VKH syndrome, including cerebral spinal fluid pleocytosis, sensory neural hearing disturbance, alopecia, poliosis, and vitiligo, may be noted although they are uncommon.

During the acute stage of the disease, FA reveals multiple hyperfluorescent sites of leakage at the level of the RPE during the venous phase, which persists into the late stage of the study (Fig 6-60). Pooling of dye is observed beneath areas of exudative neurosensory retinal detachment. Less-common fluorescein angiographic patterns are determined by the status of the overlying RPE. Dalen-Fuchs nodules appear hypofluorescent early in the study, simulating the pattern seen in APMPPE, or hyperfluorescent with late staining. ICG angiography reveals numerous hypofluorescent foci, which are best visualized during the intermediate phase of the angiogram; some of these foci may become isofluorescent in the late stage of the study (Fig 6-61). B-scan ultrasonography frequently reveals choroidal thickening.

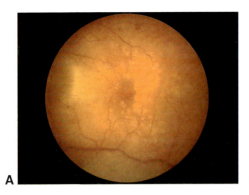
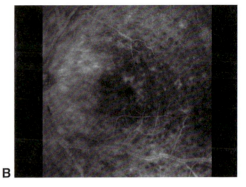

A   B

Figure 6-60 Sympathetic ophthalmia. **A,** Fundus photograph showing a multifocal choroiditis. **B,** Corresponding fluorescein angiogram disclosing multiple areas of alternating hyperfluorescence and blocked fluorescence at the level of the RPE. *(Courtesy of Albert T. Vitale, MD.)*

Figure 6-61 Sympathetic ophthalmia: indocyanine green angiogram of the same patient as in Figure 6-60. Multiple midphase hypofluorescent foci corresponding to, and more numerous than, the choroidal lesions seen on clinical examination or fluorescein angiography.

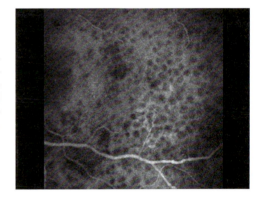

The histologic features of SO are similar for both the exciting and sympathizing eye (Figs 6-62, 6-63):

- diffuse, granulomatous, nonnecrotizing infiltration of the choroid with a predominance of lymphocytes, some epithelioid cells, few giant cells and plasma cells, and eosinophils in the inner choroid, particularly in heavily pigmented persons
- nodular clusters of epithelioid cells containing pigment, located between the RPE and the Bruch membrane, corresponding to the Dalen-Fuchs nodules; although present in one-third of patients with SO, Dalen-Fuchs nodules are not pathognomonic, as they may also be seen in patients with VKH syndrome and sarcoidosis
- absence of inflammatory involvement of the choriocapillaris and retina
- phagocytosis of uveal pigment by epithelioid cells
- extension of the granulomatous process into the scleral canals, optic disc, vessels, macula, and periphery

The precise etiology of SO is unknown; however, in the overwhelming majority of patients, there is a history of penetrating ocular injury complicated by incarceration of uveal tissue. Although it has been speculated that an infectious agent or a bacterial antigen may,

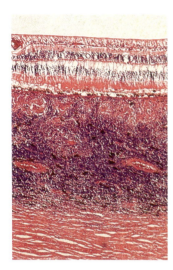

Figure 6-62 Diffuse granulomatous inflammation in sympathetic ophthalmia.

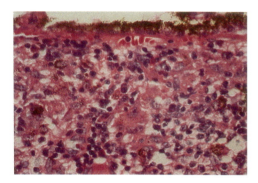

Figure 6-63 Sympathetic ophthalmia (histologic view). Note the giant cells in the choroid.

through molecular mimicry of an endogenous ocular antigen, precipitate an immune response resulting in the development of SO, no organism has been consistently isolated, and it has not been reproduced in animal models following injection of a putative infectious agent. Animal studies, however, do support the notion that SO may result from altered T-lymphocyte responses to previously sequestered ocular self-antigens such as retinal S-antigen, interphotoreceptor retinoid-binding protein, melanin-associated antigens, and antigens derived from the RPE or choroid following ocular injury. The penetrating wound itself may facilitate exposure of uveoretinal antigens to conjunctival lymphatic channels and so initiate this immunopathologic response. Furthermore, there may be a genetic predisposition to the development of the disease, as patients with SO are more likely to express HLA-DR4, -DRw53, and -DQw3 haplotypes. Recent studies from both the United Kingdom and Japan report the highest relative risk for haplotypes HLA-DRB1*04 and -DQB1*04. It should be noted that the immunogenetics of SO and VKH syndrome are virtually identical, as the same associations have been found in both diseases.

The diagnosis of SO is clinical and should be suspected in the presence of bilateral uveitis following any ocular trauma or surgery. Table 6-5 lists surgical procedures and injuries that may lead to SO. Differential diagnostic considerations include other causes of

Table 6-5 Surgical Procedures and Injuries That May Lead to Sympathetic Ophthalmia

Surgical procedures associated with sympathetic ophthalmia
Vitrectomy
Secondary intraocular lens (IOL) placement
Trabeculectomy
Iridencleisis
Contact and noncontact Nd:YAG laser cyclodestruction
Cyclocryotherapy
Proton beam and helium ion irradiation for choroidal melanoma
Cataract extraction, particularly when the iris is entrapped within the wound

Injuries associated with sympathetic ophthalmia
Perforating ulcers
Severe contusion
Subconjunctival scleral rupture
Any perforating injury, with or without direct uveal involvement or uveal prolapse

panuveitis, including tuberculosis, sarcoidosis, syphilis, and fungi, as well as traumatic or postoperative endophthalmitis. Lens-associated uveitis has been reported with SO in up to 25% of cases and may present with a similar clinical picture. The clinical presentations of SO and VKH syndrome may be strikingly similar, with systemic signs and symptoms generally present in both; however, a history of prior ocular injury is typically absent in patients with VKH syndrome.

The course of SO is chronic, with frequent exacerbations, and if left untreated SO leads to loss of vision and phthisis bulbi. Every attempt should be made to salvage eyes with a reasonable prognosis for useful vision with meticulous and prompt closure of penetrating injuries; however, enucleation within 2 weeks of injury to prevent the development of SO should be considered in patients with grossly disorganized globes with no discernible visual function. Although controversial, enucleation may still be preferred to evisceration as the operation of choice for the removal of ocular contents in severely injured eyes because it eliminates the possibility of residual uveal tissue, which may predispose to the development of sympathetic disease. BCSC Section 7, *Orbit, Eyelids, and Lacrimal System,* discusses the advantages and disadvantages of enucleation and evisceration in greater detail. Regardless of visual potential, once SO has become established, enucleation of the exciting eye has not been shown to be beneficial in altering the disease course of the sympathizing eye. In fact, the exciting eye may eventually become the better-seeing eye.

The initial treatment of SO involves systemic corticosteroids, with the frequent addition of corticosteroid-sparing agents such as azathioprine, methotrexate, mycophenolate mofetil, cyclosporine, chlorambucil, and cyclophosphamide, as extended therapy is anticipated in most patients. Topical corticosteroids, together with cycloplegic and mydriatic agents, are essential in the treatment of the acute anterior uveitis associated with SO. Periocular corticosteroids are used to manage inflammatory recurrences and CME. Intravitreal corticosteroids, including the intravitreal fluocinolone acetonide implant, represent an option for patients intolerant of systemic corticosteroid therapy. With prompt and aggressive systemic therapy, the visual prognosis of SO is good, with 60% of patients achieving a final visual acuity of 20/40, although up to 25% may become legally blind in the sympathizing eye.

Bilyk JR. Enucleation, evisceration, and sympathetic ophthalmia. *Curr Opin Ophthalmol.* 2000; 11(5):372–386.

Chan CC, Roberge RG, Whitcup SM, Nussenblatt RB. 32 cases of sympathetic ophthalmia. A retrospective study at the National Eye Institute, Bethesda, MD, from 1982 to 1992. *Arch Ophthalmol.* 1995;113(5):597–600.

Davis JL, Mittal KK, Freidlin V, et al. HLA associations and ancestry in Vogt-Koyanagi-Harada disease and sympathetic ophthalmia. *Ophthalmology.* 1990;97(9):1137–1142.

Galor A, Davis JL, Flynn HW Jr, et al. Sympathetic ophthalmia: incidence of ocular complications and vision loss in the sympathizing eye. *Am J Ophthalmol.* 2009;148(5):704–710.

Kilmartin DJ, Dick AD, Forrester JV. Prospective surveillance of sympathetic ophthalmia in the UK and Republic of Ireland. *Br J Ophthalmol.* 2000;84(3):259–263.

Lubin JR, Albert DM, Weinstein M. Sixty-five years of sympathetic ophthalmia. A clinico-pathologic review of 105 cases (1913–1978). *Ophthalmology.* 1980;87(2):109–121.

Marak GE Jr. Recent advances in sympathetic ophthalmia. *Surv Ophthalmol.* 1979;24(3): 141–156.

Shindo Y, Ohno S, Usui M, et al. Immunogenetic study of sympathetic ophthalmia. *Tissue Antigens.* 1997;49(2):111–115.

Vogt-Koyanagi-Harada Syndrome

VKH syndrome is an uncommon multisystem disease of presumed autoimmune etiology that is characterized by chronic, bilateral, diffuse, granulomatous panuveitis with accompanying integumentary, neurologic, and auditory involvement. Although the disease most commonly affects darkly pigmented ethnic groups (Asians, Asian Indians, Hispanic individuals, Native Americans, and Middle Easterners) and is uncommon among whites, VKH syndrome is also rare among sub-Saharan Africans, suggesting that other factors, in addition to skin pigmentation, are important in its pathogenesis. The incidence of VKH syndrome varies geographically, accounting for up to 4% of all uveitis referrals in the United States and 8% in Japan. In Brazil and Saudi Arabia, it is the most commonly encountered cause of noninfectious uveitis. Women appear to be affected more often than men except in the Japanese population.

The precise etiology and pathogenesis of VKH syndrome are unknown, but current clinical and experimental evidence suggests a cell-mediated autoimmune process driven by T lymphocytes directed against self-antigens associated with melanocytes of all organ systems in genetically susceptible individuals. Specifically, T helper-1 cells and up-regulation of associated cytokines (interleukin-2 and -6 and interferon gamma) are thought to play a prominent role in the pathogenesis of VKH syndrome. Recent studies suggest that interleukin-23 plays a pivotal role in the development and maintenance of the autoimmune process by inducing the differentiation of interleukin-17–producing CD4+ helper T lymphocytes. Sensitization to melanocytic antigenic peptides by cutaneous injury or viral infection has been proposed as a possible trigger of this autoimmune process. Tyrosinase or tyrosinase-related proteins, an unidentified 75-kDa protein, and S-100 protein have been implicated as target antigens on the melanocytes. A genetic predisposition for the development of the disease and an immune dysregulatory pathogenesis are further supported by the strong association with HLA-DR4 among Japanese patients with VKH syndrome; the strongest associated risk is observed with the HLA-DRB1*0405 and HLA-DRB1*0410 haplotypes. Among Hispanic patients from southern California with VKH syndrome, 84% were found to have the HLA-DR1 or HLA-DR4 haplotypes, with the former conferring a higher relative risk.

There are 4 stages of VKH syndrome: prodromal, acute uveitic, convalescent, and chronic recurrent. Histologic findings vary depending on the stage. During the acute uveitic stage, diffuse, nonnecrotizing, granulomatous inflammation virtually identical to that seen in SO consists of lymphocytes and macrophages admixed with epithelioid and multinucleate giant cells with preservation of the choriocapillaris. Proteinaceous fluid exudates are observed in the subretinal space between the detached neurosensory retina and the RPE. Although the peripapillary choroid is the predominant site for the granulomatous inflammatory infiltration, the ciliary body and iris may also be affected. Focal aggregates of epithelioid histiocytes admixed with RPE, or Dalen-Fuchs nodules, appear between the Bruch membrane and the RPE. The convalescent stage is characterized by nongranulomatous inflammation with uveal infiltration of lymphocytes, few plasma cells, and the absence of epithelioid histiocytes. The number of choroidal melanocytes decreases with loss of melanin pigment, corresponding with the characteristic clinical feature known as sunset glow fundus. In addition, the appearance of numerous small atrophic depigmented lesions in the peripheral retina, erroneously thought to be Dalen-Fuchs nodules, histologically corresponds to the focal loss of RPE cells with chorioretinal adhesions. The chronic recurrent stage is characterized by granulomatous choroiditis with damage to the choriocapillaris. Involvement of the choriocapillaris in patients with VKH syndrome, which does not occur in SO, is more a function of the stage of the disease at the time of histologic examination (acute in SO vs chronic recurrent in VKH syndrome) than a truly differentiating feature. The numerous clinical and pathological similarities between SO and VKH syndrome suggest that they share a similar immunopathogenesis, albeit with different triggering events and modes of sensitization.

The clinical features of VKH syndrome also vary depending on the stage of the disease. The prodromal stage is marked by flulike symptoms. Patients present with headache, nausea, meningismus, dysacusia, tinnitus, fever, orbital pain, photophobia, and hypersensitivity of the skin and hair to touch several days preceding the onset of ocular symptoms. Focal neurologic signs, although rare, may develop and include cranial neuropathies, hemiparesis, aphasia, transverse myelitis, and ganglionitis. Cerebrospinal fluid analysis reveals lymphocytic pleocytosis with normal levels of glucose in more than 80% of patients; this may persist for up to 8 weeks. Auditory problems are observed in 75% of patients, frequently coincident with the onset of ocular disease. Central dysacusia usually involving higher frequencies or tinnitus occurs in approximately 30% of patients early in the disease course, typically improving within 2–3 months; however, persistent deficits may remain.

The acute uveitic stage is heralded by the onset of sequential blurring of vision in both eyes, 1–2 days after the onset of CNS signs, and is marked by bilateral granulomatous anterior uveitis, a variable degree of vitritis, thickening of the posterior choroid with elevation of the peripapillary retinal choroidal layer, hyperemia and edema of the optic nerve, and multiple serous retinal detachments (Fig 6-64). The focal serous retinal detachments are often shallow, with a cloverleaf pattern around the posterior pole, but may coalesce and evolve into large bullous exudative detachments (Fig 6-65). Profound visual loss may be seen during this phase. Less commonly, mutton-fat KPs and iris nodules at the pupillary margin may be observed. IOP may be elevated; the anterior chamber may be shallow due to forward displacement of the lens–iris diaphragm from ciliary body edema or annular choroidal detachment, or it may be low, secondary to ciliary body shutdown.

The convalescent stage occurs several weeks later and is marked by resolution of the exudative retinal detachments and gradual depigmentation of the choroid, resulting in the classic orange-red discoloration, or sunset glow fundus (Fig 6-66). In addition, small, round, discrete depigmented lesions develop in the inferior peripheral fundus (Fig 6-67). Juxtapapillary depigmentation may also be seen (see Fig 6-66). In Hispanic patients, the sunset glow fundus may show focal areas of retinal hyperpigmentation or hypopigmentation. Perilimbal vitiligo (Sugiura sign) may be found in up to 85% of Japanese patients but is rarely observed among white patients (Fig 6-68). Integumentary changes, including vitiligo, alopecia, and poliosis, typically appear during the convalescent stage in about 30% of patients and correspond with the development of fundus depigmentation (Figs 6-69, 6-70). In general, skin and hair changes occur weeks to months after the onset of ocular inflammation, but in some cases they may appear simultaneously. Between 10% and 63% of patients develop vitiligo, depending on ethnic background, with the incidence of cutaneous and other extraocular manifestations being relatively low among Hispanic patients.

The chronic recurrent stage is marked by repeated bouts of granulomatous anterior uveitis, with the development of KPs, posterior synechiae, iris nodules, iris depigmentation, and stromal atrophy. Posterior segment recurrences (vitritis, papillitis, multifocal choroiditis, and exudative retinal detachment) have been reported but are uncommon during this stage. Anterior segment recurrence, however, may occur concomitantly with subclinical choroidal inflammation requiring systemic therapy. Visually debilitating

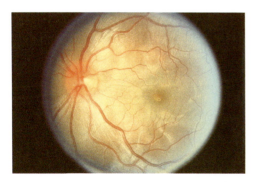

Figure 6-64 Disc hyperemia and multiple serous retinal detachments in the posterior pole of the left eye of an Hispanic patient in the acute uveitic stage of Vogt-Koyanagi-Harada (VKH) syndrome. *(Reprinted with permission from Moorthy RS, Inomata H, Rao NA. Vogt-Koyanagi-Harada syndrome.* Surv Ophthalmol. *1995;39(4):271.)*

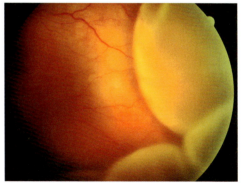

Figure 6-65 Bullous exudative retinal detachment in the acute uveitic stage of VKH syndrome. *(Courtesy of Albert T. Vitale, MD.)*

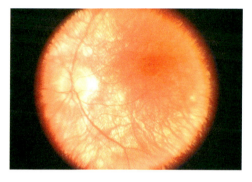

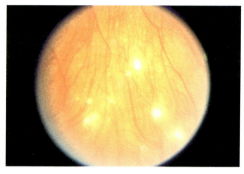

Figure 6-66 Sunset glow fundus appearance with juxtapapillary detachment in the convalescent stage of VKH syndrome in an Hispanic patient. *(Reprinted with permission from Moorthy RS, Inomata H, Rao NA. Vogt-Koyanagi-Harada syndrome. Surv Ophthalmol. 1995;39(4):272.)*

Figure 6-67 Multiple inferior peripheral punched-out chorioretinal lesions representing resolved Dalen-Fuchs nodules in the chronic stage of VKH syndrome. *(Courtesy of Ramana S. Moorthy, MD.)*

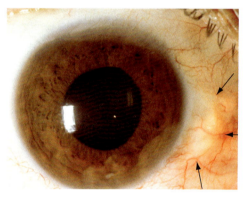

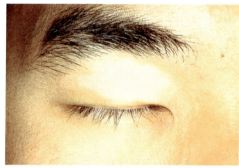

Figure 6-68 Perilimbal vitiligo of a Sugiura sign *(arrows)*. *(Courtesy of Albert T. Vitale, MD.)*

Figure 6-69 Vitiligo of the upper eyelid and marked poliosis in the chronic stage of VKH syndrome. *(Courtesy of Ramana S. Moorthy, MD.)*

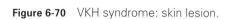

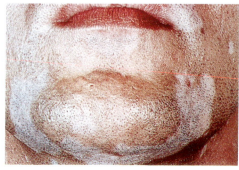

Figure 6-70 VKH syndrome: skin lesion.

sequelae of chronic inflammation develop during this stage and include posterior subcapsular cataract, glaucoma, CNV, and subretinal fibrosis.

Based on these clinical features and their distinctive appearance within the overall disease course, comprehensive diagnostic criteria for the complete, incomplete, and probable forms of VKH syndrome have been recently revised (Table 6-6). Regardless of the form of the disease, essential features for the diagnosis of VKH syndrome include bilateral involvement, no history of penetrating ocular trauma, and no evidence of other ocular or systemic disease.

Table 6-6 Revised Diagnostic Criteria for Vogt-Koyanagi-Harada Syndrome

Complete Vogt-Koyanagi-Harada syndrome
 I. No history of penetrating ocular trauma or surgery
 II. No clinical or laboratory evidence of other ocular or systemic disease
 III. Bilateral ocular disease (either A or B below must be met):
　A. Early manifestations
　　1. Diffuse choroiditis as manifested by either:
　　　a. Focal areas of subretinal fluid, or
　　　b. Bullous serous subretinal detachments
　　2. With equivocal fundus findings, then both:
　　　a. Fluorescein angiography showing focal delayed choroidal perfusion, pinpoint leakage, large placoid areas of hyperfluorescence, pooling of dye within subretinal fluid, and optic nerve staining
　　　b. Ultrasonography showing diffuse choroidal thickening without evidence of posterior scleritis
　B. Late manifestations
　　1. History suggestive of findings from IIIA, and either both 2 and 3 below, or multiple signs from 3
　　2. Ocular depigmentation
　　　a. Sunset glow fundus, or
　　　b. Sugiura sign
　　3. Other ocular signs
　　　a. Nummular chorioretinal depigmentation scars, or
　　　b. RPE clumping and/or migration, or
　　　c. Recurrent or chronic anterior uveitis
 IV. Neurologic/auditory findings (may have resolved by time of examination):
　A. Meningismus
　B. Tinnitus
　C. Cerebrospinal fluid pleocytosis
 V. Integumentary findings (not preceding central nervous system or ocular disease)
　A. Alopecia
　B. Poliosis
　C. Vitiligo

Incomplete Vogt-Koyanagi-Harada syndrome
Criteria I to III and either IV or V from above

Probable Vogt-Koyanagi-Harada syndrome
Criteria I to III from above must be present
Isolated ocular disease

Adapted from Read RW, Holland GN, Rao NA, et al. Revised diagnostic criteria for Vogt-Koyanagi-Harada disease: report of an international committee on nomenclature. *Am J Ophthalmol.* 2001;131(5):647–652.

The diagnosis of VKH syndrome is essentially clinical; exudative retinal detachment during the acute disease and sunset glow fundus during the chronic phase are highly specific to this entity. In patients presenting without extraocular changes, FA, ICG angiography, OCT, FAF imaging, lumbar puncture, and ultrasonography may be useful confirmatory tests. During the acute uveitic stage, FA typically reveals numerous punctate hyperfluorescent foci at the level of the RPE in the early stage of the study followed by pooling of dye in the subretinal space in areas of neurosensory detachment (Fig 6-71). The vast majority of patients show disc leakage, but CME and retinal vascular leakage are uncommon. In the convalescent and chronic recurrent stages, focal RPE loss and atrophy produce multiple hyperfluorescent window defects without progressive staining.

ICG angiography highlights the choroidal pathology, disclosing a delay in choriocapillaris and choroidal vessel perfusion, early choroidal stromal vessel hyperfluorescence and leakage, disc hyperfluorescence, multiple hypofluorescent spots throughout the fundus thought to correspond to foci of lymphocytic infiltration, and hyperfluorescent pinpoint changes within areas of exudative retinal detachment. These hypofluorescent spots may be present even when the funduscopic and FA findings are unremarkable and so serve as sensitive markers for the detection and follow-up of subclinical choroidal inflammation.

Ultrasonography may be helpful in establishing the diagnosis, especially in the presence of media opacity. Findings include diffuse, low to medium reflective thickening of the posterior choroid, most prominent in the peripapillary area with extension to the equatorial region; exudative retinal detachment; vitreous opacification; and posterior thickening of the sclera.

OCT may be useful in the diagnosis and monitoring of serous macular detachments, CME, and choroidal neovascular membranes. More recently, the combined use of FAF imaging and SD-OCT offers a noninvasive assessment of RPE and outer retina changes in patients with chronic VKH syndrome that may not be apparent on clinical examination.

In highly atypical cases—particularly patients presenting early in the course of the disease with prominent neurological signs and a paucity of ocular findings—a lumbar puncture, revealing lymphocytic pleocytosis, may be useful diagnostically. However, in

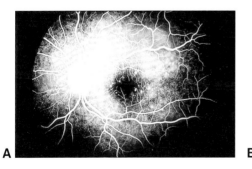
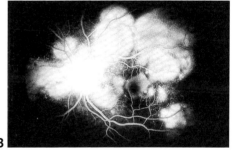

A   B

Figure 6-71 **A,** Early arteriovenous phase fluorescein angiogram showing multiple pinpoint foci of hyperfluorescence in the posterior pole of the left eye of a patient in the acute uveitic stage of VKH syndrome. **B,** Late arteriovenous phase fluorescein angiogram showing fluorescein pooling in multiple serous retinal detachments in the posterior pole in the same eye. *(Courtesy of Ramana S. Moorthy, MD.)*

the vast majority of cases, the history and clinical examination, together with FA and/or ultrasonography, are sufficient to establish the diagnosis.

The differential diagnosis of VKH syndrome includes SO, uveal effusion syndrome, posterior scleritis, primary intraocular lymphoma, uveal lymphoid infiltration, APMPPE, and sarcoidosis. These entities may be differentiated from VKH syndrome by a thorough history, review of systems, and physical examination, together with a directed laboratory evaluation.

The acute stage of VKH syndrome is exquisitely responsive to early and aggressive treatment with topical, periocular, and systemic corticosteroids and cycloplegic and mydriatic agents. Initial dosages typically are 1.0–1.5 mg/kg/day of oral prednisone or 200 mg of intravenous methylprednisolone for 3 days followed by high-dose oral corticosteroids, although the route of administration has no demonstrable effect on changes in visual acuity or the development of visually significant complications. For patients intolerant of systemic therapy, use of intravitreal corticosteroids, including the intravitreal fluocinolone acetonide implant, is an option. Systemic corticosteroids are tapered slowly according to the clinical response, on average over a 6-month period, in an effort to prevent progression of the disease to the chronic recurrent stage and to minimize the incidence and severity of extraocular manifestations. Despite adequate initial treatment with systemic corticosteroids, many patients experience recurrent episodes of inflammation. This has led many experts to initiate IMT (including cyclosporine, azathioprine, mycophenolate mofetil, chlorambucil, cyclophosphamide, and infliximab) earlier to achieve more prompt inflammatory control and to facilitate more rapid tapering of corticosteroids. The overall visual prognosis for patients treated in this fashion is fair, with up to 70% of patients retaining vision of 20/40 or better. Structural complications associated with ocular morbidity include cataract formation (50%); glaucoma (33%); CNV (up to 15%); and subretinal fibrosis, the development of which is associated with increased disease duration, more frequent recurrences, and an older age at disease onset. Recently, the use of either oral corticosteroids or IMT with extended follow-up was shown to reduce the risk of vision loss and the development of some structural complications. Specifically, oral corticosteroids reduced the risk of CNV and subretinal fibrosis by 82% and the risk of visual acuity decline to 20/200 or worse in better-seeing eyes by 67%. IMT was associated with risk reductions of 67% for vision loss to 20/50 or worse and 92% for vision loss to 20/200 or worse in better-seeing eyes.

Bykhovskaya I, Thorne JE, Kempen JH, Dunn JP, Jabs DA. Vogt-Koyanagi-Harada disease: clinical outcomes. *Am J Ophthalmol.* 2005;140(4):674–678.

Fang W, Yang P. Vogt-Koyanagi-Harada syndrome. *Curr Eye Res.* 2008;33(7):517–533.

Herbort CP, Mantovani A, Bouchenaki N. Indocyanine green angiography in Vogt-Koyanagi-Harada disease: angiographic signs and utility in patient follow-up. *Int Ophthalmol.* 2007;27(2–3):173–182.

Moorthy RS, Inomata H, Rao NA. Vogt-Koyanagi-Harada syndrome. *Surv Ophthalmol.* 1995; 39(4):265–292.

Rao NA. Pathology of Vogt-Koyanagi-Harada disease. *Int Ophthalmol.* 2007;27(2–3):81–85.

Rao NA, Gupta A, Dustin L, et al. Frequency of distinguishing clinical features in Vogt-Koyanagi-Harada disease. *Ophthalmology.* 2010;117(3):591–599.

Read RW, Holland GN, Rao NA, et al. Revised diagnostic criteria for Vogt-Koyanagi-Harada disease: report of an international committee on nomenclature. *Am J Ophthalmol.* 2001; 131(5):647–652.

Read RW, Rechodouni A, Butani N, et al. Complications and prognostic factors in Vogt-Koyanagi-Harada disease. *Am J Ophthalmol.* 2001;131(5):599–606.

Shindo Y, Ohno S, Yamamoto T, Nakamura S, Inoko H. Complete association of the HLA-DRB1*04 and -DQB1*04 alleles with Vogt Koyanagi-Harada disease. *Hum Immunol.* 1994;39(3):169–176.

Vasconcelos-Santos DV, Sohn EH, Sadda S, Rao NA. Retinal pigment epithelial changes in chronic Vogt-Koyanagi-Harada disease: fundus autofluorescence and spectral domain-optical coherence tomography findings. *Retina.* 2010;30(1):33–41.

Weisz JM, Holland GN, Roer LN, et al. Association between Vogt-Koyanagi-Harada syndrome and HLA-DR1 and -DR4 in Hispanic patients living in southern California. *Ophthalmology.* 1995;102(7):1012–1015.

Behçet Disease

Behçet disease (BD) is a chronic, relapsing, occlusive systemic vasculitis (Fig 6-72) of unknown etiology that is characterized, in part, by a uveitis that can affect both the anterior and the posterior segments of the eye, often simultaneously. The symptoms of this disease were described as early as 2500 years ago, but it was only in the early 20th century that its clinical features were more completely characterized by Adamantiades and Behçet. BD occurs in many ethnic populations all over the world. It is most common in the Northern Hemisphere in the countries of the eastern Mediterranean and on the eastern rim of Asia, particularly along the Old Silk Route. The prevalence of BD varies from as high as 80–300 cases per 100,000 inhabitants in Turkey to 8–10 per 100,000 in Japan and 0.4 per 100,000 in the United States. The "complete" type of BD (fulfilling 4 major diagnostic criteria; Table 6-7) is more common in men and the "incomplete" type (fulfilling 3 major criteria or ocular involvement with 1 other major criterion; see Table 6-7) is equally frequent in men and women. Throughout the world, the typical age of onset is between 25 and 35 years, but BD can also develop as early as age 10–15. Although there have been some familial cases of BD, most are sporadic.

The diagnosis of BD is clinical and is based on the presence of multiple systemic findings. The diagnostic system for BD given in Table 6-7 was suggested by researchers in

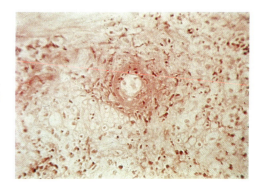

Figure 6-72 Histologic view of perivascular inflammation in a patient with Behçet disease.

Table 6-7 Diagnostic System for Behçet Disease (Japan)

Major Criteria
  Recurrent oral aphthous ulcers
  Skin lesions (erythema nodosum, acneiform pustules, folliculitis)
  Recurrent genital ulcers
  Ocular inflammatory disease

Minor Criteria
  Arthritis
  Gastrointestinal ulceration
  Epididymitis
  Systemic vasculitis or associated complications
  Neuropsychiatric symptoms

Types of Behçet Disease
  Complete (4 major criteria)
  Incomplete (3 major criteria or ocular involvement with 1 other major criterion)
  Suspect (2 major criteria with no ocular involvement)
  Possible (1 major criterion)

Adapted from Foster CS, Vitale AT. *Diagnosis and Treatment of Uveitis.* Philadelphia, PA: WB Saunders; 2002.

Japan. Another diagnostic system, which was suggested by the International Study Group for Behçet's Disease, is shown in Table 6-8. Although BD is a multisystem disease, it can have its predominant effect on a single system; thus, special clinical types of BD occur—namely, neuro-BD, ocular BD, intestinal BD, and vascular BD.

Nonocular systemic manifestations

Oral aphthae are the most frequent finding in BD (Fig 6-73). These are recurrent mucosal ulcers that produce significant discomfort and pain. They can occur on the lips, gums, palate, tongue, uvula, and posterior pharynx. They are discrete, round or oval, white ulcerations with red rims that vary in size from 2 to 15 mm. They recur every 5–10 days or every month. They last from 7 to 10 days and then heal without much scarring unless they are large.

Skin lesions can include painful or recurrent erythema nodosum, often over extensor surfaces such as the tibia, but also on the face, neck, and buttocks. They disappear with minimal, if any, scarring. Acne vulgaris or folliculitis-like skin lesions may frequently

Table 6-8 Diagnostic System for Behçet Disease (International Study Group for Behçet Disease)

Recurrent oral aphthous ulcers (at least 3 or more times per year) plus 2 of the following criteria:
  1. Recurrent genital ulcers
  2. Ocular inflammation
  3. Skin lesions
  4. Positive cutaneous pathergy test

Adapted from Foster CS, Vitale AT. *Diagnosis and Treatment of Uveitis.* Philadelphia, PA: WB Saunders; 2002.

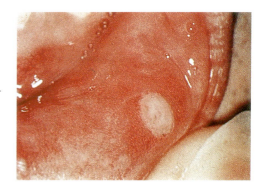

Figure 6-73 Behçet disease: mucous membrane ulcers (oral aphthae).

appear on the upper thorax and face. Nearly 40% of patients with BD exhibit cutaneous pathergy, which is characterized by the development of a sterile pustule at the site of a venipuncture or an injection but is not pathognomonic of BD.

Genital ulcers appear grossly similar to oral aphthous ulcers. In male patients, they can occur on the scrotum or penis. In female patients, they can appear on the vulva and the vaginal mucosa. These lesions are associated with variable amounts of pain.

Systemic vasculitis may also occur in up to 25% of patients with BD, and any size artery or vein in the body may be affected. Four different vascular complications can develop from the systemic vasculitis of BD: arterial occlusion, aneurysm, venous occlusion, and varices. Cardiac involvement from BD can include granulomatous endocarditis, myocarditis, endomyocardial fibrosis, coronary arteritis, and pericarditis; these can occur in up to 17% of patients. Gastrointestinal lesions can include multiple ulcers involving the esophagus, stomach, and intestines. Pulmonary involvement is mainly pulmonary arteritis with aneurysmal dilatation of the pulmonary artery. Fifty percent of patients with BD develop arthritis; in 50% of these, the knee is most affected.

Neurologic involvement is the most serious of all manifestations of BD and may occur in up to 10% of patients. Ten percent of patients with neuro-BD can have ocular disease, and 30% of patients with ocular BD may have neurologic involvement. CNS involvement mainly affects areas of motor control. Widespread vasculitis in the CNS can result in headaches. CNS symptoms such as strokes, palsies, and a confusional state may develop in 25% of patients. Mortality has been reported to be as high as 10% in patients with neuro-BD, but today it may be lower, especially with the use of IMT. More men than women appear to develop neuro-BD. Neuro-ophthalmic involvement can include cranial nerve palsies, central scotomata caused by papillitis, visual field defects, and papilledema resulting from thrombosis of the superior sagittal sinus or other venous sinuses.

Ocular manifestations

Ocular manifestations affect up to 70% of patients with BD and carry serious implications, because they are often recurrent and relapsing, resulting in permanent, often irreversible, ocular damage. Severe vision loss can occur in up to 25% of patients with BD. Ocular disease appears to be more severe in men, and more men are affected; up to 80% of cases are bilateral. Ocular involvement as an initial presenting problem is relatively uncommon, occurring in about 10% of patients. The intraocular inflammation is characterized by a nongranulo-matous necrotizing obliterative vasculitis that can affect any or all portions of the uveal tract.

Anterior uveitis may be the only ocular manifestation of BD; it presents with a transient hypopyon in up to 25% of cases (Fig 6-74). This inflammation is nongranulomatous. Redness, pain, photophobia, and blurred vision are common findings. On clinical examination, the hypopyon can shift with the patient's head position or disperse with head shaking, and it may not be visible unless viewed by gonioscopy. Although anterior uveitis may be very severe, it can spontaneously resolve even without treatment; however, the nature of ocular BD is one of explosive onset over the course of just a few hours. With relapses, posterior synechiae, iris bombé, and angle-closure glaucoma may all develop. Other less-common anterior segment findings of BD include cataract, episcleritis, scleritis, conjunctival ulcers, and corneal immune ring opacities.

The posterior segment manifestations of ocular BD are often profoundly sight threatening. The essential retinal finding is that of an obliterative, necrotizing retinal vasculitis (Fig 6-75) that affects both the arteries and the veins in the fundus. This is the most common form of uveitis seen in children and adults with BD. Posterior manifestations can include branch retinal vein occlusion, isolated branch artery occlusions, combined branch retinal vein and branch retinal artery occlusions, and vascular sheathing with variable amounts of vitritis, plus associated CME. Retinal ischemia can lead to the development of retinal neovascularization and even of neovascularization of the iris and neovascular glaucoma. After repeated episodes of retinal vasculitis and vascular occlusions, retinal vessels may become white and sclerotic. Active areas of retinal vasculitis may be accompanied by multifocal areas of chalky white retinitis. The ischemic nature of the vasculitis and accompanying retinitis may produce a funduscopic appearance that may be confused with acute retinal necrosis syndrome or other necrotizing herpetic entities (Fig 6-76; see also Chapter 7). The optic nerve is affected in 25% of patients with BD. Optic papillitis can occur, but progressive optic atrophy may occur as a result of the vasculitis affecting the arterioles that supply blood to the optic nerve.

Pathogenesis

The immunopathogenesis of BD remains unknown. Many environmental factors have been suggested as a potential cause, but none has been proven. No infectious agent or

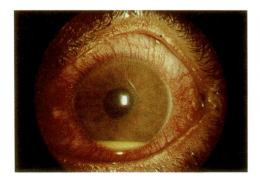

Figure 6-74 Behçet disease: hypopyon.

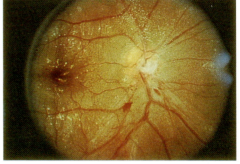

Figure 6-75 Behçet disease: retinal vasculitis.

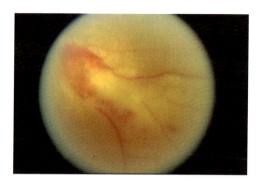

Figure 6-76 Retinitis and vasculitis with retinal hemorrhage in a patient with Behçet disease. The retinitis seen here appears similar to necrotizing herpetic retinitis with retinal whitening and occlusive retinal vasculitis. *(Courtesy of Ramana S. Moorthy, MD.)*

microorganism has been reproducibly isolated from the lesions of patients with BD. It is clinically and experimentally unlike other autoimmune diseases.

Specific HLA associations have been found in certain systemic forms of BD: HLA-B12 with mucocutaneous lesions, HLA-B27 with arthritis, and HLA-B51 with ocular lesions. These are not reproducible in all populations and are of little diagnostic value. Histologically, the lesions of BD resemble those of delayed-type hypersensitivity reactions early on; late lesions resemble those of immune-complex–type reactions.

Diagnosis

Diagnosis of BD is based on clinical findings and the diagnostic criteria given in Tables 6-7 and 6-8. HLA testing, cutaneous pathergy testing, and nonspecific serologic markers of inflammation such as ESR and C-reactive protein are of little value in confirming the diagnosis. FA demonstrates marked dilatation and occlusion of retinal capillaries with perivascular staining, evidence of retinal ischemia, leakage of fluorescein into the macula with the development of CME, and retinal neovascularization that may leak. Radiologic imaging, including chest x-ray, chest CT, and brain MRI with contrast enhancement, may be helpful, as indicated by clinical presentation.

Differential diagnosis

The differential diagnosis for BD includes HLA-B27–associated anterior uveitis, reactive arthritis syndrome, sarcoidosis, and systemic vasculitides including systemic lupus erythematosus, PAN, and Wegner granulomatosis. Necrotizing herpetic retinitis can also mimic occlusive BD retinal vasculitis.

Treatment

The goal of treatment is not only to treat the explosive onset of acute disease with systemic corticosteroids but also to control chronic inflammation and prevent or decrease the number of relapses of ocular inflammation with IMT, which is <u>essential</u>.

Corticosteroids These agents may be used to treat explosive-onset anterior segment and posterior segment inflammation, although most patients will eventually become resistant to corticosteroid therapy. Nevertheless, systemic corticosteroids (eg, 1.5 mg/kg/day of prednisone with a gradual taper) are extremely useful in controlling acute inflammation.

Immunomodulatory medications Patients who present with sight-threatening posterior segment ocular BD require prompt institution of systemic corticosteroids together with IMT, which may include azathioprine, infliximab, cyclosporine, tacrolimus, mycophenolate mofetil, chlorambucil, or cyclophosphamide. Azathioprine has been found in prospective clinical trials to be useful in preserving visual acuity in patients with established ocular BD and is a preferred first-line immunomodulatory agent. It can also be effective in controlling oral and genital ulcers and arthritis. Open-label clinical trials in Greece, Turkey, Italy, and Japan have confirmed the efficacy of infliximab in controlling inflammation, reducing relapses, and allowing corticosteroids to be tapered in up to 96% of patients with ocular BD, especially those with sight-threatening posterior segment disease such as retinal vasculitis. Because infliximab, particularly at doses of 10 mg/kg or more, carries a greater risk of long-term therapeutic complications such as disseminated tuberculosis or congestive heart failure (see Table 5-17), it is best employed for short-term induction therapy. The European League Against Rheumatism panel has recommended using azathioprine (with corticosteroids) as first-line IMT for ocular BD and cyclosporine or infliximab as second-line treatment. Cyclosporine has been used with limited success in the management of ocular BD, but is not as effective as other cytotoxic agents and may carry risks of nephrotoxicity. Tacrolimus is less toxic and may be used as a substitute for cyclosporine; it has been successfully used in Japan to treat BD. Colchicine is used for treatment of mucocutaneous disease; it is ineffective for treating ocular BD. Mycophenolate mofetil has also been successful in treating ocular BD in small case series. Chlorambucil has been found to be effective in the treatment of BD even at relatively low doses. As a single agent, chlorambucil may be the most effective of the immunomodulatory agents in achieving durable remission. Cyclophosphamide has been used with some success in Japan to treat patients with BD. It is an attractive alternative to chlorambucil, although somewhat less effective. Both chlorambucil and cyclophosphamide have been shown to be more effective than cyclosporine in the management of posterior segment ocular BD but carry a greater risk of systemic complications (see Table 5-17). Effective therapeutic reduction of white blood cell counts and proper hematologic monitoring are essential and can be quite complex with these alkylating agents. Recent reports in the European literature emphasize that interferon alfa-2a is efficacious and well tolerated; it is highly effective in Behçet uveitis and somewhat less effective in non-Behçet uveitis, with inflammation controlled in almost 90% and 60% of patients, respectively.

Prognosis

Prognosis for vision is guarded in patients with BD. Nearly 25% of patients worldwide with chronic ocular BD have visual acuity less than 20/200, most commonly caused by macular edema, occlusive retinal vasculitis, optic atrophy, and glaucoma. Adult men tend to have poorer visual outcomes. But compared to the results achieved in the 1980s, current patients appear to have better visual prognosis because of earlier and more aggressive use of IMT. Complications such as macular edema, complex cataract, glaucoma, secondary and neovascular glaucoma, retinal and optic disc neovascularization, retinal detachment, and vitreous hemorrhage may require complex medical and surgical intervention (see Chapter 10), and all have a profound impact on final visual outcomes. The presence of posterior synechiae, persistent inflammation, elevated IOP, and hypotony are all statistically significant predictive factors for vision loss. The chronic relapsing nature of this disease, with frequent exacerbations after long periods of remission, makes it difficult to predict the visual outcomes.

Accorinti M, Pirraglia MP, Paroli MP, Priori R, Conti F, Pivetti-Pezzi P. Infliximab treatment for ocular and extraocular manifestations of Behçet's disease. *Jpn J Ophthalmol.* 2007;51(3):191–196.

Gueudry J, Wechsler B, Terrada C, et al. Long-term efficacy and safety of low-dose interferon alpha2a therapy in severe uveitis associated with Behçet disease. *Am J Ophthalmol.* 2008;146(6):837–844.

Hatemi G, Silman A, Bang D, et al. EULAR recommendations for the management of Behçet disease. *Ann Rheum Dis.* 2008;67(12):1656–1662.

Kaçmaz RO, Kempen JH, Newcomb C, et al, for the Systemic Immunosuppressive Therapy for Eye Diseases Cohort Study Group. Ocular inflammation in Behçet disease: incidence of ocular complications and of loss of visual acuity. *Am J Ophthalmol.* 2008;146(6):828–836.

Keino H, Okada AA. Behçet's disease: global epidemiology of an Old Silk Road disease. *Br J Ophthalmol.* 2007;91(12):1573–1574.

Kesen MR, Goldstein DA, Tessler HH. Uveitis associated with pediatric Behçet disease in the American Midwest. *Am J Ophthalmol.* 2008;146(6):819–827.

Kitaichi N, Miyazaki A, Stanford MR, Chams H, Iwata D, Ohno S. Ocular features of Behçet's disease: an international collaborative study. *Br J Ophthalmol.* 2007;91(12):1579–1582.

Kötter I, Zierhut M, Eckstein AK, et al. Human recombinant interferon alfa-2a for the treatment of Behcet's disease with sight threatening posterior or panuveitis. *Br J Ophthalmol.* 2003;87(4):423–431.

Niccoli L, Nannini C, Benucci M, et al. Long-term efficacy of infliximab in refractory posterior uveitis of Behçet's disease: a 24-month follow-up study. *Rheumatology (Oxford).* 2007;46(7):1161–1164.

Ohno S, Nakamura S, Hori S, et al. Efficacy, safety, and pharmacokinetics of multiple administration of infliximab in Behçet's disease with refractory uveoretinitis. *J Rheumatol.* 2004;31(7): 1362–1368.

Sfikakis PP, Markomichelakis N, Alpsoy E, et al. Anti-TNF therapy in the management of Behçet's disease—review and basis for recommendations. *Rheumatology (Oxford).* 2007;46(5): 736–741.

Tugal-Tutkun I, Onal S, Altan-Yaycioglu R, Kir N, Urgancioglu M. Uveitis in Behçet disease: an analysis of 880 patients. *Am J Ophthalmol.* 2004;138(3):373–380.

Zakka FR, Chang PY, Giuliari GP, Foster CS. Current trends in the management of ocular symptoms of Adamantiades-Behçet's disease. *Clin Ophthalmol.* 2009;3:567–579.

CHAPTER 7

Infectious Ocular Inflammatory Disease

Viruses, fungi, protozoa, helminths, and bacteria can all cause infectious uveitis. Because these organisms may produce inflammation in different parts of the uveal tract, this chapter has been organized based on the causative organism and, if appropriate, subcategorized by the anatomical location of the intraocular inflammation. The most common primary site of inflammation has been identified for each entity. Some agents, such as herpes simplex virus, may cause anterior and/or posterior uveitis. Other illnesses, such as syphilis, Lyme borreliosis, and onchocerciasis, usually cause panuveitis.

Viral Uveitis

Herpesviridae Family

Herpes simplex virus and varicella-zoster virus

Anterior uveitis Acute anterior uveitis is often associated with herpetic viral disease. BCSC Section 8, *External Disease and Cornea,* extensively discusses herpes simplex virus (HSV) and varicella-zoster virus (VZV) (Figs 7-1, 7-2, 7-3). Usually, the iritis associated with herpesviruses is a keratouveitis; occasionally, anterior uveitis may occur without noticeable keratitis. In many cases, the inflammation becomes chronic. VZV infection may be considered in the differential diagnosis of chronic unilateral iridocyclitis, even if the cutaneous component of the condition occurred in the past or was minimal even when present. Some patients may develop iridocyclitis without ever having had a cutaneous component (varicella-zoster sine herpete).

Chickenpox (varicella), which is caused by the same virus responsible for secondary VZV reactivation, is frequently associated with an acute, mild, nongranulomatous, self-limiting, bilateral iritis or iridocyclitis. Cutaneous vesicles at the side of the tip of the nose (the Hutchinson sign) indicate nasociliary nerve involvement and a greater likelihood that the eye will be affected (see Fig 7-1). Most patients are asymptomatic, but as many as 40% of patients with primary VZV infection may develop iritis when examined prospectively.

Patients with intraocular viral infections, particularly with herpes group viruses, may occasionally develop stellate keratic precipitates (KPs). This morphology is also seen in Fuchs heterochromic iridocyclitis and toxoplasmosis. These stellate KPs usually assume

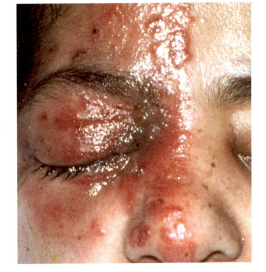

Figure 7-1 Varicella-zoster virus infection: skin lesions. *(Courtesy of Debra A. Goldstein, MD.)*

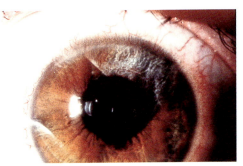

Figure 7-2 Iris stromal atrophy in a patient with varicella-zoster iridocyclitis. *(Courtesy of David Forster, MD.)*

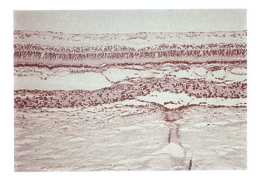

Figure 7-3 Varicella-zoster virus infection: necrosis of long ciliary nerve.

a diffuse distribution, as opposed to the usual distribution, which occurs in the inferior one-third of the cornea known as the *Arlt triangle*. In addition, the KPs are fine and fibrillar, often with a distinctly stellate pattern on high-magnification biomicroscopy. The identification of diffuse or stellate KPs is useful in the differential diagnosis of anterior segment inflammation but is not diagnostic of any particular condition. In patients with herpetic disease and concomitant keratopathy, however mild, anterior segment inflammation may also be associated with diffuse or localized decreased corneal sensation and neurotrophic keratitis.

Ocular hypertension is a frequent complication of herpetic uveitis and is thus a helpful diagnostic hallmark. Most inflammatory syndromes are associated with decreased intraocular pressure (IOP) as a result of ciliary body hyposecretion. However, just as the herpesvirus can localize to corneal, cutaneous, or conjunctival tissues, herpetic reactivation may directly cause trabeculitis and thus increase IOP, often to as high as 50–60 mm Hg. In addition, inflammatory cells may contribute to trabecular obstruction and congestion. Hyphema may occur in herpetic uveitis.

Iris atrophy is also characteristic of herpetic inflammation and can be seen with HSV-, VZV-, or cytomegalovirus (CMV)-associated iritis. The atrophy may be patchy or sectoral (see Fig 7-2) and is best demonstrated with retroillumination at the slit lamp.

Viral retinitis (discussed in the following section) may occur with these entities, particularly in immunocompromised hosts. Vasculitis commonly occurs with varicella-zoster ophthalmicus, and it may lead to anterior segment ischemia, retinal artery occlusion, and scleritis. Vasculitis in the orbit may lead to cranial nerve palsies.

Treatment for viral anterior uveitis usually includes topical corticosteroids and cycloplegic agents. Topical antiviral agents are usually ineffective in the treatment of herpetic uveitis but may be indicated in patients with herpes simplex keratouveitis to prevent dendritic keratitis during topical corticosteroid therapy. Systemic antiviral agents such as acyclovir, famciclovir, or valacyclovir are often beneficial in cases of severe uveitis. Initiation of oral antiviral therapy with the onset of VZV uveitis is now recommended. Patients with herpetic uveitis may require prolonged corticosteroid therapy with very gradual tapering. In fact, some patients with VZV infection require very long-term, albeit extremely low, doses of topical corticosteroids (as infrequent as 1 drop per week) to remain quiescent. Systemic corticosteroids are necessary at times. Long-term, suppressive, low-dose antiviral therapy may be beneficial in patients with herpetic uveitis, but controlled studies are lacking. The oral dosages are acyclovir 400 mg twice a day or valacyclovir 500 mg/day for patients with herpes simplex and acyclovir 800 mg twice a day or valacyclovir 1 g/day for VZV disease.

Barron BA, Gee L, Hauck WW, et al. Herpetic Eye Disease Study: a controlled trial of oral acyclovir for herpes simplex stromal keratitis. *Ophthalmology.* 1994;101(12):1871–1882.

Siverio Júnior CD, Imai Y, Cunningham ET Jr. Diagnosis and management of herpetic anterior uveitis. *Int Ophthalmol Clin.* 2002;42(1):43–48.

van der Lelij A, Ooijman FM, Kijlstra A, Rothova A. Anterior uveitis with sectoral iris atrophy in the absence of keratitis: a distinct clinical entity among herpetic eye diseases. *Ophthalmology.* 2000;107(6):1164–1170.

Wilhelmus KR, Gee L, Hauck WW, et al. Herpetic Eye Disease Study. A controlled trial of topical corticosteroids for herpes simplex stromal keratitis. *Ophthalmology.* 1994;101(12):1883–1895.

Acute retinal necrosis, progressive outer retinal necrosis, and nonnecrotizing herpetic retinitis Acute retinal necrosis (ARN) is part of a spectrum of necrotizing herpetic retinopathies the clinical expression of which appears to be influenced by both host and viral factors. Originally described in 1971 among otherwise healthy adults, ARN has also been reported in children and among immunocompromised patients, including those with

AIDS. Acute, fulminant disease may arise without a systemic prodrome years after primary infection or following cutaneous or systemic herpetic infection such as dermatomal zoster, chickenpox, or herpetic encephalitis. The prevalence is nearly equal between the sexes, with the majority of cases clustering in patients between the fifth and seventh decades of life. A genetic predisposition may increase the relative risk of developing ARN among patients with specific human leukocyte antigen (HLA) haplotypes, including HLA-DQw7 antigen and phenotype Bw62, DR4 in white patients in the United States and phenotypes HLA-Aw33, B44 and HLA-Aw33, DRw6 in Japanese patients. The American Uveitis Society has established mandatory and supporting criteria for the diagnosis of ARN based solely on the clinical findings and disease progression, independent of viral etiology or host immune status (Table 7-1). Retinal lesions of presumed herpetic etiology that are not characteristic of well-recognized syndromes such as CMV retinitis or progressive outer retinal necrosis are grouped under the umbrella designation *necrotizing herpetic retinopathy.*

Patients with ARN usually present with acute unilateral loss of vision, photophobia, floaters, and pain. Fellow eye involvement occurs in approximately 36% of cases, usually within 6 weeks of disease onset, but involvement may be delayed for extended periods (up to 26 years) after initial presentation. Panuveitis is observed, beginning with significant anterior segment inflammation replete with corneal edema, KPs, posterior synechiae, and elevated IOP, together with heavy vitreous cellular infiltration. Within 2 weeks, the classic triad of occlusive retinal arteriolitis, vitritis, and a multifocal yellow-white peripheral retinitis has evolved. Early on, the peripheral retinal lesions are discontinuous and have scalloped edges that appear to arise in the outer retina. Within days they coalesce to form a confluent 360° creamy retinitis that progresses in a posterior direction, leaving full-thickness retinal necrosis, arteriolitis, phlebitis, and occasional retinal hemorrhage in its wake (Figs 7-4, 7-5). Widespread necrosis of the midperipheral retina, multiple posterior retinal breaks, and proliferative vitreoretinopathy predispose to combined tractional–rhegmatogenous retinal detachments in 75% of patients (Fig 7-6). The posterior pole tends to be spared, but an exudative retinal detachment may arise with severe inflammation. The optic nerve is frequently involved, as evidenced by disc swelling and a relative afferent defect.

In most instances, the diagnosis is made clinically, with important differential diagnostic considerations, including CMV retinitis, atypical toxoplasmic retinochoroiditis, syphilis, lymphoma, leukemia, and autoimmune retinal vasculitis such as Behçet disease.

Table 7-1 American Uveitis Society Criteria for Diagnosis of Acute Retinal Necrosis

One or more foci of retinal necrosis with discrete borders, located in the peripheral retina*
Rapid progression in the absence of antiviral therapy
Circumferential spread
Occlusive vasculopathy with arteriolar involvement
Prominent vitritis, anterior chamber inflammation
Optic neuropathy/atrophy, scleritis, pain supportive but not required

*Macular lesions do not exclude diagnosis in the presence of peripheral retinitis.

Adapted from Holland GN and the Executive Committee of the American Uveitis Society. Standard diagnostic criteria for the acute retinal necrosis syndrome. *Am J Ophthalmol.* 1994;117(5):663–667.

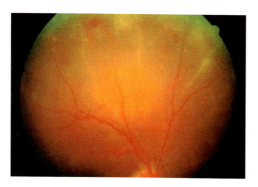

Figure 7-4 Acute retinal necrosis, vitritis, arteriolitis, and multiple peripheral "thumbprint" areas of retinitis. *(Courtesy of E. Mitchel Opremcak, MD.)*

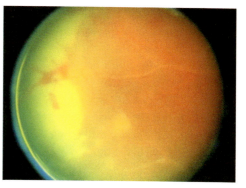

Figure 7-5 Acute retinal necrosis: confluent peripheral retinitis. *(Courtesy of E. Mitchel Opremcak, MD.)*

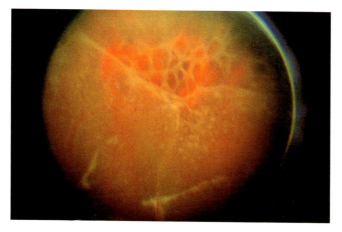

Figure 7-6 Acute retinal necrosis: retinal detachment with multiple, posterior retinal breaks. *(Courtesy of E. Mitchel Opremcak, MD.)*

ARN may also be seen in association with concurrent or antecedent herpetic encephalitis (HSV-1 or -2). When the diagnosis is uncertain, intraocular fluid analysis of aqueous and/or vitreous samples or retinal choroidal biopsy should be performed.

Intraocular antibody production as a measure of the host response to a specific microbial pathogen can be computed using the Goldmann-Witmer (GW) coefficient. (See Chapter 2 for a discussion of the GW coefficient.) A ratio of greater than 3 is considered diagnostic of local antibody production. Aqueous humor analysis is most frequently performed following anterior chamber paracentesis. It has been used more widely in Europe than in the United States as an adjunct to the diagnosis of toxoplasmosis and necrotizing herpetic retinitis caused by HSV and VZV, but it is of little value in the diagnosis of CMV retinitis. Combining the GW coefficient with polymerase chain reaction (PCR) analysis may increase diagnostic yield, especially in viral infections.

PCR is probably the most sensitive, specific, and rapid diagnostic method for detecting infectious posterior uveitis in general and ARN specifically. It has largely supplanted viral culture, intraocular antibody titers, and serology. PCR may be performed on either aqueous humor or vitreous biopsy specimens; however, for most cases of ARN, aqueous sampling is usually sufficient. Quantitative PCR may add additional information with respect to viral load, disease activity, and response to therapy. Recent studies using PCR-based assays suggest that the most common cause of ARN is VZV, followed by HSV-1, HSV-2, and, in rare instances, CMV. Patients with ARN caused by HSV-1 or VZV tend to be older (mean age 40 years), whereas those with ARN due to HSV-2 tend to be younger (under age 25). There is a higher risk of encephalitis and meningitis among patients with ARN caused by HSV-1 than by VZV. In rare instances where PCR results are negative but the clinical suspicion for herpetic necrotizing retinitis is high, endoretinal biopsy may be diagnostic.

Timely diagnosis and prompt antiviral therapy are essential given the rapidity of disease progression, the frequency of retinal detachment, and the guarded visual prognosis. Intravenous acyclovir, at 10 mg/kg/day in 3 divided doses over 10–14 days, remains the classic regimen; it is effective against HSV and VZV. Reversible elevations in serum creatinine and liver enzymes may occur; in the presence of frank renal insufficiency, the dosage will need to be reduced. For infection with VZV, oral acyclovir at 800 mg orally 5 times daily or an equivalent dose of valacyclovir (1 g orally 3 times daily) or famciclovir (500 mg orally 3 times daily) should be continued for 3 months following intravenous induction. For ARN associated with HSV-1 infection, the dose is one-half of that for VZV. Extended antiviral therapy may reduce the incidence of contralateral disease or bilateral ARN by 80% over 1 year. After 24–48 hours of antiviral therapy, systemic corticosteroids (prednisone, 1 mg/kg/day) are introduced to treat active inflammation and subsequently tapered over several weeks. Aspirin and other anticoagulants have been used to treat an associated hypercoagulable state and prevent vascular occlusions, but the results have been inconclusive.

More recently, oral valacyclovir at doses of up to 2 g 3 times daily has been used successfully as an alternative to intravenous acyclovir as induction therapy. Additionally, intravitreal ganciclovir (0.2–2.0 mg/0.1 mL) and foscarnet (1.2–2.4 mg/0.1 mL) have been used to achieve a rapid induction in combination with both intravenous and oral antivirals as first-line therapy or in patients who fail to respond to systemic acyclovir (see Chapter 11). The superiority of high-dose systemic oral therapy alone or in combination with intravitreal antiviral agents has not been demonstrated over the classic intravenous approach. Given the short intravitreal half-life of these drugs, injections may need to be repeated twice weekly until the retinitis is controlled. Effective treatment inhibits the development of new lesions and promotes lesion regression over 4 days.

Retinal detachment occurs within the first weeks to months following the onset of retinitis. Given the location and multiplicity of retinal breaks, prophylactic barrier laser photocoagulation, applied to the areas of healthy retina at the posterior border of the necrotic lesions, may prevent retinal detachment and is recommended as soon as the view permits. Early vitrectomy combined with endolaser photocoagulation has been proposed to help eliminate the contribution of vitreous traction on the necrotic retina. Due to the presence of proliferative vitreoretinopathy and multiple posterior retinal tears, internal repair using vitrectomy techniques, air–fluid exchange, endolaser photocoagulation, or long-acting gas or silicone oil tamponade is more successful in achieving a higher rate of anatomical attachment than are standard scleral buckling procedures. Untreated, approximately two-thirds of eyes obtain a final visual acuity of 20/200 or worse due to retinal detachment, concurrent optic atrophy, or macular pathology. With early recognition, aggressive antiviral therapy, and laser photocoagulation, this prognosis may be significantly improved, as shown in 1 study in which 46% of 13 eyes achieved a visual acuity of 20/40 or better and 92% a visual acuity of better than 20/400.

Progressive outer retinal necrosis (PORN) is essentially a morphologic variant of acute necrotizing herpetic retinitis, occurring most often in patients with advanced AIDS (CD4+ T lymphocytes ≤50 cells/µL) or who are otherwise profoundly immunosuppressed. The most common cause of PORN is VZV; HSV has also been isolated. As with ARN, the retinitis begins as patchy areas of outer retinal whitening that coalesce rapidly; however, in contrast to ARN, the posterior pole may be involved early in the course of the disease, vitreous inflammatory cells are typically absent, and the retinal vasculature is minimally involved, at least initially (Fig 7-7). In addition, a previous history of cutaneous zoster (67%) and eventual bilateral involvement (71%) is frequently observed in patients with PORN and human immunodeficiency virus (HIV) infection or AIDS, who have a similarly high rate (70%) of retinal detachment. The visual prognosis is poor; in the largest series reported to date, 67% of patients had a final visual acuity of no light perception. Although the disease is often resistant to intravenous acyclovir alone, successful management has been reported with combination systemic and intraocular therapy with foscarnet and ganciclovir. Long-term suppressive antiviral therapy is required in patients with HIV/AIDS who are not able to achieve immune reconstitution on highly active antiretroviral therapy (HAART). See also BCSC Section 12, *Retina and Vitreous*.

Nonnecrotizing herpetic retinitis (nonnecrotizing posterior uveitis) may occur in patients with herpetic infections, including acute retinochoroiditis with diffuse hemorrhages following acute VZV infection in children and chronic choroiditis or retinal vasculitis in adults. In a recent study using PCR-based assays and local antibody analysis of aqueous fluid samples for herpesviruses, a viral etiology was confirmed in 13% of cases deemed "idiopathic posterior uveitis." Inflammation is typically bilateral, presenting with cystoid macular edema (CME), as a birdshot-like retinochoroidopathy, or as an occlusive bilateral

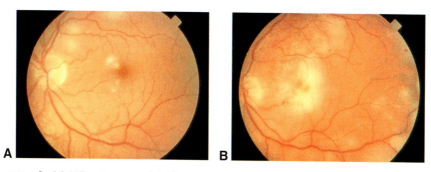

Figure 7-7 A, Multifocal areas of white retinitis in a patient with progressive outer retinal necrosis (PORN). **B,** Fundus photograph taken 5 days later showing rapid disease progression and confluence of the areas of the viral retinitis. *(Courtesy of E. Mitchel Opremcak, MD.)*

retinitis. The disease is initially resistant to conventional therapy with systemic corticosteroids and/or immunomodulatory therapy (IMT) but favorable response is achieved when patients are switched to systemic antiviral medication.

Aizman A, Johnson MW, Elner SG. Treatment of acute retinal necrosis syndrome with oral antiviral medications. *Ophthalmology.* 2007;114(2):307–312

Bodaghi B, Rozenberg F, Cassoux N, Fardeau C, LeHoang P. Nonnecrotizing herpetic retinopathies masquerading as severe posterior uveitis. *Ophthalmology.* 2003;110(9):1737–1743.

Chau Tran TH, Cassoux N, Bodaghi B, Lehoang P. Successful treatment with combination of systemic antiviral drugs and intravitreal ganciclovir injections in the management of severe necrotizing herpetic retinitis. *Ocul Immunol Inflamm.* 2003;11(2):141–144.

Crapotta JA, Freeman WR. Visual outcome in acute retinal necrosis. *Retina.* 1994;14(4):382–383.

Engstrom RE Jr, Holland GN, Margolis TP, et al. The progressive outer retinal necrosis syndrome. A variant of necrotizing herpetic retinopathy in patients with AIDS. *Ophthalmology.* 1994;101(9):1488–1502.

Ganatra JB, Chandler D, Santos C, Kuppermann B, Margolis TP. Viral causes of the acute retinal necrosis syndrome. *Am J Ophthalmol.* 2000;129(2):166–172.

Goldstein DA, Pyatetsky D. Necrotizing herpetic retinopathies. *Focal Points: Clinical Modules for Ophthalmologists.* San Francisco, CA: American Academy of Ophthalmology: 2008, module 10.

Holland GN and the Executive Committee of the American Uveitis Society. Standard diagnostic criteria for the acute retinal necrosis syndrome. *Am J Ophthalmol.* 1994;117(5):663–667.

Holland GN, Cornell PJ, Park MS, et al. An association between acute retinal necrosis syndrome and HLA-DQw7 and phenotype Bw62, DR4. *Am J Ophthalmol.* 1989;108(4):370–374.

Cytomegalovirus

Cytomegalovirus is a double-stranded DNA virus in the Herpesviridae family. It is the most common cause of congenital viral infection and causes clinically relevant disease in neonates; it also causes illness in immunocompromised patients with leukemia, lymphoma, and HIV/AIDS; transplant recipients; and those with conditions requiring systemic immunomodulation. CMV retinitis is the most common ophthalmic manifestation of both congenital CMV infection and in the context of HIV/AIDS. The clinical appearance is similar regardless of clinical context; 3 distinct variants have been described:

- a classic or fulminant retinitis with large areas of retinal hemorrhage against a background of whitened, edematous, or necrotic retina, typically appearing in the posterior pole, from the disc to the vascular arcades, in the distribution of the nerve fiber layer, and associated with blood vessels (Fig 7-8)
- a granular or indolent form found more often in the retinal periphery, characterized by little or no retinal edema, hemorrhage, or vascular sheathing, with active retinitis progressing from the borders of the lesion (Fig 7-9)
- a perivascular form often described as a variant of frosted branch angiitis, an idiopathic retinal perivasculitis initially described in immunocompetent children (Fig 7-10)

Early CMV retinitis may present as a small white retinal infiltrate masquerading as a cotton-wool spot, commonly seen as part of HIV-related microvasculopathy, and is distinguished from the latter by its inevitable progression without treatment.

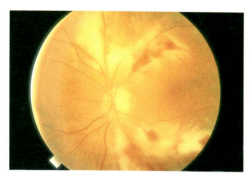

Figure 7-8 Cytomegalovirus (CMV) retinitis. *(Courtesy of E. Mitchel Opremcak, MD.)*

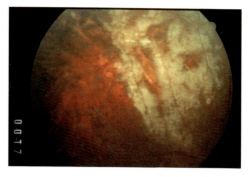

Figure 7-9 Granular CMV retinitis. *(Courtesy of Careen Lowder, MD.)*

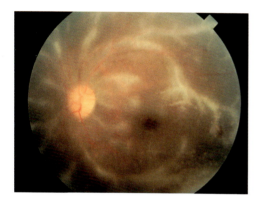

Figure 7-10 "Frosted branch" CMV perivasculitis. *(Courtesy of Albert T. Vitale, MD.)*

The diagnosis of congenital disease is suggested by the clinical appearance of the lesions, coupled with evidence of viral inclusion bodies in urine, saliva, and subretinal fluid, and associated systemic disease findings. The complement-fixation test for cytomegalic inclusion disease is of value 5–24 months after the loss of the maternal antibodies transferred during pregnancy. Likewise, the diagnosis of CMV retinitis in the setting of HIV/AIDS or IMT is essentially clinical, based on the features just described. In immunocompromised patients with atypical lesions or those not responding to anti-CMV therapy, PCR-based analysis of the aqueous or vitreous samples may provide critical diagnostic information of high sensitivity and specificity that allows the clinician to differentiate CMV from other herpetic causes of necrotizing retinitis, and from toxoplasmic retinochoroiditis.

CMV reaches the eye hematogenously, with passage of the virus across the blood–ocular barrier, infection of retinal vascular endothelial cells, and cell-to-cell transmission of the virus within the retina. The histologic features of both congenital and acquired disease include a primary, full-thickness, coagulative necrotizing retinitis and secondary diffuse choroiditis. Infected retinal cells show pathognomonic cytomegalic changes consisting of large eosinophilic intranuclear inclusions and small multiple basophilic cytoplasmic inclusions (Fig 7-11A). Viral inclusions may also be seen in the retinal pigment epithelium (RPE) and vascular endothelium. Electron microscopy of infected retinal tissue reveals viral particles with the typical morphology of the herpes family (Fig 7-11B).

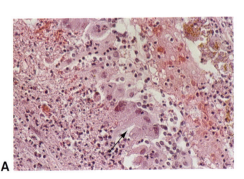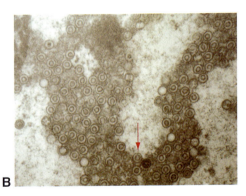

Figure 7-11 **A,** Photomicrograph of a retinal biopsy specimen demonstrating a necrotic retina and giant (megalo) cells with eosinophilic intracytoplasmic inclusions *(arrow)* consistent with CMV retinitis (hematoxylin and eosin stain). **B,** Electron photomicrograph of the same specimen showing intranuclear inclusions containing scattered nucleocapsids, relative electron lucency of the central core *(arrow)*, and the typical envelope consistent with CMV. *(Part A courtesy of Careen Lowder, MD. Part B reproduced with permission from Spaide RF, Vitale AT, Toth IR, Oliver JM. Frosted branch angiitis associated with cytomegalovirus retinitis. Am J Ophthalmol. 1992;113(5):525; courtesy of Albert T. Vitale, MD.)*

Congenital CMV retinitis is usually associated with other systemic manifestations of disseminated infection, including fever, thrombocytopenia, anemia, pneumonitis, and hepatosplenomegaly, with a reported prevalence in children with congenital CMV infection of between 11% and 22%. However, CMV retinitis has been reported to occur later in life among children with no discernible lesions ophthalmoscopically and no evidence of systemic disease reactivation. This suggests that even asymptomatic children with evidence of congenital CMV infection should be followed up at regular intervals for potential ocular involvement later into childhood. Resolution of the retinitis leaves both pigmented and atrophic lesions, with retinal detachment occurring in up to one-third of children. Optic atrophy and cataract formation are not uncommon sequelae.

Prior to the introduction of HAART, an estimated 30% of patients with HIV/AIDS, typically with CD4$^+$ T lymphocyte counts ≤50 cells/μL, developed CMV retinitis at some point during their disease. Rhegmatogenous retinal detachments with multiple breaks, particularly in areas of peripheral retinal necrosis, occurred at a rate of approximately 33% per eye per year. The availability of HAART in the industrialized world has resulted not only in a significant decline in HIV/AIDS–associated mortality, but also in an 80% decline in new cases per year of CMV retinitis and its associated complications, including retinal detachment, which is itself associated with CMV lesion size. This decrease appears to have stabilized, and new cases of CMV retinitis continue to occur among patients in whom HAART fails and those who experience immune reconstitution but fail to develop CMV-specific immunity.

Successful management of CMV retinitis requires not only HAART but also appropriate anti-CMV therapy. This is particularly important given that CMV retinitis itself confers a twofold increased risk in mortality among patients with a CD4$^+$ T-cell count <100 cells/μL (an effect not seen with counts ≥100 cells/μL) and also given the clear mortality benefit associated with systemic anti-CMV therapy. Resistant CMV infection is further associated with increased mortality among patients with HIV/AIDS being treated for CMV retinitis. Options for systemic coverage include high-dose induction with either intravenous ganciclovir (5 mg/kg twice daily) or foscarnet (90 mg/kg twice daily) for 2 weeks followed by low-dose daily maintenance therapy or oral valganciclovir (900 mg twice daily) for 3 weeks followed by maintenance therapy (900 mg/day). Intravitreal injection of ganciclovir or foscarnet, and the ganciclovir implant, which delivers therapeutic concentrations of drug for 8 months, are highly effective in treating intraocular disease and may be useful alternatives in patients who cannot tolerate intravenous systemic therapy because of myelotoxicity; however, extraocular systemic CMV and the fellow eye remain uncovered. Combination treatment with oral valganciclovir may obviate this limitation and be particularly effective for patients with vision-threatening posteriorly located retinitis. In patients on HAART with CMV retinitis who experience sustained immune recovery (CD4$^+$ T lymphocytes ≥100 cells/μL for 3–6 months), systemic anti-CMV maintenance therapy may be safely discontinued. HAART-naive patients may require only 6 months of anti-CMV therapy with good immune reconstitution, whereas HAART-treated patients may require long-term maintenance therapy. Moreover, aggressive anti-CMV therapy initiated at the same time as HAART may decrease the incidence of immune recovery uveitis. Despite immune recovery, patients with a history of CMV retinitis who discontinue maintenance anti-CMV therapy remain at risk for recurrence and should be followed up at 3-month intervals.

Anterior uveitis Although uncommon, CMV infection may produce a chronic or recurrent unilateral anterior uveitis associated with ocular hypertension and variable degrees of sectoral iris atrophy among immunocompetent adults. This association is based on the demonstration of both CMV DNA by PCR and intraocular antibodies directed against CMV by enzyme-linked immunosorbent assay (ELISA), together with corresponding negative study results for HSV and VZV upon aqueous analysis. CMV anterior uveitis requires specific, prolonged, systemic anti-CMV treatment, most often with valganciclovir, as relapses are common with discontinuation of therapy. Consultation with an infectious disease specialist may be appropriate.

Chee SP, Bascal K, Jap A, Se-Thoe SY, Cheng CL, Tan BH. Clinical features of cytomegalovirus anterior uveitis in immunocompetent patients. *Am J Ophthalmol.* 2008;145(5):834–840.

Coats DK, Demmler GJ, Paysse EA, Du LT, Libby C. Ophthalmologic findings in children with congenital cytomegalovirus infection. *J AAPOS.* 2000;4(2):110–116.

Istas AS, Demmler GJ, Dobbins JG, Stewart JA. Surveillance for congenital cytomegalovirus disease: a report from the National Congenital Cytomegalovirus Disease Registry. *Clin Infect Dis.* 1995;20(3):665–670.

Jabs DA, Holbrook JT, Van Natta ML, et al, and the Studies of Ocular Complications of AIDS Research Group. Risk factors for mortality in patients with AIDS in the era of highly active antiretroviral therapy. *Ophthalmology.* 2005;112(4):771–779.

Jabs DA, Martin BK, Forman MS. Mortality associated with resistant cytomegalovirus among patients with cytomegalovirus retinitis and AIDS. *Ophthalmology.* 2010;117(1):128–131.

Kedhar SR, Jabs DA. Cytomegalovirus retinitis in the era of highly active antiretroviral therapy. *Herpes.* 2007;14(3):66–71.

Kempen JH, Jabs DA. Ocular complications of human immunodeficiency virus infection. In: Johnson GJ, Minassian DC, Weale RA, West SK, eds. *The Epidemiology of Eye Disease.* 2nd ed. London: Hodder Arnold; 2003:318–340.

Kempen JH, Jabs DA, Wilson LA, Dunn JP, West SK, Tonascia J. Mortality risk for patients with cytomegalovirus retinitis and acquired immune deficiency syndrome. *Clin Infect Dis.* 2003;37(10):1365–1373.

Epstein-Barr virus

Epstein-Barr virus (EBV) is a ubiquitous double-stranded DNA virus with a complex capsid and envelope belonging to the subfamily Gammaherpesvirinae. It is the viral agent commonly associated with infectious mononucleosis (IM) and has also been implicated in the pathogenesis of Burkitt lymphoma (especially among African children), nasopharyngeal carcinoma, Hodgkin disease, and Sjögren syndrome. EBV has a tropism for B lymphocytes, the only cells known to have surface receptors for the virus.

Ocular manifestations may arise as a consequence of either congenital EBV infection or, much more commonly, during primary infection in the context of IM. Cataract has been reported in association with congenital EBV infection; a mild, self-limiting follicular conjunctivitis, usually appearing early in the course of the disease, is most common with acquired IM. Other, less frequently reported anterior ocular manifestations of acquired IM include epithelial or stromal keratitis; episcleritis; bilateral, granulomatous iridocyclitis; dacryoadenitis; and, less frequently, cranial nerve palsies and Parinaud oculoglandular syndrome.

A variety of posterior segment manifestations have been reported in association with EBV infection, including isolated optic disc edema and optic neuritis, macular edema, retinal hemorrhages, retinitis, punctate outer retinitis, choroiditis, multifocal choroiditis and panuveitis (MCP), pars planitis and vitritis, progressive subretinal fibrosis, uveitis, and secondary choroidal neovascularization (CNV) (Fig 7-12). Evidence for an association between these ocular findings and the presence of antibodies against a variety of EBV-specific capsid antigens indicative of active or persistent EBV infection is not well established, especially given the very high seroprevalence of EBV (90%) in the adult population.

Most ocular disease is self-limiting and does not require treatment; however, the presence of iridocyclitis may necessitate the use of topical corticosteroids and cycloplegia; systemic corticosteroids may be required to treat posterior segment inflammation. The efficacy of systemic antiviral therapy for EBV infection has not been established.

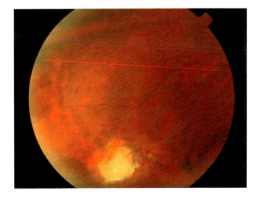

Figure 7-12 Epstein-Barr virus–related retinitis and vasculitis. *(Reproduced with permission from Vitale AT, Foster CS. Uveitis affecting infants and children: infectious causes. In: Hartnett ME, Trese M, Capone A, Keats B, Steidl SM, eds. Pediatric Retina. Philadelphia, PA: Lippincott Williams & Wilkins; 2004:269; courtesy of Albert T. Vitale, MD.)*

Kelly ST, Rosenthal AR, Nicholson KG, Woodward CG. Retinochoroiditis in acute Epstein-Barr virus infection. *Br J Ophthalmol.* 1989;73(12):1002–1003.

Matoba AY. Ocular disease associated with Epstein-Barr virus infection. *Surv Ophthalmol.* 1990;35(2):145–150.

Raymond LA, Wilson CA, Linnemann CC Jr, Ward MA, Bernstein DI, Love DC. Punctate outer retinitis in acute Epstein-Barr virus infection. *Am J Ophthalmol.* 1987;104(4):424–426.

Spaide RS, Sugin S, Yannuzzi LA, DeRosa JT. Epstein-Barr virus antibodies in multifocal choroiditis and panuveitis. *Am J Ophthalmol.* 1991;112(4):410–413.

Usui M, Sakai J. Three cases of EB virus-associated uveitis. *Int Ophthalmol.* 1990;14(5–6): 371–376.

Rubella

Rubella is the prototypical teratogenic viral agent. It consists of single-stranded RNA surrounded by a lipid envelope, or "toga"; hence its inclusion in the Togaviridae family. Although rubella is still an important cause of blindness in developing nations, the epidemic pattern of the disease was interrupted in the United States by the introduction of a vaccine in 1969. The peak age incidence shifted from 5–9 years (young children) in the prevaccine era to 15–19 years (older children) and 20–24 years (young adults) today. Approximately 5%–25% of women of childbearing age who lack rubella antibodies are susceptible to primary infection. Rubella may involve the retina as a part of the congenital rubella syndrome (CRS) or during acquired infection (German measles).

The fetus is infected with the rubella virus transplacentally, secondary to maternal viremia during the course of primary infection. The frequency of fetal infection is highest during the first 10 weeks and during the final month of pregnancy, with the rate of congenital defects varying inversely with gestational age. Although obvious maternal infection during the first trimester of pregnancy may end in spontaneous abortion, stillbirth, or severe fetal malformations, seropositive asymptomatic maternal rubella may also result in severe fetal disease.

The classic features of CRS include cardiac malformations (patent ductus arteriosus, interventricular septal defects, and pulmonic stenosis), ocular findings (chorioretinitis, cataract, corneal clouding, microphthalmia, strabismus, and glaucoma), and deafness (Fig 7-13). Hearing loss is the most common systemic finding. Individuals with CRS are at greater risk for developing diabetes mellitus and subsequent diabetic retinopathy later in life.

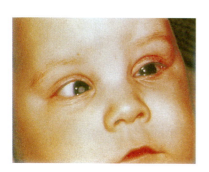

Figure 7-13 Patient with congenital rubella syndrome, with cataract, esotropia, mental retardation, congenital heart disease, and deafness. *(Courtesy of John D. Sheppard, Jr, MD.)*

A unilateral or bilateral pigmentary retinopathy is the most common ocular mani-festation of CRS (25%–50%), followed by cataract (15%) and glaucoma (10%). The pig-mentary disturbance, often described as "salt-and-pepper" fundus, shows considerable variation, ranging from finely stippled, bone spicule–like, small, black, irregular masses to gross pigmentary irregularities with coarse, blotchy mottling (Fig 7-14). It can be sta-tionary or progressive. Despite loss of the foveal light reflex and prominent pigmentary changes, neither vision nor the electroretinogram is typically affected. Congenital (nu-clear) cataracts and microphthalmia are the most frequent causes of poor visual acuity and, rarely, CNV. Unless otherwise compromised by glaucoma, the optic nerve and the retinal vessels are typically normal in appearance.

Histologic studies of the lens reveal retained cell nuclei in the embryonic nucleus as well as anterior and posterior cortical degeneration. Poor development of the dilator muscle, necrosis of the iris pigment epithelium, and chronic nongranulomatous inflam-mation are present in the iris. The RPE displays alternating areas of atrophy and hyper-trophy. The anterior chamber angle appears similar to that seen in congenital glaucoma. Although the mechanism of rubella embryopathy is not known at a cellular level, it is thought that the virus inhibits cellular multiplication and establishes a chronic, persistent infection during organogenesis. The persistence of viral replication after birth, with ongo-ing tissue damage, is central to the pathogenesis of CRS and may explain the appearance of hearing and neurologic and/or ocular deficits long after birth.

Acquired infection (German measles) presents with a prodrome of malaise and fever in adolescents and adults prior to the onset of the rubella exanthem. An erythematous, macu-lopapular rash appears first on the face, spreads toward the hands and feet, involves the en-tire body within 24 hours, and disappears by the third day. Although the rash is not always prominent and the occurrence of fever is variable, lymphadenopathy is invariably present.

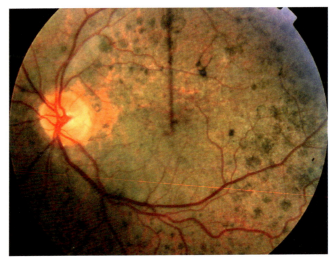

Figure 7-14 Congenital rubella syndrome with diffuse retinal pigment epithelial mottling with "salt-and-pepper" appearance. *(Courtesy of Albert T. Vitale, MD.)*

The most frequent ocular complication of acquired rubella infection is conjunctivitis (70%), followed by the infrequent occurrence of epithelial keratitis and retinitis. Acquired rubella retinitis has been described in adults presenting with acute-onset decreased vision and multifocal chorioretinitis, with large areas of bullous neurosensory detachment, underlying pigment epithelial detachment involving the entire posterior pole, anterior chamber and preretinal vitreous cells, dark gray atrophic lesions of the RPE, normal appearance of the retinal vessels and optic nerve, and absence of retinal hemorrhage. The neurosensory detachments resolve spontaneously and visual acuity returns to normal. Most recently, chronic rubella virus infection has been implicated in the pathogenesis of Fuchs heterochromic iridocyclitis, as evidenced by the presence of rubella-specific intraocular antibody production and the intraocular persistence of the virus.

The pathognomonic retinal findings, associated systemic findings, and a history of maternal exposure to rubella suggest the diagnosis of CRS. Serologic criteria for rubella infection include a fourfold increase in rubella-specific IgG in paired sera 1–2 weeks apart or the new appearance of rubella-specific IgM. Because the fetus is capable of mounting an immune response to the rubella virus, specific IgM or IgA antibodies to rubella in the cord blood confirm the diagnosis.

The differential diagnosis of congenital rubella retinitis consists of those entities constituting the TORCHES syndrome (toxoplasmosis, other agents, rubella, cytomegalovirus, herpesviruses [including EBV], and syphilis). See also BCSC Section 6, *Pediatric Ophthalmology and Strabismus*. Other viral illnesses, such as mumps, exanthema subitum, postvaccination encephalitis, and infection with HSV, VZV, and CMV, should be considered and ruled out by appropriate serologic tests. There is no specific antiviral therapy for congenital rubella and treatment is supportive. Similarly, uncomplicated acquired rubella does not require specific therapy; however, rubella retinitis and postvaccination optic neuritis may respond well to systemic corticosteroids.

Arnold J, McIntosh ED, Martin FJ, Menser MA. A fifty-year follow up of ocular defects in congenital rubella: late ocular manifestations. *Aust N Z J Ophthalmol.* 1994;221(1):1–6.

Givens KT, Lee DA, Jones T, Ilstrup DM. Congenital rubella syndrome: ophthalmic manifestations and associated systemic disorders. *Br J Ophthalmol.* 1993;77(6):358–363.

McEvoy RC, Fedun B, Cooper LZ, et al. Children at high risk of diabetes mellitus: New York studies of families with diabetes in children with congenital rubella syndrome. *Adv Exp Med Biol.* 1988;246:221–227.

Quentin CD, Reiber H. Fuchs heterochromic cyclitis: rubella virus antibodies and genome in aqueous humor. *Am J Ophthalmol.* 2004;138(1):46–54.

Lymphocytic Choriomeningitis Virus

Lymphocytic choriomeningitis virus (LCMV) is an under-recognized fetal teratogen that should probably be listed among the "other agents" in the TORCHES group of congenital infections. The microbe is a single-stranded RNA virus of the Arenaviridae family; rodents are the natural hosts and reservoir. Transmission is thought to be airborne, from contamination of food by infected rodent excreta, or possibly from the bite of an infected animal. Symptomatic maternal illness occurs in approximately two-thirds of cases, with vertical transmission to the fetus occurring during episodes of maternal viremia. As with other congenital infections, transmission earlier in gestation results in more serious sequelae.

Systemic findings include macrocephaly, hydrocephalus, and intracranial calcifications. Neurologic abnormalities, seizures, and mild mental retardation are not uncommon. Ocular findings include both macular and chorioretinal peripheral scarring, similar in morphology and distribution to that seen in congenital toxoplasmosis. Other findings include optic atrophy, strabismus, and nystagmus.

LCMV infection is differentiated from congenital toxoplasmosis by serologic testing of both the mother and the infant and by the pattern of intracerebral calcifications, which tend to be diffuse in toxoplasmosis compared to a periventricular distribution in congenital LCMV disease. Immunofluorescent antibody tests, Western blot, and ELISA are available for detecting both the IgM and IgG antibodies that, together with the clinical findings, establish the diagnosis.

Mets MB, Barton LL, Khan AS, Ksiazek TG. Lymphocytic choriomeningitis virus: an under-diagnosed cause of congenital chorioretinitis. *Am J Ophthalmol.* 2000;130(2):209–215.

Measles (Rubeola)

Congenital and acquired measles infection is caused by a single-stranded RNA virus of the genus *Morbillivirus* in the Paramyxoviridae family. The virus is highly contagious and is transmitted either directly or via aerosolization of nasopharyngeal secretions to the mucous membranes of the conjunctiva or respiratory tract of susceptible individuals, or from a pregnant woman to her fetus transplacentally.

Despite the existence of a safe, effective, and inexpensive vaccine for over 40 years, measles remains the fifth leading cause of mortality worldwide among children younger than 5 years; in the United States, however, measles is now quite rare.

Ocular manifestations of congenital measles infection include cataract, optic nerve head drusen, and bilateral diffuse pigmentary retinopathy involving both the posterior pole and retinal periphery. The retinopathy may also be associated with either normal or attenuated retinal vessels, retinal edema, and macular star formation. Electroretinographic results and visual acuity are typically normal.

The most common ocular complications of measles are keratitis and a mild, papillary, nonpurulent conjunctivitis. Although both keratitis and conjunctivitis resolve without sequelae in the vast majority of cases in the United States, postmeasles blindness, a severe visual impairment arising specifically as a consequence of the corneal complications of the disease, is a significant problem worldwide. Measles retinopathy is more common in acquired than in congenital disease, presenting with profound visual loss 6–12 days after the appearance of the characteristic exanthem, and may or may not be accompanied by encephalitis. It is characterized by attenuated arterioles, diffuse retinal edema, macular star formation, scattered retinal hemorrhages, blurred disc margins, and clear media. With resolution of systemic symptoms and of the acute retinopathy, arteriolar attenuation with or without perivascular sheathing, optic disc pallor, and a secondary pigmentary retinopathy with either a bone spicule or "salt-and-pepper" appearance may evolve.

The electroretinogram is usually extinguished during the acute phase of measles retinopathy but activity may return with visual improvement as the inflammation resolves.

Visual field testing may reveal severe constriction, ring scotomata, or small peripheral islands of vision. Resolution of acquired measles retinopathy over a period of weeks to months is generally associated with a return of useful vision, although the extended visual prognosis is guarded because of the possibility of permanent visual field constriction.

The differential diagnosis of congenital measles retinopathy includes the entities making up the TORCHES syndrome, atypical retinitis pigmentosa, and neuroretinitis; that of acquired disease includes central serous chorioretinopathy, Vogt-Koyanagi-Harada (VKH) syndrome, toxoplasmic retinochoroiditis, retinitis pigmentosa, neuroretinitis, and other viral retinopathies.

The diagnosis of measles and its attendant ocular sequelae and its differentiation from the aforementioned entities are made clinically by means of an accurate history and review of systems; observation of the sequence of signs, symptoms, and lesion progression; and serologic testing. The virus may be recovered from the nasopharynx, conjunctiva, lymphoid tissues, respiratory mucous membranes, urine, and blood for a few days prior to and several days after the rash. Leukopenia is frequently seen during the prodromal phase. A variety of tests are available for serologic confirmation of measles infection, including complement fixation, ELISA, and immunofluorescent and hemagglutination inhibition assays.

Supportive treatment of the systemic manifestations of measles is normally sufficient, because the disease is usually self-limiting. In certain high-risk populations, including pregnant women, children younger than age 1 year, and immunocompromised individuals, infection may be prevented by prophylactic treatment with gamma globulin, 0.25 mL/kg, administered within 5 days of exposure. Likewise, the ocular manifestations of measles are treated symptomatically, with topical antivirals or antibiotics to prevent secondary infections in patients with keratitis or conjunctivitis. The use of systemic corticosteroids should be considered for cases of acute measles retinopathy.

Foxman SG, Heckenlively JR, Sinclair SH. Rubeola retinopathy and pigmented paravenous retinochoroidal atrophy. *Am J Ophthalmol.* 1998;99(5):605–606.

Yoser SL, Forster DJ, Rao NA. Systemic viral infections and their retinal and choroidal manifestations. *Surv Ophthalmol.* 1993;37(5):313–352.

Subacute sclerosing panencephalitis

Subacute sclerosing panencephalitis (SSPE) is a rare late complication of acquired measles infection most often arising in unvaccinated children 6–8 years following primary infection. Children infected with measles before the age of 1 carry a 16 times greater risk than those infected at age 5 or later. Onset is usually in late childhood or adolescence and is characterized by the insidious onset of visual impairment, behavioral disturbances, and memory impairment, followed by myoclonus and progression to spastic paresis, dementia, and death within 1–3 years.

Ocular findings are reported in up to 50% of patients with SSPE and may precede the neurologic manifestations by several weeks to 2 years. The most consistent finding is a maculopathy, consisting of focal retinitis and RPE changes, occurring in 36% of patients (Fig 7-15). Retinitis may progress within several days to involve the posterior pole and peripheral retina. Other ophthalmoscopic findings include disc swelling and papilledema, optic atrophy, macular edema, macular pigment epithelial disturbances, small intraretinal

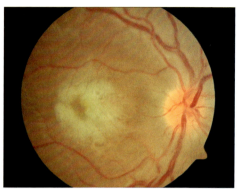

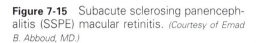
Figure 7-15 Subacute sclerosing panenceph-alitis (SSPE) macular retinitis. *(Courtesy of Emad B. Abboud, MD.)*

hemorrhages, gliotic scar, whitish retinal infiltrates, serous macular detachment, drusen, preretinal membranes, macular hole, cortical blindness, hemianopsia, horizontal nystag-mus, and ptosis. Characteristically, there is little, if any, vitritis. Mottling and scarring of the RPE occurs as the retinitis resolves.

The diagnosis is made based on clinical manifestations; the presence of characteristic, periodic electroencephalographic discharges; the demonstration of raised IgG antibody titer against measles in the plasma and cerebrospinal fluid (CSF); and/or histology sugges-tive of panencephalitis on brain biopsy.

The differential diagnosis of the posterior segment findings associated with SSPE in-cludes necrotizing viral retinitis caused by HSV, VZV, and CMV infection as well multiple sclerosis (MS). In contrast to SSPE, MS is not a panencephalitis; magnetic resonance im-aging (MRI) shows focal periventricular white matter lesions in the latter. Furthermore, CME and retinal vasculitis are prominent features of MS but have not been seen in pa-tients with SSPE.

Definitive treatment of SSPE remains undetermined. A combination of oral isoprin-osine and intraventricular interferon alpha appears to be the most effective treatment; patients who respond to this regimen require lifelong therapy.

Garg RK. Subacute sclerosing panencephalitis. *Postgrad Med J.* 2002;78(916):63–70.

Robb RM, Watters GV. Ophthalmic manifestations of subacute sclerosing panencephalitis. *Arch Ophthalmol.* 1970;83(4):426–435.

West Nile Virus

West Nile virus (WNV) is a single-stranded RNA virus of the family Flaviviridae, first isolated in 1937 in the West Nile district of Uganda. It belongs to the Japanese encephalitis virus serocomplex and is endemic to Europe, Australia, Asia, and Africa. WNV first ap-peared in the United States in 1999 during an outbreak in New York City and subsequently spread westward across the country, southward into Central America, and northward into Canada, resulting in the largest epidemics of neuroinvasive WNV disease ever reported. Of the 663 cases reported to the Centers for Disease Control and Prevention (CDC) dur-ing 2009, 335 (51%) were reported as West Nile meningitis or encephalitis (neuroinvasive disease), 302 (46%) were reported as West Nile fever (milder disease), and 26 (4%) were clinically unspecified. Thirty cases (4.5%) were fatal.

WNV is maintained in an enzootic cycle mainly involving birds and the *Culex* genus of mosquitoes. Birds are the natural host of the virus, which is transmitted from them to humans and other vertebrates through the bite of an infected mosquito. The peak onset of the disease occurs in late summer, but onset can occur anytime between July and December. The incubation period ranges from 3 to 14 days with the vast majority of WNV infections being subclinical (80%) or presenting as a febrile illness (20%) often accompanied by myalgia, arthralgia, headache, conjunctivitis, lymphadenopathy, and a maculopapular or roseolar rash. Severe neurologic disease (meningitis or encephalitis), frequently seen in association with diabetes and advanced age, was initially reported to occur in only 1 of 150 infections, but the severity of WNV infection has increased over time.

Since the first description of intraocular involvement secondary to WNV in 2003, multiple ophthalmic sequelae have been recognized. Presenting ocular symptoms include pain, photophobia, conjunctival hyperemia, and blurred vision. A characteristic multifocal chorioretinitis is seen in the majority of patients, together with nongranulomatous anterior uveitis and vitreous cellular infiltration. Chorioretinal lesions vary in size (200–1000 μm) and number, being distributed throughout the midperiphery, frequently (80%) in linear arrays, following the course of retinal nerve fibers, with or without involvement of the posterior pole (Fig 7-16). Active chorioretinal lesions appear whitish to yellow, are flat and deep, and evolve with varying degrees of pigmentation and atrophy. Fluorescein angiography (FA) reveals central hypofluorescence with late staining of active lesions, and early hyperfluorescence with late staining of inactive lesions. Many inactive lesions exhibit a targetlike appearance angiographically, with central hypofluorescence caused by blockage from pigment and peripheral hyperfluorescence due to atrophy (Fig 7-17). Indocyanine green (ICG) angiography reveals hypofluorescent spots, more numerous than those seen on FA or funduscopy. Other findings include anterior uveitis, vitritis, intraretinal hemorrhages, disc edema, optic atrophy, and, less commonly, focal retinal vascular sheathing and occlusion, cranial nerve VI palsy, and nystagmus. Congenital WNV infection has been reported in an infant presenting without intraocular inflammation but with chorioretinal scarring in each eye.

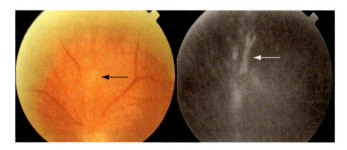

Figure 7-16 West Nile virus chorioretinitis. Fundus photograph with corresponding fluorescein angiogram of active chorioretinitis with lesions distributed in a linear array *(arrows)*. *(Reproduced with permission from Garg S, Jampol LM. Systemic and intraocular manifestations of West Nile virus infection. Surv Ophthalmol. 2005;50(1):8.)*

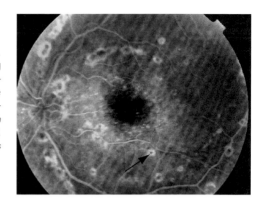

Figure 7-17 West Nile virus chorioretinitis. Midphase fluorescein angiogram showing chorioretinal lesions with central hypofluorescence and peripheral hyperfluorescence *(arrow)*. Capillary leakage is present from underlying diabetic maculopathy. *(Reproduced with permission from Khairallah M, Ben Yahia S, Ladjimi A, et al. Chorioretinal involvement in patients with West Nile virus infection. Ophthalmology. 2004;111(11):2068.)*

In the majority of patients, intraocular inflammation associated with WNV infection has a self-limiting course, with a return of visual acuity to baseline after several months. Persistent visual loss may occur because of CNV, foveal scar, ischemic maculopathy, vitreous hemorrhage, tractional retinal detachment, optic nerve pathology, and retrogeniculate damage. Diabetes has been implicated as a risk factor for WNV-related death and has been observed with significantly increased frequency, together with nonproliferative retinopathy, among patients with WNV-associated ocular involvement.

The presence of the unique pattern of multifocal chorioretinal lesions in patients with systemic symptoms suggestive of WNV infection can help to establish the diagnosis while serologic test results are pending. Conversely, a systemic ocular evaluation including dilated funduscopy and FA may be very helpful in suggesting the diagnosis of WNV infection in patients presenting with meningoencephalitis. The most commonly used laboratory method for diagnosis is demonstration of IgM antibody to the virus using IgM antibody-capture ELISA, which can be confirmed by plaque-reduction neutralization testing (PRNT). The differential diagnosis includes syphilis, MCP, histoplasmosis, sarcoidosis, and tuberculosis, all of which may be distinguished on the basis of medical history, systemic signs and symptoms, serology, and the pattern of chorioretinitis.

There is no currently proven treatment for WNV infection, and in patients with severe disease therapy is supportive. Treatment of anterior uveitis with topical corticosteroids is certainly indicated, but the efficacy of systemic and periocular corticosteroids for the chorioretinal manifestations of WNV infection is unknown. Public health strategies directed at prevention are the mainstays of WNV infection control.

Chan CK, Limstrom SA, Tarasewicz DG. Lin SG. Ocular features of West Nile virus infection in North America: a study in 14 eyes. *Ophthalmology.* 2006;113(9):1539–1546.

Garg S, Jampol LM. Systemic and intraocular manifestations of West Nile virus infection. *Surv Ophthalmol.* 2005;50(1):3–13.

Khairallah M, Ben Yahia S, Attia S, et al. Indocyanine green angiographic features in multifocal chorioretinitis associated with West Nile virus infection. *Retina.* 2006;26(3):358–359.

Khairallah M, Ben Yahia S, Attia S, Zaouali S, Ladjimi A, Messaoud R. Linear pattern of West Nile virus-associated chorioretinitis is related to retinal nerve fibers organization. *Eye (Lond).* 2007;21(7):952–955.

Khariallah M, Ben Yahia S, Letaief M, et al. A prospective evaluation of factors associated with chorioretinitis in patients with West Nile virus infection. *Ocul Immunol Inflamm.* 2007;15(6):435–439.

Rift Valley Fever

Rift Valley fever (RVF) is an acute, epizootic, febrile viral illness caused by arthropod-borne Bunyaviridae of the *Phlebovirus* genus. While primarily affecting domestic animals (sheep, goats, camels, and cattle), the disease may be transmitted to humans, most often through direct contact with the blood or organs of infected animals or by the inhalation of aerosols released during their slaughter. Humans may also develop RVF by ingesting the unpasteurized milk of infected animals or as a result of bites from infected mosquitoes. The incubation period in humans ranges from 3 to 7 days followed by 1 of 3 clinical syndromes: an uncomplicated, febrile, influenza-like illness; hemorrhagic fever; or neurologic involvement with encephalitis, which carries a mortality rate of 1%. The virus was first identified in 1931 in the Rift Valley of Kenya and has caused several major outbreaks in Kenya (1950), Egypt (1977), and most recently Saudi Arabia (2000).

Ocular disease has been reported to occur in up to 20% of individuals with RVF, with visual symptoms appearing within 2 weeks of disease onset. Bilateral macular or paramacular retinitis was identified in all affected eyes at the time of initial assessment during the most recent outbreak in Saudi Arabia (Fig 7-18). Additional posterior segment manifestations included intraretinal hemorrhages (40%), vitritis (26%), optic nerve edema (15%), and retinal vasculitis (7%); an anterior uveitis was observed in 31% of patients. FA revealed delayed filling of the retinal and choroidal circulation with early hypofluorescence and late staining of the inflammatory retinal lesions. Spontaneous resolution of RVF retinitis, retinal hemorrhages, and vitritis was observed within 10–12 weeks, leaving in its wake optic atrophy, ischemic retina, and attenuated, occluded retinal vessels. Although glaucoma, posterior synechiae, and cataract were uncommon complications,

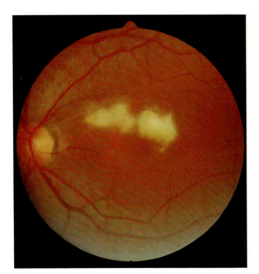

Figure 7-18 Rift Valley fever. Fundus photograph of a 44-year-old male farmer from Saudi Arabia presenting with decreased vision and macular retinitis sparing the fovea following a history of fever and contact with animal abortus. *(Courtesy of Albert T. Vitale, MD.)*

macular (60%) or paramacular (9%) scarring, vascular occlusion (23%), and optic atrophy (20%) were important causes of ocular morbidity and permanent visual loss. Visual acuity was profoundly reduced at presentation (less than 20/200 in 80% of affected eyes); vision remained the same or deteriorated in 87%.

The diagnosis of RVF is made both clinically and serologically, with the demonstration of antibodies, either IgM in a single serum sample or by a rising IgG titer in samples from acutely ill and convalescent patients. The RVF virus may be isolated from the blood in the acute phase of the illness or detected in either serum or tissue by reverse transcription PCR.

The differential diagnosis includes other viral entities such as measles, rubella, influenza, dengue fever, and WNV infection as well as bacterial illnesses such as brucellosis, Lyme disease, toxoplasmosis, cat-scratch disease, and rickettsial diseases. In most instances, these diseases can be differentiated from RVF by clinical history and serologic testing.

Treatment of systemic disease consists of general supportive therapy, as most cases of RVF are relatively mild and of short duration. For those patients developing encephalitis or hemorrhagic fever, early recognition and aggressive critical care support are essential to reduce mortality. While topical steroids may be helpful in the treatment of anterior uveitis, the role of systemic antiviral and anti-inflammatory therapy for the retinal manifestations of RVF is unknown. An inactivated vaccine has been developed for human use, but it is at present neither licensed nor commercially available. Public health measures including mosquito control, increased disease awareness among residents and visitors to endemic areas, and education regarding modes of disease transmission are essential for the control and prevention of RVF outbreaks.

Al-Hazmi A, Al-Rajhi AA, Abboud EB, et al. Ocular complications of Rift Valley fever outbreak in Saudi Arabia. *Ophthalmology.* 2005;112(2):313–318.

Human T-Cell Lymphotropic Virus Type 1

Human T-cell lymphotropic virus type 1 (HTLV-1), a retrovirus of the Oncovirinae subfamily, is endemic in Japan, the Caribbean islands, and parts of Central and South America; it accounts for approximately 1% of uveitis cases in Japan. It is transmitted transplacentally, by sexual contact and blood transfusion, and through breast feeding. The diagnosis of HTLV-1 infection is made by serologic testing with confirmatory Western blot analysis. Molecular analysis of selected tissue specimens for HTLV-1–related disease employing microdissection and PCR may be diagnostic in selected cases.

As with HIV, the major target cell of HTLV-1 is the CD4$^+$ T cell. HTLV-1 infection is the established cause of adult T-cell leukemia/lymphoma (ATL), HTLV-1–associated myelopathy/tropical spastic paralysis (HAM/TSP), and HTLV-1 uveitis (HU), defined as uveitis of undetermined origin in an HTLV-1 carrier. Additional ocular manifestations of HTLV-1 infection include retinal infiltrates caused by secondary ATL, retinal degeneration, optic neuropathy, and keratopathy, as well as keratoconjunctivitis sicca in patients with HAM/TSP.

Most cases of HU (75%) are classified anatomically as an intermediate uveitis. Women are affected more often than men, although the mean age of onset is earlier in men (35 years) than women (48 years). Patients present with blurred vision and floaters caused by a mild granulomatous anterior uveitis (20%), unilateral vitritis (60%), membranous vitreous opacities, or snowballs. Retinal vasculitis (60%), exudative retinal lesions (25%), optic disc abnormalities (20%), and CME (3%) may also be observed. Retinal vasculitis noted clinically and on FA is a salient feature of HU and is exquisitely responsive to corticosteroid therapy. For cases that progress despite adequate therapy, the clinician must consider a masquerade syndrome, as both retinal infiltration caused by ATL and retinal degeneration associated with HAM/TSP have been shown to mimic HU. This underscores the importance of including HTLV-1 infection in the differential diagnosis of retinal vasculitis, particularly in patients from endemic areas. ICG angiography of patients with HU suggests choroidal inflammatory involvement in addition to retinal vasculitis. HTLV-1–associated keratopathy is a newly described finding in Brazilian and Caribbean patients with HTLV-1 infection but has not been found among Japanese patients. Previously referred to as *HTLV-1–related chronic interstitial keratitis*, these corneal lesions are uniformly asymptomatic and do not affect vision. They result most likely from asymptomatic lymphoplasmacytic infiltrates.

While many cases of HU respond to topical, periocular, or systemic steroid therapy and resolve completely within 1–2 months, up to one-half of patients experience recurrent disease. HU can be associated with sight-threatening ocular complications including cataract and epiretinal membrane formation, glaucoma, persistent vitreous opacification, retinal vascular occlusion, retinochoroidal degeneration, and optic atrophy; these complications may occur in up to one-third of cases, with poor visual outcomes in up to 10% of affected eyes.

Buggage RR. Ocular manifestations of human T-cell lymphotropic virus type 1 infection. *Curr Opin Ophthalmol.* 2003;14(6):420–425.

Goto H, Mochizuki M, Yamaki K, Kotake S, et al. Epidemiological survey of intraocular inflammation in Japan. *Jpn J Ophthalmol.* 2007;51(1):41–44.

Dengue Fever

Dengue fever is the most common mosquito-borne viral disease in humans, caused by a member of the Flaviviridae family and transmitted by the *Aedes aegypti* mosquito. It is endemic to more than 100 countries in the tropical and subtropical regions of the globe, affecting predominantly young individuals (age range 11–61 years) with no sex predilection. Systemic signs and symptoms include fever, headache, myalgia, purpuric rash, and other bleeding manifestations secondary to thrombocytopenia. The most common ocular manifestation is petechial subconjunctival hemorrhage, although a maculopathy involving both the retinal and choroidal vessels may develop in approximately 10% of patients 1 month after the onset of systemic disease, presenting with a sudden decrease in vision and central scotoma. The maculopathy associated with dengue fever is bilateral (73%), albeit asymmetric, with a mean best-corrected visual acuity of 20/40 in the affected eye. Intraretinal hemorrhages, usually in combination with periphlebitis, are seen most frequently (45%), followed by yellow subretinal dots (28%), RPE mottling (17%), fovealitis (16%), disc hyperemia (14%) and edema (11%), and arteriolar sheathing (4%). A variable degree of anterior and vitreous cells are also observed. FA demonstrates venous occlusive disease in 25% of eyes as well as arteriolar and/or venular leakage; ICG angiography reveals more numerous hypofluorescent spots corresponding to yellow subretinal lesions not visualized by FA or seen on clinical examination. Optical coherence tomography (OCT) is valuable in identifying fovealitis as the cause of decreased visual acuity in eyes with no apparent lesions on examination and is helpful for monitoring clinical progress. The diagnosis is made based on observation of the typical clinical findings together with serology results positive for dengue IgM. Although topical, periocular, and systemic steroids and immunoglobulins have been employed with variable success, the optimal treatment modality is unknown as the disease may be self-limiting.

Bacsal K, Chee S-P, Cheng C-L, Flores JVP. Dengue-associated maculopathy. *Arch Ophthalmol.* 2007;125(4):501–510.

Chikungunya Fever

Chikungunya fever is a potentially fatal illness that resembles dengue fever, caused by an arthropod-borne *Alphavirus* in the family Togaviridae. In addition to fever, patients present with headache, fatigue, nausea, vomiting, myalgia, arthralgia, and skin rash. The ocular manifestations in a 2006 epidemic in India have been reported and included iridocyclitis and retinitis most commonly and nodular episcleritis less frequently, each with a typically benign course. The bilateral anterior uveitis may be granulomatous or nongranulomatous and associated with diffuse pigmented KPs, iris pigment release, elevated IOP, and, infrequently, posterior synechiae. Chikungunya retinitis may resemble herpetic retinitis in an immunocompetent host, in that both appear several weeks after the primary illness; however, the former is characterized by focal, multifocal, or confluent retinochoroiditis in the posterior pole with retinal hemorrhage, edema, and minimal vitritis in contrast to peripheral retinal involvement and more intense vitreous reaction in the latter.

The diagnosis is suggested when individuals from endemic areas present with a history of fever and arthralgia as well as anterior uveitis with pigmented KPs or posterior pole retinochoroiditis or neuroretinitis. Diagnosis may be confirmed serologically by the demonstration of Chikungunya-specific IgM antibodies, virus isolation, or reverse transcription PCR. Although confluent retinitis has been treated with systemic acyclovir and prednisone, there is no evidence to suggest that this improves visual outcome or affects the clinical course. Topical steroids and antihypertensive agents are useful in the treatment of anterior uveitis and elevated intraocular pressure.

Mahendradas P, Ranganna SK, Shetty R, et al. Ocular manifestations associated with Chikungunya. *Ophthalmology.* 2008;115(2):287–291.

Other Viral Diseases

Acute iritis may occur with other viral infectious entities. The iritis seen in influenza, adenovirus infection, and IM is mild and transient. Synechiae and ocular damage seldom occur. Iritis associated with adenovirus infection is usually secondary to corneal disease (see BCSC Section 8, *External Disease and Cornea*).

Fungal Uveitis

Ocular Histoplasmosis Syndrome

Ocular histoplasmosis syndrome (OHS) is a multifocal chorioretinitis presumed to be caused by infection with *Histoplasma capsulatum,* a dimorphic fungus with both yeast and filamentous forms early in life. The yeast form is the cause of both systemic and ocular disease; primary infection occurs after inhalation of the fungal spores into the lungs. Ocular disease is thought to arise as a consequence of hematogenous dissemination of the organism to the spleen, liver, and choroid following the initial pulmonary infection. Acquired histoplasmosis is usually asymptomatic or may result in a benign illness, typically during childhood.

OHS is most frequently found in endemic areas of the United States such as the Ohio and Mississippi River valleys, where 60% of individuals react positively to histoplasmin skin testing. However, OHS has also been reported in nonendemic areas in this country (Maryland) and sporadically throughout Europe (the United Kingdom and Netherlands). Although no serologic confirmation of histoplasmosis infection in patients with OHS has been reported, a causal relationship is strongly suggested by epidemiologic evidence linking an increased prevalence of ocular disease among patients who live or formerly resided in endemic areas. Furthermore, *H capsulatum* DNA has been detected in chronic choroidal lesions of a patient with OHS, and individuals with disciform scars are more likely than control subjects to react positively to histoplasmin skin testing. Men and women are affected equally, and the vast majority of patients are of northern European extraction.

The diagnosis of OHS is based on the clinical triad of multiple white, atrophic choroidal scars (so-called *histo spots*); peripapillary pigment changes; and a maculopathy caused by CNV in the absence of vitreous cells. Histo spots may appear in the macula or periphery, are discrete and punched out (arising from a variable degree of scarring in the choroid and adjacent outer retina), and are typically asymptomatic (Fig 7-19). Approximately 1.5% of patients from endemic areas exhibit typical peripheral histo spots, first appearing during adolescence. Linear equatorial streaks can be seen in 5% of patients (Fig 7-20). In contrast, metamorphopsia and a profound reduction in central vision herald macular involvement from CNV and bring the patient to the attention of the ophthalmologist. The mean age of patients presenting with vision-threatening maculopathy is 41 years. Funduscopy of active neovascular lesions reveals a yellow-green subretinal membrane typically surrounded by a pigment ring; overlying neurosensory detachment; and subretinal hemorrhage, frequently arising at the border of a histo scar in the disc–macula area. Cicatricial changes characterize advanced disease, with subretinal fibrosis and disciform scarring of the macula.

The pathogenesis of OHS is thought to involve a focal infection of the choroid at the time of initial systemic infection. This choroiditis may subside and leave an atrophic scar and depigmentation of the RPE, or it may result in disruption of the Bruch membrane, choriocapillaris, and RPE, with subsequent proliferation of subretinal vessels originating from the choroid. Lacking tight junctions, these neovascular complexes leak fluid, lipid,

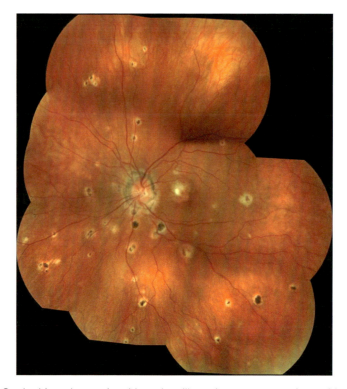

Figure 7-19 Ocular histoplasmosis with peripapillary pigmentary scarring, midperipheral chorioretinal scars (some pigmented and fibrotic), and spontaneously regressed nasal juxtafoveal choroidal neovascular membrane in the absence of vitreous cells. Visual acuity: 20/25. *(Courtesy of Ramana S. Moorthy, MD.)*

Figure 7-20 Ocular histoplasmosis: linear equatorial streaks. *(Courtesy of E. Mitchel Opremcak, MD.)*

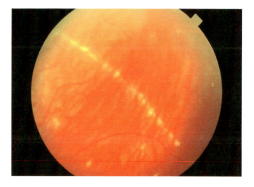

and blood, resulting in loss of macular function. The initiating stimulus for the growth of new subretinal vessels is unknown; however, immune mechanisms in patients with an underlying genetic predisposition for the development of this disease have been implicated. HLA-DRw2 is twice as common among patients with histo spots alone, whereas both HLA-B7 and HLA-DRw2 are 2 to 4 times more common among patients with disciform scars caused by OHS as compared to control subjects. Similarly, HLA-DR2 was absent in a group of patients with MCP, a disease that simulates OHS in many respects, whereas the antigen was present among those with CNV due to OHS.

The differential diagnosis includes entities other than age-related macular degeneration (AMD) that are frequently associated with CNV, including angioid streaks, choroidal rupture, idiopathic CNV, MCP, punctate inner choroidopathy, and granulomatous fundus lesions that may mimic the scarring seen in OHS (as in toxoplasmosis, tuberculosis, coccidioidomycosis, syphilis, sarcoidosis, and toxocariasis). The atrophic spots and maculopathy of myopic degeneration and disciform scarring in AMD may also be confused with OHS.

Over time, new choroidal scars develop in more than 20% of patients; however, only 3.8% of these progress to CNV. If histo spots appear in the macular area, the patient has a 25% chance of developing maculopathy within 3 years; if no spots are observed, the chances fall to 2%. The risk of developing CNV in the contralateral eye is high, ranging from 8% to 24% over a 3-year period. Massive subretinal exudation and hemorrhagic retinal detachments may occur and result in permanent loss of macular function. Although some cases of spontaneous resolution with a return to normal vision have been reported, the visual prognosis of untreated OHS-associated CNV is poor, with 75% of eyes reaching a final visual acuity of 20/100 or worse over a 3-year period.

The early, acute granulomatous lesions of OHS are rarely observed but may be treated with oral or regional (periocular) corticosteroids (Fig 7-21). In the early stages of FA, foci of active choroiditis block the dye and appear hypofluorescent; later in the study, these lesions stain, becoming hyperfluorescent. In contrast, areas of active CNV appear hyperfluorescent early in the angiogram and leak later in the study. Choroidal neovascular membranes may arise outside the vascular arcades, but typically do not reduce vision and may be safely managed with observation only. Treatment options for vision-threatening juxtafoveal or subfoveal CNV include thermal laser photocoagulation (Fig 7-22), photodynamic therapy (PDT) using verteporfin with or without intravitreal triamcinolone, submacular surgery for membrane removal, and intravitreal injection of anti–vascular endothelial growth factor (anti-VEGF) agents.

The Macular Photocoagulation Study (MPS) group conducted 2 multicenter, randomized, controlled clinical trials that showed a beneficial effect of argon blue-green and

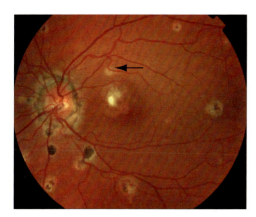

Figure 7-21 Ocular histoplasmosis: macular choroiditis *(arrow)* with multiple yellow elevated lesions. *(Courtesy of Ramana S. Moorthy, MD.)*

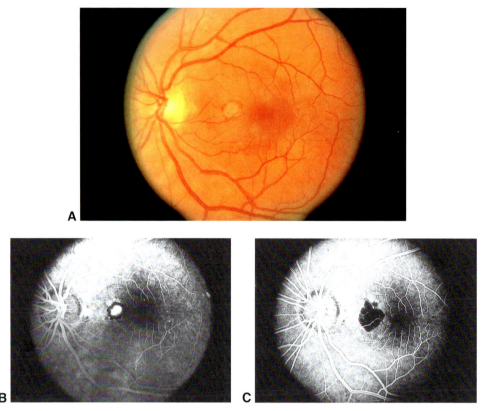

Figure 7-22 Ocular histoplasmosis. **A,** Extrafoveal subretinal neovascularization. **B,** Fluorescein angiogram of an extrafoveal subretinal neovascular membrane. **C,** Fluorescein angiogram of a subretinal neovascular membrane following laser photocoagulation. *(Courtesy of E. Mitchel Opremcak, MD.)*

krypton red laser photocoagulation for well-defined, classic extrafoveal, juxtafoveal, and peripapillary CNV secondary to OHS (see Fig 7-22). (See BCSC 12, *Retina and Vitreous,* Chapter 4.) The proportion of eyes experiencing severe visual loss was significantly reduced with photocoagulation. Disease progression was seen in 12% of treated individuals compared with 42% of control patients. A high rate of persistent or recurrent CNV was observed following photocoagulation, in 26% of extrafoveal and in 33% of juxtafoveal lesions. Thermal laser photocoagulation is not used in the treatment of subfoveal CNV in the context of OHS, given the profound and immediate loss of central vision that results from the destructive effects of this modality.

PDT with verteporfin has been advocated for the treatment of subfoveal OHS-associated CNV based on small, prospective, uncontrolled case series. The Verteporfin in Ocular Histoplasmosis study reported that after 2 years, 45% of patients experienced moderate visual gain and 82% avoided visual loss, with an increase in the median contrast sensitivity score of 3.5 letters. There were no serious adverse events. Moreover, at 48 months, 60% of patients gained ≥7 letters from baseline while only 7% lost >15 letters.

Similarly, intravitreal triamcinolone was shown to be relatively safe and effective in the management of OHS-associated juxtafoveal and subfoveal CNV in small retrospective case studies.

A number of anti-VEGF agents currently being used in the management of neovascular AMD are available for the off-label treatment of OHS-associated CNV. These include the ribonucleic acid aptamer pegaptanib; ranibizumab, the active fragment of a humanized anti-VEGF monoclonal antibody; and the related full-length molecule, bevacizumab. Intravitreal anti-VEGF therapy has been shown to be superior to PDT in patients with neovascular AMD in visual acuity outcome, but no such randomized, prospective study comparing these modalities has been conducted in OHS-associated CNV. A recent retrospective study of 24 eyes with OHS-associated CNV treated with intravitreal bevacizumab monotherapy demonstrated that at least 50% of eyes with subfoveal or juxtafoveal CNV experienced ≥3 lines of visual gain and up to 100% patients had improved or stable visual acuity after 3–12 months of follow-up. Final visual acuity was 20/40 or better in 58% of eyes, compared with 21% at baseline. As with neovascular AMD, combination approaches with PDT and intravitreal corticosteroids or anti-VEGF agents may prove fruitful, especially in treating entities with an underlying inflammatory etiology.

Selected patients with an active subretinal neovascular membrane located under the foveal avascular zone may benefit from submacular surgery and removal of the membrane (Fig 7-23). However, although short-term visual outcomes were initially encouraging, longer follow-up and the subsequent publication of the Submacular Surgery Trials (SST) Group H results showing CNV recurrence rates approaching 50% within the first 12 months have muted the enthusiasm for this approach. While the study indicated that surgery may be of benefit for patients with a visual acuity worse than 20/100, a clear recommendation for surgery even for this subgroup may be overshadowed by the not-infrequent occurrence of complications, including intraoperative retinal breaks (12.5% peripheral and 2% posterior pole), cataract (39%), and retinal detachment (4.5%). In selected cases of extensive peripapillary CNV associated with OHS, surgical removal may provide a more definitive visual benefit with low recurrence rates and be preferable to

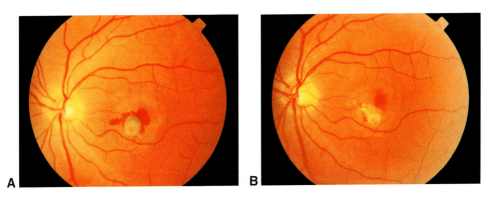

Figure 7-23 Ocular histoplasmosis. **A,** Subfoveal neovascularization. **B,** Subfoveal neovascular membrane following submacular surgical removal. *(Courtesy of E. Mitchel Opremcak, MD.)*

photoablation, given the likelihood of multiple PDT and anti-VEGF treatments. Thermal laser photocoagulation, PDT, anti-VEGF agents, intravitreal corticosteroids, and submacular surgery for the treatment of CNV are discussed in greater detail in BCSC Section 12, *Retina and Vitreous.*

For a discussion of the ocular manifestations of candidiasis, aspergillosis, cryptococcosis, and coccidioidomycosis and their treatments, please see Chapter 8.

Almony A, Thomas MA, Atebara NH, Holekamp NM, Del Priore LV. Long-term follow-up of surgical removal of extensive peripapillary choroidal neovascularization in presumed ocular histoplasmosis syndrome. *Ophthalmology.* 2008;115(3):540–545.

Brown DM, Kaiser PK, Michels M, et al, for the ANCHOR Study Group. Ranibizumab versus verteporfin for neovascular age-related macular degeneration. *N Eng J Med.* 2006;355(14):1432–1444.

Ehrlich R, Ciulla TA, Maturi R, et al. Intravitreal bevacizumab for choroidal neovascularization secondary to presumed ocular histoplasmosis syndrome. *Retina.* 2009;29(10):1418–1423.

Hawkins BS, Bressler NM, Bressler SB, et al. Surgical removal vs observation for subfoveal choroidal neovascularization, either associated with the ocular histoplasmosis syndrome or idiopathic: I. Ophthalmic findings from a randomized clinical trial. Submacular Surgery Trials (SST) Group H trial. SST: report no. 9. *Arch Ophthalmol.* 2004;122(11):1597–1612.

Macular Photocoagulation Study Group. Five-year follow-up of fellow eyes of individuals with ocular histoplasmosis and unilateral extrafoveal or juxtafoveal choroidal neovascularization. *Arch Ophthalmol.* 1996;114(6):677–688.

Rechtman E, Allen VD, Danis RP, Pratt LM, Harris A, Speicher MA. Intravitreal triamcinolone for choroidal neovascularization in ocular histoplasmosis syndrome. *Am J Ophthalmol.* 2003;136(4):739–741.

Rosenfeld PJ, Saperstein DA, Bressler NM, et al. Photodynamic therapy with verteporfin in ocular histoplasmosis: uncontrolled, open-label 2-year study. *Ophthalmology.* 2004;111(9):1725–1733.

Saperstein DA, Rosenfeld PJ, Bressler NM, Rosa RH, et al. Verteporfin therapy for CNV secondary to OHS. *Ophthalmology.* 2006;113(12):2371.e1-3.

Spencer WH, Chan C-C, Shen DF, Rao NA. Detection of *Histoplasma capsulatum* DNA in lesions of chronic ocular histoplasmosis syndrome. *Arch Ophthalmol.* 2003;121(11):1551–1555.

Protozoal Uveitis

Toxoplasmosis

Toxoplasmosis is the most common cause of infectious retinochoroiditis in both adults and children. It is caused by the parasite *Toxoplasma gondii,* a single-cell obligate intracellular protozoan parasite with a worldwide distribution (Fig 7-24). Cats are the definitive hosts of *T gondii,* and humans and a variety of other animals serve as intermediate hosts. *T gondii* has a complex life cycle and exists in 3 major forms:

- the oocyst, or soil form (10–12 µm)
- the tachyzoite, or infectious form (4–8 µm; Fig 7-25)
- the tissue cyst, or latent form (10–200 µm), which contains as many as 3000 bradyzoites

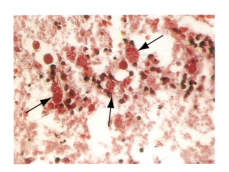

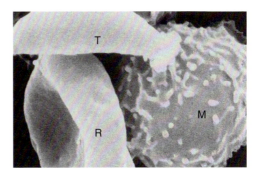

Figure 7-24 *Toxoplasma gondii,* histologic view. Note the cysts *(arrows)* in the necrotic retina.

Figure 7-25 Scanning electron microscope view of toxoplasmal tachyzoite *(T)* parasitizing a macrophage *(M)* while a red blood cell *(R)* looks on. *(Courtesy of John D. Sheppard, Jr, MD.)*

Transmission of *T gondii* to humans and other animals may occur with all 3 forms of the parasite through a variety of vectors. The oocysts, which reproduce sexually and are found uniquely in the intestinal mucosa of cats, are shed in infected cats' feces in large numbers, contaminating the environment, where they undergo a sporulation process. These oocysts may then be ingested by the intermediate hosts or reingested by cats. Tachyzoites are found in the circulatory system and may invade nearly all host tissue; however, in the immunocompetent host, the replication of tachyzoites eventually ceases and most organisms are removed, although a small number remain as dormant bradyzoites within intercellular tissue cysts.

Recent studies have identified 3 distinct clonal lineages of *T gondii* in humans and in animals that vary in their virulence but are antigenically similar. These 3 genotypes, designated types I, II, and III, plus recombinant or atypical genotypes, can be distinguished serologically. Most human infections in North America and Europe have been attributed to type II parasites, which are less virulent than type I parasites and the atypical genotypes in animal models. In the United States, the prevalence of *T gondii* infection is 22.5% among the general population, whereas that of ocular toxoplasmosis among infected persons is estimated to be only 2%. In sharp contrast, an estimated 85% of the population in southern Brazil is infected with *T gondii,* and approximately 18% of these individuals manifest evidence of retinochoroiditis. Recent studies have demonstrated a greater heterogeneity of parasites in Brazil than in North America. It is postulated that variance in disease severity and ocular involvement in different regions around the world seen in both acquired and congenital infections may be due to genotypic differences of the infecting parasite, with more severe disease and higher rates of ocular involvement related to the presence of type I alleles or atypical genotypes.

Human infection by *T gondii* may be either acquired or congenital. The principal modes of transmission include:

- ingestion of undercooked, infected meat containing *Toxoplasma* cysts; contaminated water, fruit, or vegetables; or unpasteurized goat milk from a chronically infected animal

- inadvertent contact with cat feces, cat litter, or soil containing oocysts
- transplacental transmission with primary infection during pregnancy
- introduction of tachyzoites through a break in the skin
- blood transfusion or organ transplantation

At least a dozen outbreaks of toxoplasmosis have been reported from around the world in the past 40 years. Five of the more recent epidemics occurring between 1979 and 2003 have been well studied, and contaminated water supplies or inhaled/ingested sporulated oocysts in dirt have been implicated as the source of infection. Moreover, the rate of ocular involvement in these outbreaks was disproportionately high, which may be attributable to the genotype of the infecting parasite and possibly host immunologic or genetic factors.

The reported seropositivity rates among healthy adults vary considerably throughout the world, ranging from 3% to 10.8% in the United States to between 50% and 80% in France. Among patients with HIV infection in the United States, the reported seropreva-lence of *T gondii* varies from 15% to 40%.

It has been estimated that between 70% and 80% of women of childbearing age in the United States lack antibodies to *T gondii,* which places them at risk for contracting the disease; however, the incidence of toxoplasmosis acquired during pregnancy is only 0.2%–1%. In southern Brazil, where the prevalence of toxoplasmosis is extremely high, the prevalence of congenital infection was recently reported at 1/770 births, with a cor-respondingly high prevalence of ocular involvement. Overall, 40% of primary maternal infections result in congenital infection; transplacental transmission is greatest during the third trimester. The risk of severe disease developing in the fetus is inversely proportional to gestational age: disease acquired early in pregnancy often results in spontaneous abor-tion, stillbirth, or severe congenital disease, whereas that acquired later in gestation may produce an asymptomatic, normal-appearing infant with latent infection. Chronic or re-current maternal infection during pregnancy is not thought to confer a risk of congenital toxoplasmosis because maternal immunity protects against fetal transmission. Pregnant women without serologic evidence of prior exposure to the *T gondii* should take sanitary precautions when cleaning up after cats and avoid undercooked meats.

The classic presentation of congenital toxoplasmosis includes retinochoroiditis, hy-drocephalus, and intracranial calcification. Retinochoroiditis, which occurs in up to 80% of cases, is the most common abnormality in patients with congenital infections and is bilateral in approximately 85% of affected individuals, with a predilection for the posterior pole and macula (Fig 7-26). In children with mild infection, posterior segment involve-ment may be subclinical and chronic, and as many as 85% develop chorioretinitis after a mean of 3.7 years, with 25% of these becoming blind in 1 or both eyes. It is now the standard of care to treat newborns with toxoplasmosis with antiparasitic therapy for the first year of life to reduce the rate and severity of ocular involvement. BCSC Section 6, *Pediatric Ophthalmology and Strabismus,* discusses maternal transmission and congenital toxoplasmosis in greater detail.

Although toxoplasmosis after infancy was once considered to be exclusively the result of reactivation of congenital disease, acquired infection is now thought to play an impor-tant role in the development of ocular toxoplasmosis in children and adults. In 1 study,

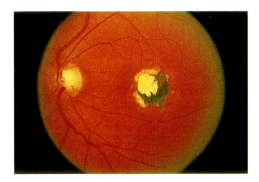

Figure 7-26 Congenital quiescent, mature, hyperpigmented toxoplasmal macular scar. Patient has 20/400 acuity. *(Courtesy of John D. Sheppard, Jr, MD.)*

acquired postnatal infection was thought to represent up to two-thirds of cases of toxo-plasmic ocular disease. A recent report of epidemic toxoplasmosis from India confirmed previous observations suggesting that postnatally acquired *T gondii* infection occurs in all age groups, including children, and that ocular disease can arise after infection with-out concurrent systemic signs or symptoms. This has significant public health implica-tions with respect to primary prevention strategies, which must target not only pregnant women but also children and adults at risk for acquiring the disease. In the United States, previous studies indicated that toxoplasmosis may account for up to 38% of all cases of posterior uveitis, although this figure appears to be decreasing and varies with geography and referral bias.

Presenting symptoms, although dependent on the location of the lesion, frequently include unilateral blurred or hazy vision and floaters. A mild to moderate granulomatous anterior uveitis is frequently observed, and up to 20% of patients have acutely elevated IOP at presentation. Classically, ocular toxoplasmosis appears as a focal, white retinitis with overlying moderate vitreous inflammation ("headlight in the fog"), often adjacent to a pigmented chorioretinal scar (Figs 7-27, 7-28). These lesions occur more commonly in the posterior pole but may occasionally be seen immediately adjacent to or directly involving the optic nerve; they are sometimes mistaken for optic papillitis. Retinal vessels in the vicinity of an active lesion may show perivasculitis with diffuse venous sheathing and segmental arterial sheathing (Kyrieleis arteriolitis). Additional ocular complications

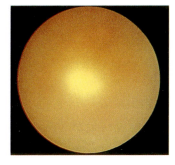

Figure 7-27 Toxoplasmic retinochoroiditis: "headlight in the fog."

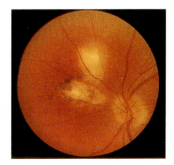

Figure 7-28 Toxoplasmosis: satellite retinitis around old scar.

include cataract, CME, serous retinal detachment, and CNV (Fig 7-29). Focal retinitis in the absence of chorioretinal scarring should raise the suspicion of acquired disease or another cause for the necrotizing retinitis (Fig 7-30). Retinochoroiditis developing in immunocompromised and older patients may present with atypical findings, including large, multiple, and/or bilateral lesions, with or without associated chorioretinal scars. Other atypical presentations include unilateral neuroretinitis, punctate outer retinal toxoplasmosis (PORT), unilateral pigmentary retinopathy simulating retinitis pigmentosa, scleritis, rhegmatogenous and serous retinal detachments, retinal vascular occlusions, and a presentation in association with Fuchs uveitis syndrome. PORT is characterized by small, multifocal lesions at the level of the deep retina with scant overlying vitreous inflammation (Fig 7-31).

Diagnosis

In most instances, the diagnosis of toxoplasmic retinochoroiditis is made clinically, on the basis of the appearance of the characteristic lesion on indirect ophthalmoscopy. Serologic evaluation using indirect fluorescent antibody and ELISA tests to detect specific anti–*T gondii* antibodies is commonly used to confirm exposure to the parasite. IgG antibodies appear within the first 2 weeks after infection; typically remain detectable for life, albeit at low levels; and may cross the placenta. IgM antibodies, however, rise early during the acute phase of the infection, typically remain detectable for less than 1 year, and do not cross the placenta. The presence of anti–*T gondii* IgG antibodies supports the diagnosis of toxoplasmic retinochoroiditis in the appropriate clinical context, whereas a negative antibody titer essentially rules out the diagnosis. The presence of IgM in newborns confirms congenital infection and is indicative of acquired disease when present in adults. Measurement of IgA antibody titers may also be useful in a diagnosis of congenital toxoplasmosis in a fetus or newborn, because IgM production is often weak during this period and the presence of IgG antibodies may indicate passive transfer of maternal antibodies in utero. IgA antibodies, however, usually disappear by 7 months. Intraocular production of

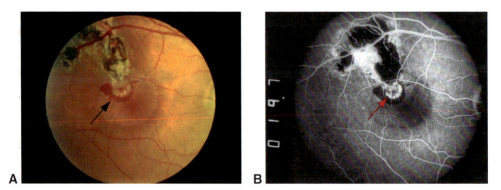

Figure 7-29 Toxoplasmic retinochoroiditis–associated choroidal neovascularization. **A,** Fundus photograph showing a choroidal neovascular membrane (CNVM) with intraretinal hemorrhage and subretinal fluid adjacent to an old toxoplasmic scar *(arrow)*. **B,** Early-phase fluorescein angiogram showing blocked fluorescence associated with scar and lacy hyperfluorescence that corresponds to CNVM *(arrow)*. *(Courtesy of Albert T. Vitale, MD.)*

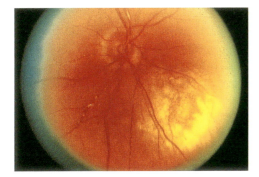

Figure 7-30 Recently acquired large, non-pigmented, inactive toxoplasmal retinal scar. *(Courtesy of John D. Sheppard, Jr, MD.)*

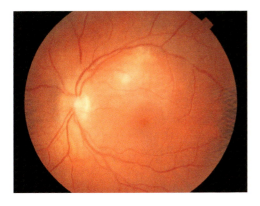

Figure 7-31 Punctate outer retinal toxoplasmosis (PORT). *(Courtesy of E. Mitchel Opremcak, MD.)*

specific anti-*Toxoplasma* antibodies may be computed using the GW coefficient. A ratio of greater than 3 is considered diagnostic of local antibody production. More recently, highly sensitive and specific PCR-based techniques have been used to detect *T gondii* DNA in both the aqueous humor and vitreous fluid of patients with ocular toxoplasmosis; these techniques are of particular value in cases with atypical presentations.

Treatment

Ocular toxoplasmosis is a progressive and recurrent disease, with new lesions occurring at the margins of old scars as well as elsewhere in the fundus. In the immunocompetent patient, the disease has a self-limiting course; the borders of the lesions become sharper and less edematous over a 6- to 8-week period without treatment, and RPE hypertrophy occurs gradually over a period of months. In the immunocompromised patient, the disease tends to more severe and progressive. Treatment is aimed at shortening the duration of the parasitic replication, which leads to more rapid cicatrization of the lesions and thereby limits chorioretinal scarring and progression, reduces the frequency of inflammatory recurrences, and minimizes structural complications associated with intraocular inflammation.

Numerous agents have been used to treat toxoplasmosis over the years, but no single drug or combination can be applied categorically to every patient, and there is no consensus as to the most efficacious regimen. There is, in fact, little firm evidence that antimicrobial therapy alters the natural history of toxoplasmic retinochoroiditis in immunocompetent patients. In this setting, the decision to treat is influenced by the number, size, and location of the lesions relative to the macula and optic disc, as well as the severity and duration of the vitreous inflammation. Some clinicians may elect to observe small lesions in the retinal periphery that are not associated with a significant decrease in vision or vitritis; others treat virtually all patients in an effort to reduce the number of subsequent recurrences. Relative treatment indications include

- lesions threatening the optic nerve or fovea
- decreased visual acuity
- lesions associated with moderate to severe vitreous inflammation
- lesions greater than 1 disc diameter in size
- persistence of disease for more than 1 month
- the presence of multiple active lesions

Treatment is almost always indicated in immunocompromised patients (those with HIV/AIDS, neoplastic disease, or undergoing IMT), patients with congenital toxoplasmosis, and pregnant women with acquired disease.

The classic regimen for the treatment of ocular toxoplasmosis consists of triple therapy: pyrimethamine (loading dose: 50–100 mg; treatment dose: 25–50 mg/day), sulfadiazine (loading dose: 2–4 g; treatment dose: 1.0 g 4 times daily), and prednisone (treatment dose: 0.5–1.0 mg/kg/day, depending on the severity of the inflammation). Because sulfonamides and pyrimethamine inhibit folic acid metabolism, folinic acid (5 mg every other day) is added to try to prevent the leukopenia and thrombocytopenia that may result from the pyrimethamine therapy. Leukocyte and platelet counts should be monitored weekly. Potential side effects of sulfa compounds include skin rash, kidney stones, and Stevens-Johnson syndrome. Some clinicians advocate adding clindamycin (300 mg 4 times daily) to this regimen as "quadruple" therapy or in the instance of sulfa allergy. Clindamycin, either alone or in combination with other agents, has been effective in managing acute lesions, but pseudomembranous colitis is a potential complication of its use.

Systemic corticosteroids are generally begun either at the time of antimicrobial therapy or within 48 hours in immunocompetent patients. The use of systemic corticosteroids without appropriate antimicrobial cover or the use of long-acting periocular and intraocular corticosteroid formulations such as triamcinolone acetonide is contraindicated because of the potential for severe, uncontrollable intraocular inflammation and loss of the eye (Fig 7-32). Topical corticosteroids, however, are used liberally in the presence of prominent anterior segment inflammation. In general, treatment lasts from 4 to 6 weeks, at which time inflammation begins to subside and the retinal lesion shows signs of consolidation. This period may be extended if there is persistent disease activity.

Many ophthalmologists have begun to use trimethoprim-sulfamethoxazole (treatment dose: 160 mg/80 mg twice daily) and prednisone as an alternative to the classic therapy for reasons of cost, the frequent unavailability of sulfadiazine, and the presumption that trimethoprim-sulfamethoxazole has a better safety profile. However, a prospective randomized trial of trimethoprim-sulfamethoxazole versus pyrimethamine and sulfadiazine in the treatment of ocular toxoplasmosis showed no major differences in efficacy between the 2 regimens and did not convincingly demonstrate that trimethoprim-sulfamethoxazole

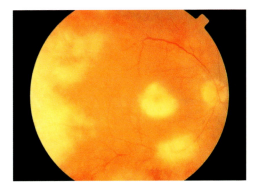

Figure 7-32 Toxoplasmosis: acute retinal necrosis following periocular corticosteroid injection. *(Courtesy of E. Mitchel Opremcak, MD.)*

had a superior safety profile. Azithromycin (250 mg/day) has been used successfully to treat ocular toxoplasmosis in immunocompetent patients alone and in combination with pyrimethamine (50 mg/day), demonstrating efficacy similar to that of the standard treatment of pyrimethamine and sulfadiazine. The treatment combination of azithromycin and pyrimethamine may be better tolerated and have fewer side effects.

Newborns with congenital toxoplasmosis are commonly treated with pyrimethamine and sulfonamides for 1 year, in consultation with a pediatric infectious disease specialist.

In cases of newly acquired toxoplasmosis during pregnancy, treatment is given to prevent infection of the fetus and to limit fetal damage if infection has already occurred, as well as to limit the destructive sequelae of intraocular disease in the mother. Spiramycin (treatment dose: 400 mg 3 times daily) may be used safely without undue risk of teratogenicity and may reduce the rate of tachyzoite transmission to the fetus. Because this agent is commonly unavailable in the United States, alternative medications may be needed; these include azithromycin, clindamycin, and atovaquone (treatment dose: 750 mg every 6 hours). Sulfonamides may be used safely in the first 2 trimesters of pregnancy. Alternatively, local treatment involving intraocular injections of clindamycin and short-acting periocular corticosteroids (eg, dexamethasone) has been advocated in pregnant women in an effort to reduce systemic side effects and the risk of teratogenicity.

Patients with HIV/AIDS require extended systemic treatment given the frequent association of ocular disease with cerebral involvement (56%) and the frequency of recurrent ocular disease when antitoxoplasmic medication is discontinued (Fig 7-33). The best

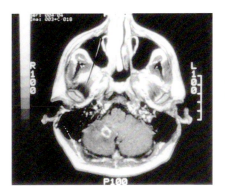

Figure 7-33 Central nervous system toxoplasmosis presenting with ataxia in a patient with AIDS: cerebellar lesion in enhanced computed tomography (CT) scan. *(Courtesy of John D. Sheppard, Jr, MD.)*

regimen for secondary prophylaxis remains to be determined; however, atovaquone acts synergistically with pyrimethamine and sulfadiazine and may be useful in reducing the dose and toxicity of these drugs in the treatment of patients with AIDS and toxoplasmosis. The management of ocular toxoplasmosis in association with HIV/AIDS is also covered in Chapter 11.

Long-term intermittent trimethoprim-sulfamethoxazole treatment (1 tablet taken every 3 days) was shown to decrease the risk of reactivation among patients with recurrent toxoplasmic retinochoroiditis observed for a 20-month period. A similar strategy may be useful as prophylaxis in patients with ocular toxoplasmosis and HIV/AIDS.

Similarly, the utility of prophylactic antimicrobial treatment shortly before and after intraocular surgery in patients with inactive toxoplasmic scars, particularly those that threaten the optic disc or fovea, was raised by a recent report describing an association between cataract surgery and an increased risk of reactivation of otherwise inactive toxoplasmic retinochoroiditis. There is, however, no consensus with respect to this treatment approach or to the optimal antibiotic regimen in this clinical situation.

Balasundaram MB, Andavar R, Palaniswamy M, Venkatapathy N. Outbreak of acquired ocular toxoplasmosis involving 248 patients. *Arch Ophthalmol.* 2010;128(1):28–32.

Bosch-Driessen LE, Berendschot TT, Ongkosuwito JV, Rothova A. Ocular toxoplasmosis: clinical features and prognosis of 154 patients. *Ophthalmology.* 2002;109(5):869–878.

Bosch-Driessen LH, Plaisier MB, Stilma JS, van der Lelij A, Rothova A. Reactivations of ocular toxoplasmosis after cataract extraction. *Ophthalmology.* 2002;109(1):41–45.

Grigg ME, Ganatra J, Boothroyd JC, Margolis TP. Unusual abundance of atypical strains associated with human ocular toxoplasmosis. *J Infect Dis.* 2001;184(5):633–639.

Holland GN. Ocular toxoplasmosis: a global reassessment. Part I: epidemiology and course of disease. *Am J Ophthalmol.* 2003;136(6):973–988.

Holland GN. Ocular toxoplasmosis: a global reassessment. Part II: disease manifestations and management. *Am J Ophthalmol.* 2004;137(1):1–17.

Khan A, Jordan C, Muccioli C, et al. Genetic divergence of *Toxoplasma gondii* strains associated with ocular toxoplasmosis, Brazil. *Emerg Infect Dis.* 2006;12(6):942–949.

Kishore K, Conway MD, Peyman GA. Intravitreal clindamycin and dexamethasone for toxoplasmic retinochoroiditis. *Ophthalmic Surg Lasers.* 2001;32(3):183–192.

Kump LI, Androudi SN, Foster CS. Ocular toxoplasmosis in pregnancy. *Clin Experiment Ophthalmol.* 2005;33(5):455–460.

Montoya JG, Parmley S, Liesenfeld O, Jaffe GJ, Remington JS. Use of the polymerase chain reaction for diagnosis of ocular toxoplasmosis. *Ophthalmology.* 1999;106(8):1554–1563.

Silveira C, Belfort R Jr, Muccioli C, et al. The effect of long-term intermittent trimethoprim/sulfamethoxazole treatment on recurrences of toxoplasmic retinochoroiditis. *Am J Ophthalmol.* 2002;134(1):41–46.

Smith JR, Cunningham ET Jr. Atypical presentations of ocular toxoplasmosis. *Curr Opin Ophthalmol.* 2002;13(6):387–392.

Soheilian M, Sadoughi MM, Ghajarnia M, et al. Prospective randomized trial of trimethoprim/sulfamethoxazole versus pyrimethamine and sulfadiazine in the treatment of ocular toxoplasmosis. *Ophthalmology.* 2005;112(11):1876–1882.

Stanford MR, See SE, Jones LV, Gilbert RE. Antibiotics for toxoplasmic retinochoroiditis: an evidence-based systematic review. *Ophthalmology.* 2003;110(5):926–931.

Library and eLearning Centre
Gartnavel General Hospital

Vasconcelos-Santos DV, Machado Azevedo DOM, Campos WR, et al, for the UFMG Congenital Toxoplasmosis Brazilian Group. Congenital toxoplasmosis in southeastern Brazil:
results of early ophthalmologic examination of a large cohort of neonates. *Ophthalmology.*
2009;116(11):2199–2205.

Helminthic Uveitis

Toxocariasis

Ocular toxocariasis is an uncommon disease of children and young adults that may produce significant visual loss. Non-Hispanic whites are affected most commonly; there is
no sexual predisposition. Its prevalence was recently estimated to be 1% of a large uveitic
population seen at tertiary care centers in northern California.

Human toxocariasis results from tissue invasion by the second-stage larvae of *Toxocara canis* or *Toxocara cati,* roundworm parasites that complete their life cycles in the
small intestines of dogs and cats, respectively. Transmission occurs through geophagia,
ingestion of contaminated food, or the oral-fecal route. Pica and contact with puppies or
kittens are common among children with toxocariasis. The organisms grow in the small
intestine, enter the portal circulation, disseminate throughout the body by hematogenous
and lymphatic routes, and ultimately reside in target tissues, including the eye. Maturation of the adult worm does not occur in humans; consequently, ova are not shed in the al-
imentary tract, rendering stool analysis for larvae unproductive. Ocular toxocariasis and
the systemic disease visceral larvae migrans (VLM) rarely present contemporaneously.
VLM typically affects children younger than age 3, possibly because of an increased rate
of pica among this group, whereas ocular toxocariasis is seen most often in older children
or young adults. Finally, there is a direct relationship between the degree of peripheral eosinophilia and the parasitic burden in the systemic disease but not in ocular toxocariasis.

Patients present with unilateral decreased vision that may be accompanied by pain,
photophobia, floaters, strabismus, or leukocoria. Bilateral disease is exceedingly rare. The
anterior segment is typically white and quiet. However, nongranulomatous anterior inflammation and posterior synechiae may be present with severe disease. Posterior segment findings include 3 recognizable ocular syndromes:

- leukocoria resulting from moderate to severe vitreous inflammation and chronic
  endophthalmitis: 25% of cases (Fig 7-34)
- localized macular granuloma: 25% of cases (Fig 7-35)
- peripheral granuloma: 50% of cases (Fig 7-36)

Uncommon variants include unilateral pars planitis with diffuse peripheral inflammatory exudates and granulomas involving the optic nerve. Table 7-2 lists the characteristics of each presentation.

Determinants of the visual prognosis are multifactorial and include the degree of intraocular inflammation and the location of the inflammatory foci with respect to the foveal
center; the presence or absence of CME; and the development of tractional membranes

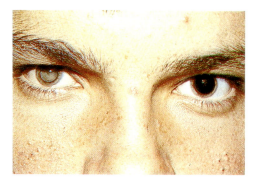

Figure 7-34 Toxocariasis: leukocoria.

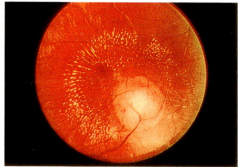

Figure 7-35 Toxocariasis: macular granuloma.

Figure 7-36 Toxocariasis: peripheral granuloma.

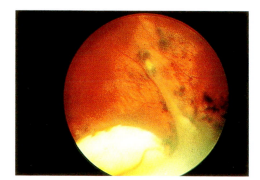

involving the optic nerve, macula, and ciliary body. In the absence of foveal involvement, vision at presentation is usually best when the granulomas are located in the posterior pole, as these eyes are less likely than those with peripheral granulomas to have macular traction. Eyes with endophthalmitis have the worst vision at presentation.

The diagnosis of ocular toxocariasis is essentially clinical, based on the characteristic lesion morphology, supportive laboratory data, and findings on imaging studies. The serum ELISA titer of 1:8 is 91% sensitive and 90% specific for prior exposure to the organism; however, any positive titer should be considered significant in the appropriate clinical context. On the other hand, the absence of serum antibodies does not rule out

Table 7-2 Ocular Toxocariasis

Syndrome	Age of Onset	Characteristic Lesion
Chronic endophthalmitis	2–9	Chronic unilateral uveitis, cloudy vitreous cyclitic membrane
Localized granuloma	6–14	Present in the macula and peripapillary region Solitary, white, elevated in the retina; minimal reaction; 1–2 disc diameters in size
Peripheral granuloma	6–40	Peripheral hemispheric masses with dense connective tissue strands in the vitreous cavity that may connect to the disc Rarely bilateral

the diagnosis. In these cases, examination of intraocular fluids with ELISA may reveal specific *T canis* antibodies and a positive GW coefficient, providing evidence of primary ocular involvement. *Toxocara* larvae have been recovered from the vitreous during pars plana vitrectomy (Fig 7-37). Finally, B-scan ultrasonography and computed tomography (CT) are useful in the presence of media opacity; they may reveal vitreous membranes and tractional retinal detachment and confirm the absence of calcium, a characteristic finding in retinoblastoma.

The most important differential diagnostic consideration is that of sporadic unilateral retinoblastoma. Factors that may be helpful in making this distinction include the distinctly younger age at presentation, the paucity of inflammatory stigmata, and the demonstration of lesion growth in children with retinoblastoma. Other differential diagnostic entities include infectious endophthalmitis, toxoplasmosis, and pars planitis, as well as congenital retinovascular abnormalities such as retinopathy of prematurity, persistent fetal vasculature, Coats disease, and familial exudative vitreoretinopathy.

Although there is no uniformly satisfactory treatment for ocular toxocariasis, medical therapy with periocular and systemic corticosteroids is aimed at reducing the inflammatory response in an effort to prevent structural complications. The utility of antihelminthic therapy has not been established. Vitreoretinal surgical techniques have been successfully used to manage tractional and rhegmatogenous complications. Laser photocoagulation of live, motile larvae may be considered if identified on clinical examination, and may be used to treat the rare occurrence of CNV arising in association with inactive *Toxocara* granulomas.

Stewart JM, Cubillan LD, Cunningham ET Jr. Prevalence, clinical features, and causes of vision loss among patients with ocular toxocariasis. *Retina.* 2005;25(8):1005–1013.

Cysticercosis

Cysticercosis is the most common ocular tapeworm infection; it occurs especially in underdeveloped areas where hygiene is poor. Human infection is caused by *Cysticercus cellulosae,* the larval stage of the cestode *Taenia solium,* which is endemic to Mexico, Africa, Southeast Asia, eastern Europe, Central and South America, and India. Although the eye is more commonly affected than any other organ, neural cysticercosis is associated with significant morbidity and a mortality of 40%.

Human cysticercosis is caused by ingestion of water or foods contaminated by the pork tapeworm. The eggs mature into larvae, penetrate the intestinal mucosa, and spread

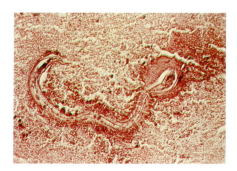

Figure 7-37 Toxocariasis: eosinophilic vitreous abscess. The organism is in the center of the abscess.

hematogenously to the eye via the posterior ciliary arteries into the subretinal space in the region of the posterior pole. Larvae within the subretinal space may cause an exudative retinal detachment or may perforate the retina, causing a retinal break that may or may not be self-sealing or associated with retinal detachment, and gain access to the vitreous cavity.

Ocular cysticercosis is a disorder of the young, occurring most frequently between the ages of 10 and 30 years, without sexual predilection. Although cysticercosis may involve any structure of the eye and its adnexae (orbit, eyelid, subconjunctiva, or anterior chamber), the posterior segment is involved most often, with the subretinal space harboring the parasite more often than the vitreous body. Depending on the location of the intraocular cyst, patients may present asymptomatically with relatively good vision or may complain of floaters, moving sensations, ocular pain, photophobia, redness, and very poor visual acuity. Epileptiform seizures may be the first sign of cerebral cysticercosis, occurring in patients with concomitant ocular involvement. Biomicroscopy of the anterior segment and vitreous body reveals variable degrees of inflammatory activity, with vitreous infiltration being most pronounced during the early stages of the disease. Larvae death produces a severe inflammatory reaction characterized by zonal granulomatous inflammation surrounding necrotic larvae on histologic examination.

Larvae may be seen in the vitreous or subretinal space in up to 46% of infected patients. The characteristic clinical appearance is that of a globular or spherical, translucent, white cyst with a head, or scolex, that undulates in response to the examining light within the vitreous or subretinal space. The cyst itself varies in size from 1.5 to 6 disc diameters. RPE atrophy may be observed surrounding the presumptive entry site of the cysticercus into the subretinal space; retinal detachment has been observed with high frequency in some series.

The characteristic appearance of a motile cysticercus in the anterior chamber, intravitreous, or subretinal space is pathognomonic (Figs 7-38, 7-39). Anticysticercus antibodies are detected by ELISA in approximately 50% and 80% of patients with ocular and neural cysticercosis, respectively. Anterior chamber paracentesis may reveal a large number of eosinophils; peripheral eosinophilia may also be present. If a patient is a definitive host, with an adult tapeworm in the gastrointestinal tract, stool examination may find the

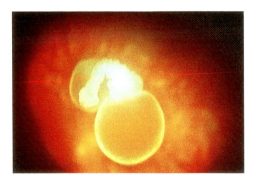

Figure 7-38 Intraocular cysticercus.

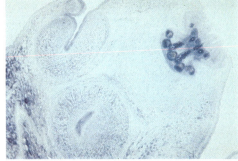

Figure 7-39 Pathology of cysticercus, showing the protoscolex, or head, of the larva.

eggs of *T solium*. B-scan ultrasonography may also be helpful diagnostically in the presence of intraocular cysticerci, revealing a characteristic picture of a sonolucent zone with a well-defined anterior and posterior margin. A central echo-dense, curvilinear, highly reflective structure within the cyst is suggestive of a scolex, further narrowing the diagnosis. CT may reveal intracerebral calcification or hydrocephalus in the setting of neural cysticercosis.

The differential diagnosis includes conditions associated with leukocoria (retinoblastoma, Coats disease, retinopathy of prematurity, persistent fetal vasculature, toxocariasis, retinal detachment, and so on) and diffuse unilateral subacute neuroretinitis (see the following section).

Left untreated, intravitreal or subretinal cysticercosis can cause blindness, atrophy, and phthisis within 3 to 5 years. Antihelminthic drugs such as praziquantel and albendazole have been used successfully in the medical management of active neural cysticercosis; however, these agents are generally not effective for intraocular disease. They are frequently used in combination with systemic corticosteroids, because larvae death is accompanied by worsening of the ocular disease and panuveitis. Similarly, laser photocoagulation has been advocated for small subretinal cysticerci; however, most authors report poor results when the dead parasite is allowed to remain within the eye. For this reason, early removal of the larvae from the vitreous cavity or subretinal space with vitreoretinal surgical techniques has been advocated and successfully employed.

Cardenas F, Quiroz H, Plancarte A, Meza A, Dalma A, Flisser A. *Taenia solium* ocular cysticercosis: findings in 30 cases. *Ann Ophthalmol.* 1992;24(1):25–28.

Kaliaperumal S, Rao VA, Parija SC. Cysticercosis of the eye in South India—a case series. *Indian J Med Microbiol.* 2005;23(4):227–230.

Kruger-Leite E, Jalkh AE, Quiroz H, Schepens CL. Intraocular cysticercosis. *Am J Ophthalmol.* 1985;99(3):252–257.

Diffuse Unilateral Subacute Neuroretinitis

Diffuse unilateral subacute neuroretinitis (DUSN) is an uncommon but important disease believed to be caused by nematode infection. It should be considered in the differential diagnosis of posterior uveitis occurring among otherwise healthy, young patients (mean age 14 years; range 11–65 years), because early recognition and prompt treatment may preserve vision. Evidence to date suggests that DUSN is caused by solitary nematodes of 2 different sizes, apparently related to geographic region, that migrate through the subretinal space. The smaller worm, measuring 400–1000 µm in length, has been proposed to be either *Ancylostoma caninum* (the dog hookworm) or *T canis,* the latter being endemic to the southeastern United States, Caribbean islands, and Brazil. The larger worm is believed to be *Baylisascaris procyonis* (the raccoon roundworm), which measures 1500–2000 µm in length and has been found in the northern midwestern United States and Canada. DUSN has also been reported in Germany and China.

The clinical course of DUSN is characterized by the insidious onset of unilateral visual loss from recurrent episodes of focal, multifocal, and diffuse inflammation of the retina, RPE, and optic nerve. The early stages of the disease are marked by moderate to severe vitritis; optic disc swelling; and multiple, focal, gray-white lesions in the postequatorial fundus that vary in size from 1200 μm to 1500 μm (Fig 7-40). These lesions are evanescent and may be associated with overlying serous retinal detachment. It is at this stage that the worms are most easily visualized in the subretinal space. Differential diagnostic considerations at this phase of the disease include sarcoidosis-associated uveitis, MCP, acute posterior multifocal placoid pigment epitheliopathy (APMPPE), multiple evanescent white dot syndrome (MEWDS), serpiginous choroidopathy, Behçet disease, ocular toxoplasmosis, OHS, nonspecific optic neuritis, and papillitis. The later stages are typified by retinal arteriolar narrowing, optic atrophy, diffuse pigment epithelial degeneration, and abnormal electroretinographic results (Fig 7-41). These findings may be confused with posttraumatic chorioretinopathy, occlusive vascular disease, toxic retinopathy, and retinitis pigmentosa. Although highly unusual, bilateral cases have been reported, as have cases of DUSN associated with neurologic disease (neural larvae migrans).

The diagnosis is made in the aforementioned clinical setting and is most strongly supported by the observation of a worm in the subretinal space. Results of systemic and laboratory evaluations are typically negative for patients with DUSN. Electroretinographic abnormalities may be present even when the test is performed early in the disease course.

Direct laser photocoagulation of the worm in the early phases of the disease may be highly effective in halting progression of the disease and improving visual acuity, and has not been associated with a significant exacerbation of inflammation (Fig 7-42). Medical therapy with corticosteroids may achieve transient control of the inflammation, but that is followed by recurrence of symptoms and progression of visual loss. Initial experience

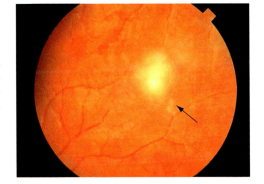

Figure 7-40 Diffuse unilateral subacute neuroretinitis (DUSN). Note the multiple white retinal lesions and the S-shaped nematode in the subretinal space *(arrow)*. *(Courtesy of E. Mitchel Opremcak, MD.)*

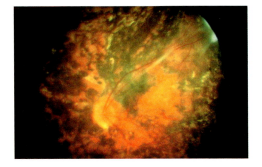

Figure 7-41 DUSN, or unilateral wipeout. *(Courtesy of E. Mitchel Opremcak, MD.)*

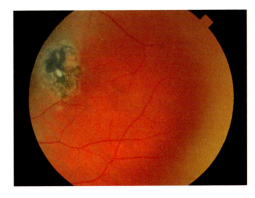

Figure 7-42 Retinal scar following laser photocoagulation of a nematode in a patient with DUSN. *(Courtesy of E. Mitchel Opremcak, MD.)*

with antihelminthic therapy was disappointing; however, successful treatment with oral thiabendazole (22 mg/kg twice daily for 2–4 days with a maximum dose of 3 g) has been reported in patients with moderate to severe inflammation. Treatment with albendazole (200 mg twice daily for 30 days) may be a better-tolerated alternative. Immobilization of the subretinal nematode has been observed following systemic antihelminthic therapy, and so it has been recommended that patients with DUSN in whom the worm cannot be initially identified receive a course of such therapy in order to maximize the chances of identifying and treating the offending organism. Furthermore, a second nematode, presumably from reinfection, may occasionally be observed in patients who have undergone a successful previous photocoagulation. These patients may also benefit from a course of systemic antihelminthic therapy, particularly if inflammation does not abate promptly following laser photocoagulation.

Cortez R, Denny JP, Muci-Mendoza R, Ramirez G, Fuenmayor D, Jaffe GJ. Diffuse unilateral subacute neuroretinitis in Venezuela. *Ophthalmology.* 2005;112(12):2110–2114.

Onchocerciasis

One of the leading causes of blindness in the world, onchocerciasis is endemic in many areas of sub-Saharan Africa and in isolated foci in Central and South America. It is rarely seen or diagnosed in the United States. Worldwide, at least 18 million people are infected, of whom almost 300,000 are blind. In hyperendemic areas, everyone over the age of 15 is infected, and half will become blind before they die.

Humans are the only host for *Onchocerca volvulus,* the filarial parasite that causes the disease. The larvae of *O volvulus* are transmitted through the bite of female black flies of the *Simulium* genus. The flies breed in fast-flowing streams; hence, the disease is commonly called *river blindness.* The larvae develop into mature adult worms that form subcutaneous nodules. The adult female releases millions of microfilariae that migrate throughout the body, particularly to the skin and the eye. Microfilariae probably reach the eye by multiple routes:

- direct invasion of the cornea from the conjunctiva
- penetration of the sclera, both directly and through the vascular bundles
- hematogenous spread (possibly)

Live microfilariae are usually well tolerated, but dead microfilariae initiate a focal inflammatory response.

Anterior segment signs of onchocerciasis are common. Microfilariae can be observed swimming freely in the anterior chamber. Live microfilariae can be seen in the cornea; dead microfilariae cause a small stromal punctate inflammatory opacity that clears with time. Mild uveitis and limbitis are common, but severe anterior uveitis may also occur and lead to synechiae, secondary glaucoma, and secondary cataract. Chorioretinal changes are also common and vary widely in severity. Early disruption of the RPE is typical, with pigment dispersion and focal areas of atrophy. Later, severe chorioretinal atrophy occurs, predominantly in the posterior pole. Optic atrophy is common in advanced disease.

Diagnosis is based on clinical appearance and a history of pathogen exposure in an endemic area and is confirmed by finding microfilariae in small skin biopsies or in the eye. Ivermectin, a macrolytic lactone, is the treatment of choice for onchocerciasis. Although not approved for sale in the United States, ivermectin is available on a compassionate basis for individual treatment. Ivermectin safely kills the microfilariae but does not have a permanent effect on the adult worms. A single oral dose of 150 µg/kg should be repeated annually, probably for 10 years. Topical corticosteroids can be used to control any anterior uveitis.

Although annual ivermectin treatment reduces the microfilarial load in the anterior chamber and the development of new anterior chamber lesions, it does not reduce the macrofilarial load even at doses as high as 1600 µg/kg. Ivermectin does not appear to prevent the development of new chorioretinal lesions or resolve existing lesions, although it does appear to slow progression of visual field loss and optic atrophy, even in advanced disease. Nodules containing adult worms can be removed surgically, but this approach does not usually cure the disease because many nodules are deeply buried and cannot be found. The adult worm is infected with the parasitic bacterium *Wolbachia,* an organism crucial to the sexual development of the worm. Targeting Wolbachia with a 6-week course of doxycycline, in addition to ivermectin, has become the treatment of choice because it can cause long-term sterilization of adult worms and early worm death.

Awadzi K, Attah SK, Addy ET, Opoku NO, Quartey BT. The effects of high-dose ivermectin regimens on *Onchocerca volvulus* in onchocerciasis patients. *Trans R Soc Trop Med Hyg.* 1999;93(2):189–194.

Ejere H, Schwartz E, Wormald R. Ivermectin for onchocercal eye disease (river blindness). *Cochrane Database Syst Rev.* 2001;1(1):CD002219.

Winthrop KL, Furtado JM, Silva JC, Resnikoff S, Lansingh VC. River blindness: an old disease on the brink of elimination and control. *J Glob Infect Dis.* 2011;3(2):151–155.

Bacterial Uveitis

Syphilis

Syphilis is a multisystem, chronic bacterial infection caused by the spirochete *Treponema pallidum* and is associated with multiple ocular manifestations that occur in both the acquired and congenital forms of the disease. Transmission occurs most often during sexual contact; however, transplacental infection of the fetus may occur after the tenth week of pregnancy. Having reached an all-time low in the year 2000 in the United States, the incidence rate of syphilis is currently 4.5 cases per 100,000 persons per year and is increasing, especially among men and African Americans, where the rate is 5 times greater than among non-Hispanic whites. In contrast, the rate of congenital syphilis was reported to be 10.1 per 100,000 live births in 2001, reflecting sharp declines in both primary and secondary syphilis among women over the past decade.

Although syphilis is thought to be responsible for less than 2% of all uveitis cases, it is one of the great masqueraders of medicine and should always be considered in the differential diagnosis of any intraocular inflammatory disease. It is one of the few entities that can be cured with appropriate antimicrobial therapy, even in patients with HIV/AIDS. Delay in the diagnosis of syphilitic uveitis may lead not only to permanent visual loss but also to significant neurologic and cardiac morbidity, which may have been averted with early treatment.

Centers for Disease Control and Prevention. *Sexually Transmitted Disease Surveillance 2008.* Atlanta, GA: US Department of Health and Human Services; November 2009.

Congenital syphilis

Congenital syphilis persists in the United States largely because a significant number of women do not receive serologic testing until late in pregnancy, if at all, which in turn is related to absent or late prenatal care. Systemic findings in patients with early congenital syphilis (age 2 years or younger) include hepatosplenomegaly, characteristic changes of the long bones on radiographic examination, abdominal distention, desquamative skin rash, low birth weight, pneumonia, and severe anemia. Late manifestations (age 3 or older) result from scarring during early systemic disease and include Hutchinson teeth, Mulberry molars, abnormal facies, cranial nerve VIII deafness, bony changes such as saber shins and perforations of the hard palate, cutaneous lesions such as rhagades, and neurosyphilis. Cardiovascular complications are unusual in late congenital syphilis.

Ocular inflammatory signs of syphilis may present at birth or decades later and include uveitis, interstitial keratitis, optic neuritis, glaucoma, and congenital cataract. A multifocal chorioretinitis and, less commonly, retinal vasculitis are the most frequent uveitic manifestations of early congenital infection. They may result in a bilateral "salt-and-pepper" fundus, which affects the peripheral retina, posterior pole, or a single quadrant. These changes are not progressive, and the patient may have normal vision. A less commonly described funduscopic variation is that of a bilateral secondary degeneration of the RPE, which may mimic retinitis pigmentosa with narrowing of the retinal and choroidal vessels, optic disc pallor with sharp margins, and morphologically variable deposits of pigment.

Nonulcerative stromal interstitial keratitis, often accompanied by anterior uveitis, is the most common inflammatory sign of untreated late congenital syphilis, occurring in up to 50% of cases, most commonly in girls (Fig 7-43). Keratouveitis is thought to be an allergic response to *T pallidum* in the cornea. Symptoms include intense pain and photophobia. The cornea may be diffusely opaque, with reduced vision, even to the level of light perception only. Blood vessels invade the cornea, and when they meet in the center of the visual axis after several months, the inflammation subsides and the cornea partially

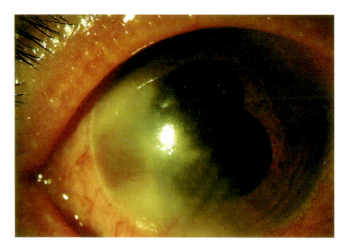

Figure 7-43 Active syphilitic interstitial keratitis.

clears. Late stages show deep ghost (nonperfused) stromal vessels and opacities. Although the iritis accompanying interstitial keratitis may be difficult to observe because of corneal haze, secondary guttata and hyaline strands projecting into the angle provide evidence of anterior segment inflammation. Glaucoma may also occur. The constellation of interstitial keratitis, cranial nerve VIII deafness, and Hutchinson teeth is called the *Hutchinson triad.*

Acquired syphilis

The natural history of untreated acquired syphilis has been well described. *Primary syphilis* follows an incubation period of approximately 3 weeks and is characterized by a chancre, a painless, solitary lesion that originates at the site of inoculation, resolving spontaneously within 12 weeks regardless of treatment. The central nervous system may be seeded with treponemes during this period, although there is an absence of neurologic findings. *Secondary syphilis* occurs 6–8 weeks later and is heralded by the appearance of lymphadenopathy and a generalized maculopapular rash that may be prominent on the palms and soles. Uveitis occurs in approximately 10% of cases. This is followed by a latent period ranging from 1 year (early latency) to decades (late latency). Approximately one-third of untreated patients develop *tertiary syphilis,* which may be further subcategorized as benign tertiary syphilis (the characteristic lesion being gumma, most frequently found on the skin and mucous membranes but also appears in the choroid and iris), cardiovascular syphilis, and neurosyphilis. Although uveitis may occur in up to 5% of patients who have progressed to tertiary syphilis, it can occur at any stage of infection, including primary disease. Because the eye is an extension of the CNS, ocular syphilis is best regarded as a variant of neurosyphilis, a notion that has important diagnostic and therapeutic implications.

The ocular manifestations of syphilis are protean and affect all structures, including the conjunctiva, sclera, cornea, lens, uveal tract, retina, retinal vasculature, optic nerve, cranial nerves, and pupillomotor pathways. Patients present with pain, redness, photophobia, blurred vision, and floaters. Intraocular inflammation may be granulomatous or nongranulomatous, unilateral or bilateral, and it may affect the anterior, intermediate, or posterior segments. Iridocyclitis may be associated with iris roseola, vascularized papules (iris papulosa), larger red nodules (iris nodosa), and gummata. Interstitial keratitis, posterior synechiae, lens dislocation, and iris atrophy are additional anterior segment findings seen in association with acquired syphilitic uveitis.

Posterior segment findings of acquired syphilis include vitritis, chorioretinitis, focal retinitis, necrotizing retinitis, retinal vasculitis, exudative retinal detachment, isolated papillitis, and neuroretinitis. A focal or multifocal chorioretinitis, usually associated with a variable degree of vitritis, is the most common manifestation (Fig 7-44). These lesions are typically small, grayish yellow, and located in the postequatorial fundus, but they may become confluent. Retinal vasculitis and disc edema, with exudates appearing around the disc and the retinal arterioles, together with serous retinal detachment, may accompany the chorioretinitis. A syphilitic posterior placoid chorioretinitis has been described, the clinical appearance and angiographic characteristics of which are thought to be pathognomonic of secondary syphilis (Fig 7-45). Solitary or multifocal, macular or papillary, placoid, yellowish gray lesions at the level of the RPE, often with accompanying vitritis, display corresponding early hypofluorescence and late staining, along with retinal perivenous staining on FA.

Less common posterior segment involvement includes focal retinitis, periphlebitis, and, infrequently, exudative retinal detachment. Syphilis may present as a focal retinitis (Fig 7-46) or as a peripheral necrotizing retinitis that may resemble ARN or PORN (Fig 7-47). Although the foci of retinitis may become confluent and are frequently associated with retinal vasculitis, syphilitic retinitis is more slowly progressive and responds dramatically to therapy with intravenous penicillin, often with a good visual outcome. Isolated retinal vasculitis that affects the retinal arterioles, capillaries, and larger arteries or veins (or both) is another feature of syphilitic intraocular inflammation that may best be appreciated on FA. Focal retinal vasculitis may masquerade as a branch retinal vein occlusion.

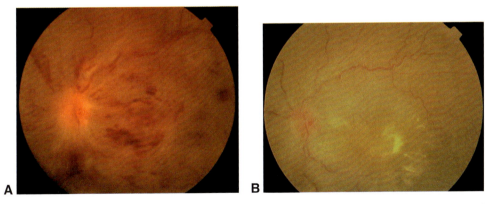

Figure 7-44 **A,** Acute syphilitic chorioretinitis. Note the diffuse disc edema, retinal edema, and choroidal edema in the posterior pole. **B,** Healed chorioretinitis after 2 weeks of intravenous penicillin therapy. Note the subretinal hard exudate that is organizing, as well as the reduction in disc edema and choroidal inflammation. *(Courtesy of Ramana S. Moorthy, MD.)*

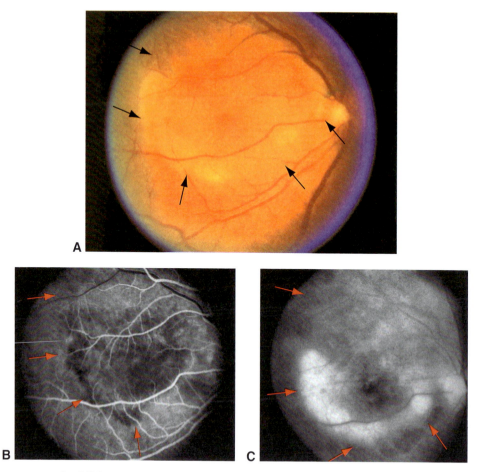

Figure 7-45 Syphilitic posterior placoid chorioretinitis. **A,** Fundus photograph of the right eye showing a large, geographic lesion involving the central macula *(arrows)*. **B,** Fluorescein angiogram disclosing early, irregular hypofluorescence *(arrows)* followed by **(C)** late staining at the level of the pigment epithelium *(arrows)*. *(Reproduced with permission from Gass JDM, Braunstein RA, Chenoweth RG. Acute syphilitic posterior placoid chorioretinitis. Ophthalmology. 1990;97(10):1289–1290.)*

Syphilis is an important entity to consider in the differential diagnosis of patients with neuroretinitis and papillitis who present with macular star formation. Patients with syphilis who are immunocompromised or who have HIV/AIDS may have atypical or more fulminant ocular disease patterns. Optic neuritis and neuroretinitis are more common in the initial presentation of these patients, and disease recurrences are noted even after appropriate antibacterial therapy.

Neuro-ophthalmic manifestations of syphilis include the Argyll Robertson pupil, ocular motor nerve palsies, optic neuropathy, and retrobulbar optic neuritis, which all appear most often in patients with tertiary syphilis or in neurosyphilis. (See BCSC Section 5, *Neuro-Ophthalmology,* for a more complete discussion.)

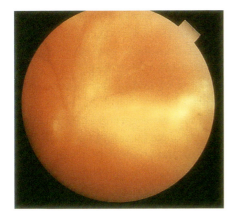

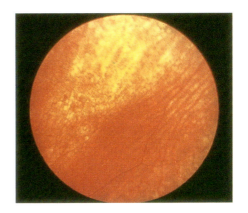

Figure 7-46 Acute syphilitic retinitis.

Figure 7-47 Syphilitic uveitis, acute retinitis.

Diagnosis

The diagnosis of syphilitic uveitis is usually based on history and clinical presentation and is supported by serologic testing. Primary syphilis may be diagnosed by direct visualization of spirochetes with dark-field microscopy and by direct fluorescent antibody tests of lesion exudates or tissue. Serodiagnosis is normally based on the results of both nontreponemal antigen tests, such as the Venereal Disease Research Laboratory (VDRL) and rapid plasma reagin evaluations, and treponemal antigen tests, such as the fluorescent treponemal antibody absorption (FTA-ABS) assay and the microhemagglutination assay for *T pallidum* antibodies (MHA-TP). Nontreponemal antibody titers correlate with disease activity, generally increasing during primary or secondary syphilis and dropping when the spirochetes are not active, such as during latent syphilis or after adequate antibiotic treatment. They are useful barometers for monitoring therapy for both systemic and ocular disease. The FTA-ABS test result becomes positive during the secondary stage of syphilis and remains positive, with rare exceptions, throughout the patient's life; as such, it is not useful in assessing a therapeutic response. Testing for HIV should be performed in all patients with syphilis, given the high frequency of coinfection. As a result of the passive transfer of immunoglobulin (IgG) across the placenta, the VDRL and FTA-ABS test results are positive among infants born to mothers with syphilis. For this reason, serodiagnosis of congenital syphilis is made using the IgM FTA-ABS test, because this antibody does not cross the placenta and its presence indicates infection in the infant.

False-positive nontreponemal test results are seen in a variety of medical conditions, including systemic lupus erythematosus (SLE), leprosy, advanced age, intravenous drug abuse, bacterial endocarditis, tuberculosis, vaccinations, infectious mononucleosis, HIV infection, atypical pneumonia, malaria, pregnancy, rickettsial infections, and other spirochetal infections (eg, Lyme disease). Likewise, false-positive treponemal test results may be seen with other spirochetal infections (leptospirosis), autoimmune disease (SLE, primary biliary cirrhosis, and rheumatoid arthritis), leprosy, malaria, and advanced age. Although nontreponemal tests are appropriate for screening large populations with a relatively lower risk for syphilis, specific treponemal tests, such as FTA-ABS, have a higher predictive value in the setting of uveitis and should be used in conjunction with nontreponemal tests in diagnosing and treating ocular syphilis. Both the false-positive and false-negative rates of serologic testing may be greater in HIV-infected patients.

A lumbar puncture with examination of CSF is warranted in every case of syphilitic uveitis. A positive CSF VDRL result is diagnostic for neurosyphilis, but it may be nonreactive in some cases of active central nervous system involvement. Although less specific, the CSF FTA-ABS test is highly sensitive and may be useful in excluding neurosyphilis. Follow-up for patients with chorioretinitis and abnormal CSF findings requires spinal fluid examination every 6 months until the cell count, protein, and VDRL results return to normal. Finally, specific ELISA- and PCR-based DNA amplification techniques are being used with increasing frequency in the serodiagnosis of syphilis. Given their high sensitivity and specificity, these techniques, particularly PCR analysis of intraocular and/or cerebrospinal fluids, may be valuable in confirming the diagnosis in atypical cases.

Treatment

Parenteral penicillin G is the preferred treatment for all stages of syphilis (Table 7-3). Although the formulation, dose, route of administration, and duration of therapy vary with the stage of the disease, patients with syphilitic uveitis should be considered as having a central nervous system disease, requiring neurologic dosing regimens regardless of immune status. The current CDC recommendation for the treatment of neurosyphilis is

Table 7-3 Treatment of Syphilis

Stage of Disease	Primary Treatment Regimen	Alternative Treatment Regimen
Congenital syphilis	Crystalline penicillin G 100,000–150,000 MU/kg/d given IV as 50,000 MU/kg every 12 hours during the first 7 days of life and every 8 hours thereafter, for a total of 10 days	Procaine penicillin G 50,000 MU/kg IM as a single dose × 10 days
Primary, secondary, or early latent disease	Benzathine penicillin G 2.4 MU IM as a single dose	Doxycycline 100 mg po bid × 2 weeks or tetracycline 500 mg po qid × 2 weeks
Late latent or latent syphilis of uncertain duration, tertiary disease in the absence of neurosyphilis	Benzathine penicillin G 2.4 MU IM, weekly × 3 doses	Doxycycline 100 mg po bid × 4 weeks or tetracycline 500 mg po qid × 4 weeks
Neurosyphilis	Aqueous penicillin G 18–24 MU/d given IV as 3–4 MU every 4 hours × 10–14 days	Procaine penicillin 2.4 MU/d IM × 10–14 days and probenecid 500 mg po qid × 10–14 days

MU = million units.

Adapted with permission from Centers for Disease Control and Prevention. Sexually transmitted diseases treatment guidelines 2002. *MMWR Recomm Rep.* 2002;51(RR-6):1–78.

18–24 million units (MU) of aqueous crystalline penicillin G per day, administered as 3–4 MU intravenously every 4 hours or as a continuous infusion for 10–14 days. This may be supplemented with intramuscular benzathine penicillin G, 2.4 MU weekly for 3 weeks. Alternatively, neurosyphilis may be treated with 2.4 MU/day of intramuscular procaine penicillin plus probenecid 500 mg 4 times a day, both for 10–14 days.

The recommended treatment regimen for congenital syphilis in infants during the first months of life is intravenous crystalline penicillin G at 100,000–150,000 units/kg/day, administered as 50,000 units/kg/day every 12 hours during the first 7 days of life and every 8 hours thereafter, for a total of 10 days. Alternatively, intramuscular procaine penicillin G, 50,000 units/kg in a single daily dose for 10 days, may be given.

There are no proven alternatives to penicillin for the treatment of neurosyphilis, congenital infection, or disease in pregnant women or patients coinfected with HIV; for that reason, patients with penicillin allergy require desensitization and then treatment with penicillin. Alternative treatments in penicillin-allergic patients who show no signs of neurosyphilis and who are HIV-negative include doxycycline or tetracycline. Ceftriaxone and chloramphenicol have been reported to be effective alternatives in patients with ocular syphilis who are penicillin-allergic and HIV coinfected.

Patients should be monitored for the development of the Jarisch-Herxheimer reaction, a hypersensitivity response of the host to treponemal antigens that are released in large numbers as spirochetes are killed during the first 24 hours of treatment. Patients present with constitutional symptoms but may also experience a concomitant increase in the severity of ocular inflammation that may require local and/or systemic corticosteroids. In the vast majority of cases, however, supportive care and observation are sufficient.

Topical, periocular, and/or systemic corticosteroids, under appropriate antibiotic cover, may be useful adjuncts for treating the anterior and posterior segment inflammation associated with syphilitic uveitis. Finally, the sexual contacts of the patient must be identified and treated, as a high percentage of these individuals are at risk for developing and transmitting this disease.

Aldave AJ, King JA, Cunningham ET Jr. Ocular syphilis. *Curr Opin Ophthalmol.* 2001;12(6): 433–441.

Browning DJ. Posterior segment manifestations of active ocular syphilis, their response to a neurosyphilis regimen of penicillin therapy, and the influence of human immunodeficiency virus status on response. *Ophthalmology.* 2000;107(11):2015–2023.

Centers for Disease Control and Prevention. Sexually transmitted diseases treatment guidelines 2002. *MMWR Recomm Rep.* 2002;51(RR-6):1–78.

Gass JD, Braunstein RA, Chenoweth RG. Acute syphilitic posterior placoid chorioretinitis. *Ophthalmology.* 1990;97(10):1288–1297.

Jumper JM, Machemer R, Gallemore RP, Jaffe GJ. Exudative retinal detachment and retinitis associated with acquired syphilitic uveitis. *Retina.* 2000;20(2):190–194.

Mendelsohn AD, Jampol LM. Syphilitic retinitis. A cause of necrotizing retinitis. *Retina.* 1984; 4(4):221–224.

Tamesis RR, Foster CS. Ocular syphilis. *Ophthalmology.* 1990;97(10):1281–1287.

Villanueva AV, Sahouri MJ, Ormerod LD, Puklin JE, Reyes MP. Posterior uveitis in patients with positive serology for syphilis. *Clin Infect Dis.* 2000;30(3):479–485.

Lyme Disease

Lyme disease (LD) is the most common tick-borne illness in the United States. It has protean systemic and ocular manifestations and is caused by the spirochete *Borrelia burgdorferi*. Animal reservoirs include deer, horses, cows, rodents, birds, cats, and dogs. The spirochete is transmitted to humans through the bite of infected ticks, *Ixodes scapularis* in the northeast, mid-Atlantic, and midwestern United States and *Ixodes pacificus* in the western United States. In 2008, the national incidence rate was 9.4 cases per 100,000 persons per year. The disease affects men (53%) slightly more often than women and has a bimodal distribution, with peaks in children aged 5–14 years and in adults aged 50–59 years. There is a seasonal variation, with most cases occurring between May and August. LD may be found worldwide, but outside the United States it is caused by different species of *Borrelia*, such as *B afzelli* and *B garinii*.

Clinical features

The clinical manifestations of LD have been divided into 3 stages; ocular findings vary within each stage. The most characteristic feature of stage 1, or local disease, is a macular rash known as *erythema chronicum migrans* at the site of the tick bite; it appears within 2–28 days in approximately 70% of patients. As the lesion enlarges and becomes papular, the paracentral area may clear, forming a bull's eye, with the site of the bite marking the center (Figs 7-48, 7-49). Constitutional symptoms appear at this stage and include fever, malaise, fatigue, myalgias, and arthralgias.

Stage 2, or disseminated disease, occurs several weeks to 4 months following exposure. Spirochetes spread hematogenously to the skin, central nervous system, joints, heart, and eyes. A secondary erythema chronicum migrans rash may be seen at sites remote from the site of tick bite. Left untreated, up to 80% of patients with erythema chronicum migrans in the United States develop joint manifestations, most commonly a monoarthritis or oligoarthritis involving the large joints, typically the knee (Fig 7-50). Joint involvement may be the only clinical manifestation of Lyme disease in children, in whom the differential diagnosis of juvenile idiopathic arthritis (JIA) must be considered.

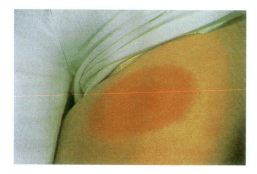 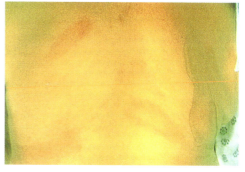

Figure 7-48 Erythema chronicum migrans in a patient with Lyme disease, with a single dense erythematous lesion. *(Courtesy of Alan B. MacDonald, MD.)*

Figure 7-49 Erythema chronicum migrans: multiple bull's-eye lesions in a patient with Lyme disease. *(Courtesy of Alan B. MacDonald, MD.)*

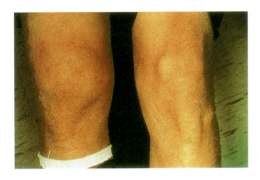

Figure 7-50 Lyme disease arthritis. *(Courtesy of Alan B. MacDonald, MD.)*

Neurologic involvement, which occurs in up to 40% of patients, may include meningitis, encephalitis, painful radiculitis, or unilateral or bilateral Bell palsy. In endemic areas, as many as 25% of new-onset cranial nerve VII palsies may be attributed to *B burgdorferi* infection.

The most frequent systemic manifestation of stage 3, or persistent disease, which occurs 5 months or more after the initial infection, is episodic arthritis that may become chronic. Chronic arthritis has been associated with the HLA-DR4 and -DR2 haplotypes in North America; individuals expressing HLA-DR4 have a poorer response to antibiotics. Acrodermatitis chronica atrophicans, a bluish red lesion on the extremities that may progress to fibrous bands and nodules, can occur in some patients, as may chronic neurologic syndromes including neuropsychiatric disease, radiculopathy, chronic fatigue, peripheral neuropathy, and memory loss.

Ocular disease

The spectrum of ocular findings in patients with LD is expanding and varies with disease stage. The most common ocular manifestation of early stage 1 disease is a follicular conjunctivitis, which occurs in approximately 11% of patients; less commonly seen is episcleritis. (See BCSC Section 8, *External Disease and Cornea*, for further discussion and the differential diagnosis.)

Intraocular inflammatory disease is reported most often in stage 2 and, less frequently, in stage 3 disease; this may manifest as anterior uveitis, intermediate uveitis, posterior uveitis, or panuveitis. Intermediate uveitis is one of the most common intraocular presentations. Vitritis may be severe and may be accompanied by a granulomatous anterior chamber reaction, papillitis, neuroretinitis, choroiditis, retinal vasculitis, and exudative retinal detachment (Figs 7-51, 7-52).

A distinct clinical entity of peripheral multifocal choroiditis has been described in patients with LD; it is characterized by multiple, small, round, punched-out lesions associated with vitritis, similar to those seen with sarcoidosis. Choroidal involvement may lead to pigment epithelial clumping resembling the inflammatory changes seen with syphilis or rubella. Retinal vasculitis, seen in association with peripheral multifocal choroiditis or vasculitic branch retinal vein occlusion, may be more common than previously known.

Neuro-ophthalmic manifestations include multiple cranial nerve involvement (II, III, IV, V, VI, and, most commonly, VII) unilaterally or bilaterally, either sequentially or

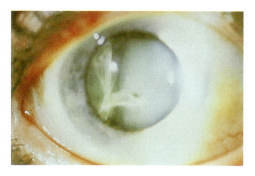

Figure 7-51 Dense anterior vitreous debris causing floaters and blurring in ocular Lyme disease. *(Courtesy of William W. Culbertson, MD.)*

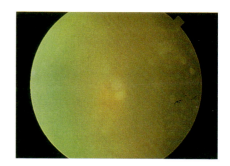

Figure 7-52 Grade III vitreous opacification in Lyme disease vitritis, as seen by indirect ophthalmoscopy, is reminiscent of severe pars planitis. *(Courtesy of John D. Sheppard, Jr, MD.)*

simultaneously. Optic nerve findings include optic neuritis, papilledema associated with meningitis, and papillitis most commonly seen with Lyme uveitis. Horner syndrome has also been reported.

Keratitis is the most common ocular manifestation of stage 3 disease; much less common is episcleritis. Both may present months to years after the onset of infection. Typically, infiltrates are bilateral, patchy, focal, and stromal, or they are subepithelial infiltrates with indistinct borders. However, infiltrates may also present as a peripheral keratitis with stromal edema and corneal neovascularization. The keratitis is thought to represent an immune phenomenon rather than an infectious process because it responds to topical corticosteroids alone.

Diagnosis

The diagnosis of LD is based on history, clinical presentation, and supportive serology. In the appropriate clinical context, erythema chronicum migrans is diagnostic. However, interpreting serologic data is problematic because of the lack of standardization of the values by which a positive test is defined—the degree of cross-reactivity with other spirochetes—thus leading to frequent false-positive and false-negative test results. The CDC recommends a 2-step protocol for the diagnosis of active disease or previous infection:

1. ELISA for IgM and IgG, followed by
2. Western immunoblot testing

PCR-based assays have been successfully used to amplify both genomic and plasmid *B burgdorferi* DNA from a variety of tissues, including ocular fluids, with the highest yields being obtained from the skin.

Treatment

The current treatment recommendations for the various clinical manifestations of LD are listed in Table 7-4. For patients with ocular involvement, the route and duration of antibiotic treatment has not been established; however, as with syphilitic uveitis, intraocular inflammation associated with LD is best regarded as a manifestation of central nervous

Table 7-4 Treatment of Lyme Disease

	Drug	Adult Dosage	Pediatric Dosage
Early localized Lyme disease			
Erythema chronicum migrans	Doxycycline*	100 mg po bid × 10–21 d	≥8 yrs: 1–2 mg/kg bid
	or Amoxicillin	500 mg po tid × 14–21 d	25–50 mg/kg/d divided tid
	or Cefuroxime axetil	500 mg po bid × 14–21 d	30 mg/kg/d divided bid
Acute neurologic or cardiac disease			
Facial nerve palsy	Doxycycline*	100 mg po bid × 14–21 d	≥8 yrs: 1–2 mg/kg bid
	or Amoxicillin	500 mg po tid × 14–21 d	25–50 mg/kg/d divided tid
Meningitis, radiculopathy, or third-degree heart block	Ceftriaxone†	2 g/d IV qd × 14–28 d	75–100 mg/kg qd IV
Late disease			
Arthritis without neurologic disease	Doxycycline*	100 mg po bid × 28 d	≥8 yrs: 1–2 mg/kg bid
	or Amoxicillin	500 mg po tid × 28 d	25–50 mg/kg/d divided tid
Recurrent arthritis, CNS or peripheral nervous system disease	Ceftriaxone†	2 g qd IV × 14–28 d	50–100 mg/kg qd IV

*Should not be used in children younger than age 8 or in pregnant or lactating women.
†Or cefotaxime 2 g IV q8h × 14–28 d for adults and 150–200 mg/kg/d in 3–4 doses for children.

Adapted with permission from Wormser GP, Nadelman RB, Dattwyler RJ, et al. Guidelines from the Infectious Diseases Society of America. Practice guidelines for the treatment of Lyme disease. *Clin Infect Dis.* 2000;31(suppl 1):1–14.

system involvement and warrants careful neurologic evaluation, including a lumbar puncture. Patients with severe posterior segment manifestations—and certainly those with confirmed central nervous system involvement—require intravenous antibiotic therapy with neurologic dosing regimens. Likewise, patients with less-severe disease who respond incompletely or relapse when oral antibiotics are discontinued should probably be treated with intravenous agents as outlined. Patients who present with symptomatic Lyme carditis or who have atrioventricular block should be hospitalized and monitored with cardiac telemetry in addition to receiving treatment with intravenous antibiotics.

Following the initiation of appropriate antibiotic therapy, anterior segment inflammation may be treated with topical corticosteroids and mydriatics. The use of systemic corticosteroids has been described as part of the management of LD; however, the routine use of corticosteroids is controversial, as it has been associated with an increase in antibiotic treatment failures. As with syphilis, the Jarisch-Herxheimer reaction may complicate antibiotic therapy. Patients may become reinfected with *B burgdorferi* following successful antibiotic therapy, especially in the endemic areas, or they may experience a more severe or chronic course by virtue of concomitant babesiosis (an intraerythrocytic parasitic infection caused by protozoa of the genus *Babesia*, which is also transmitted by the *Ixodes* tick) or human granulocytic anaplasmosis (previously known as *human granulocytic ehrlichiosis*) and require retreatment with antibiotics. Prevention strategies include avoiding tick-infested habitats, using tick repellents, wearing protective outer garments, removing ticks promptly, and reducing tick populations.

Centers for Disease Control and Prevention (CDC). Lyme disease—United States 2003–2005. *MMWR Morb Mortal Wkly Rep.* 2007;56(23):573–576.

Hilton E, Smith C, Sood S. Ocular Lyme borreliosis diagnosed by polymerase chain reaction on vitreous fluid. *Ann Intern Med.* 1996;125(5):424–425.

Mikkilä HO, Seppälä IJ, Viljanen MK, Peltomaa MP, Karma A. The expanding clinical spectrum of ocular Lyme borreliosis. *Ophthalmology.* 2000;107(3):581–587.

Winterkorn JM. Lyme disease: neurologic and ophthalmic manifestations. *Surv Ophthalmol.* 1990;35(3):191–204.

Wormser GP, Dattwyler RJ, Shapiro ED, et al. The clinical assessment, treatment, and prevention of Lyme disease, human granulocytic anaplasmosis, and babesiosis: clinical practice guidelines by the Infectious Diseases Society of America. *Clin Infect Dis.* 2006;43(9):1089–1134.

Wormser GP, Nadelman RB, Dattwyler RJ, et al. Guidelines from the Infectious Diseases Society of America. Practice guidelines for the treatment of Lyme disease. *Clin Infect Dis.* 2000; 31(suppl 1):1–14.

Leptospirosis

Leptospirosis, a zoonotic infection with a worldwide distribution, occurs most frequently in tropical and subtropical regions and is caused by the gram-negative spirochete *Leptospira interrogans*. The natural reservoirs for *Leptospira* organisms are animals, including livestock, horses, dogs, and rodents, which excrete the organism in their urine. Humans contract the disease upon exposure to contaminated soil, water, tissues, or infected animals; the organism gains systemic access through mucous membranes or abraded skin surfaces. The disease is not known to be spread from person to person, but maternal-fetal transmission may occur, albeit uncommonly. Occupational groups at risk include agricultural workers, sewer workers, veterinarians, fish workers, slaughterhouse workers, and military personnel, as well as individuals participating in activities such as swimming, wading, whitewater rafting, and even triathlon competitions. An estimated 100 to 200 cases are identified annually in the United States, with about half occurring in Hawaii.

Over 200 pathologic strains belong to the species *L interrogans*. Leptospirosis is frequently a biphasic disease with the initial, or leptospiremic phase, following an incubation period of 2–4 weeks, heralded by the abrupt onset of fever, chills, headache, myalgias, vomiting, and diarrhea. Circumcorneal conjunctival congestion commonly appears on the third to fourth day of the illness and is considered pathognomonic for severe systemic leptospirosis. The initial febrile attack varies in its severity, with approximately 90% of patients experiencing a self-limiting anicteric illness; about 10% develop severe septicemic leptospirosis, also known as *Weil disease*. Weil disease is characterized by renal and hepatocellular dysfunction; it occurs approximately 6 days after infection and carries a mortality of up to 30% because of multiorgan failure. Leptospires may be isolated from the blood and CSF up to 10 days after infection but are cleared rapidly from most host tissues as the patient progresses to the second, or immune, phase of the illness. The organism may persist for longer periods of time in immunologically privileged sites such as the brain and the eye. The clinical course of the immune phase is variable, the most important features being meningitis and leptospiruria. Other manifestations include the development of cranial nerve palsies, myelitis, and uveitis, all of which may appear many months after the acute stage of the illness.

The burden of ocular disease caused by leptospirosis is undoubtedly underestimated because the disease itself is underdiagnosed and there is a prolonged interval between systemic and ocular disease. Circumcorneal conjunctival hyperemia is the earliest and most common sign of ocular leptospirosis, but the development of intraocular inflammation, either anterior or diffuse uveitis (in 10% and 44% of patients, respectively), is the more serious, potentially vision-threatening complication.

The onset of predominantly anterior uveitis is marked by blurred vision, photophobia, and pain, but it may be insidious and mild and escape detection. The presentation of panuveitis, however, is often acute, severe, and relapsing, with 1 or both eyes being affected. A recent case series reported panuveitis to be distinctly more common than isolated anterior disease. The hallmarks include nongranulomatous anterior uveitis, with hypopyon in 12% of cases; moderate to dense vitritis with membranous veil-like opacities; optic disc edema; and retinal periphlebitis. Associated complications include glaucoma and rapid maturation of cataract, with the uncommon occurrence of spontaneous absorption of cataractous lens material. Macular edema, epiretinal membrane formation, and intermediate uveitis are uncommon.

The differential diagnosis includes HLA-B27–associated seronegative spondyloarthropathies, idiopathic pars planitis, Behçet disease, Eales disease, sarcoidosis, tuberculosis, and syphilis. Appropriate history and laboratory evaluation help distinguish syphilis, tuberculosis, and sarcoidosis from leptospiral uveitis. The high prevalence of bilaterality and vitreal inflammation, the infrequency of CME, and the absence of occlusive retinal vasculitis and peripheral retinal neovascularization differentiate this entity from HLA-B27–associated uveitis, idiopathic pars planitis, Behçet disease, and Eales disease, respectively.

A definitive diagnosis requires isolation of the organism from bodily fluids, but this is seldom possible given that the acute phase of the disease, when leptospires may be isolated from blood and CSF, is very short, and that the process itself is very resource intensive. A presumptive diagnosis is made on the basis of serologic assays such as the microagglutination test with seroconversion, or on a fourfold or greater rise in paired serum samples in the appropriate clinical context. Although the microagglutination test is considered the gold standard, it is labor intensive and not widely available. Recently, rapid serologic assays such as ELISA and complement-fixation tests for the detection of IgM antibodies against leptospiral antigens have been developed that are highly sensitive and specific. In addition, lipoprotein L2 and lipopolysaccharide antigen for serodiagnosis of uveitis associated with leptospirosis have been identified, and PCR-based assays are under evaluation for rapid diagnostic evaluation. Leptospirosis may cause a positive rapid plasma reagin or FTA-ABS test result.

Intravenous antibiotic therapy with 1.5 MU of penicillin G every 6 hours for 1 week beginning within the first 4 days of the appearance of acute illness provides the greatest benefit for severe systemic leptospirosis. Oral doxycycline, 100 mg twice daily for 1 week, may be used for mild or moderate cases. It is not known whether systemic antibiotic treatment during the leptospiremic phase is protective with respect to long-term complications such as uveitis; however, because pathogenic leptospires may survive and multiply in the blood and anterior chamber for long periods, systemic antibiotic treatment should be considered for ocular disease that occurs even months after onset of the acute systemic disease. In addition, topical, periocular, or systemic corticosteroids, together with mydriatic and cycloplegic agents, are routinely used to suppress intraocular inflammation. The visual prognosis of leptospiral uveitis is quite favorable despite severe panuveal inflammation.

Rathinam SR. Ocular manifestations of leptospirosis. *J Postgrad Med.* 2005;51(3):189–194.

Rathinam SR. Ocular leptospirosis. *Curr Opin Ophthalmol.* 2002;13(6):381–386.

Ocular Nocardiosis

Although ocular involvement in patients with *Nocardia asteroides* infection is rare, ocular disease may be the presenting complaint in this potentially lethal but treatable systemic disease characterized by pneumonia and disseminated abscesses. The responsible organism is commonly found in soil, and initial infection occurs by ingestion or inhalation. Ocular involvement occurs by hematogenous spread of the bacteria, and symptoms may vary from the mild pain and redness of iridocyclitis to the severe pain and decreased vision of panophthalmitis. Findings range from an isolated, unilateral chorioretinal mass with minimal vitritis to diffuse iridocyclitis with cell and flare, vitritis, and multiple choroidal abscesses with overlying retinal detachment.

Diagnosis can be established with a culture of the organism taken from tissue or fluid, by vitreous aspiration for Gram stain and culture, or, occasionally, by enucleation and microscopic identification of organisms. Treatment of systemic *N asteroides* infection with systemic sulfonamide may be required for protracted periods of time. Combination therapy with additional antibiotics may be required.

Ameen M, Arenas R, Vásquez del Mercado E, Fernández R, Torres E, Zacarias R. Efficacy of imipenem therapy for *Nocardia* actinomycetomas refractory to sulfonamides. *J Am Acad Dermatol.* 2010;62(2):239–246.

Ng EW, Zimmer-Galler IE, Green WR. Endogenous *Nocardia asteroides* endophthalmitis. *Arch Ophthalmol.* 2002;120(2):210–213.

Tuberculosis

Tuberculosis (TB) was once considered the most common cause of uveitis; today ocular involvement caused by TB is uncommon in the United States. Worldwide, however, it remains the most important systemic infectious disease, with more than 9.4 million new cases and 1.8 million deaths reported in 2008. Nearly one-third of the world's population is infected, and 95% of cases occur in developing countries. In the United States, following many years of annual decline, the incidence of TB began to increase coincident with the

AIDS epidemic, and the disease has reemerged as an important public health problem. Although the frequency of ocular disease parallels the prevalence of TB in general, it remains relatively uncommon both in endemic areas and among institutionalized populations with unequivocal systemic disease. In the United States, the incidence of uveitis attributable to TB at a large tertiary care facility was only 0.6%, whereas at major referral centers in India, it ranged from 0.6% to 10%, and in similar institutions in Japan and Saudi Arabia, was 7.9% and 10.5%, respectively.

Tuberculosis is caused by *Mycobacterium tuberculosis,* an acid-fast–staining, obligate aerobe, most commonly transmitted by aerosolized droplets. The organism has an affinity for highly oxygenated tissues, and tuberculous lesions are commonly found in the apices of the lungs as well as in the choroid, which has the highest blood flow rate in the body. Systemic infection may occur primarily, as a result of recent exposure; in the vast majority (90%) of patients, however, it occurs secondarily, with reactivation of the disease caused by compromised immune function. Widespread hematogenous dissemination of TB, known as *miliary disease,* likewise occurs most often in the setting of immunocompromise. High-risk groups include health care professionals, recent immigrants from endemic areas, the indigent, immunocompromised patients (chronic disease, HIV/AIDS, or IMT), and older adults.

Pulmonary TB develops in approximately 80% of patients, whereas extrapulmonary disease is seen in about 20%, with one-half of these patients exhibiting a normal-appearing chest radiograph and up to 20% having a negative result on the purified protein derivative (PPD) skin test. Patients coinfected with HIV present more often with extrapulmonary disease, the frequency of which increases with deteriorating immune function. Only 10% of infected individuals develop symptomatic disease; one-half of these manifest illness within the first 1–2 years. The vast majority, however, remain infected but asymptomatic. The classic presentation of symptomatic disease—fever, night sweats, and weight loss—is seen with both pulmonary and extrapulmonary infection. This is important to keep in mind when conducting a review of systems in patients suspected of tuberculous uveitis because histologically proven intraocular TB has been found in patients with both asymptomatic and extrapulmonary disease.

Ocular disease

The ocular manifestations of TB may result from either active infection or an immunologic reaction to the organism. *Primary ocular TB* is defined as TB in which the eye is the primary portal of entry, and it manifests mainly as conjunctival, corneal, and scleral disease. *Secondary ocular TB,* of which uveitis is the most common manifestation, occurs by virtue of hematogenous dissemination or by contiguous spread from adjacent structures. External ocular and anterior segment findings include scleritis, phlyctenulosis, interstitial keratitis, corneal infiltrates, anterior chamber and iris nodules, and isolated granulomatous anterior uveitis; the last is exceedingly uncommon in the absence of posterior segment disease.

Tuberculous uveitis is classically a chronic granulomatous disease that may affect the anterior and/or posterior segments; it is replete with mutton-fat KPs, iris nodules, posterior synechiae, and secondary glaucoma, although a nongranulomatous uveitis may also occur. Patients typically experience a waxing and waning course, with long-term degradation of the blood–aqueous barrier, an accumulation of vitreous opacities, and CME (Figs 7-53, 7-54).

Disseminated choroiditis is the most common presentation and is characterized by deep, multiple, discrete, yellowish lesions between 0.5 and 3.0 mm in diameter, numbering from 5 to several hundred (Fig 7-55). These lesions, or tubercles, are located predominantly in the posterior pole and may be accompanied by disc edema, nerve fiber hemorrhages, and varying degrees of vitritis and granulomatous anterior uveitis. Alternatively, they may present as a single, focal, large, elevated choroidal mass (tuberculoma) that varies in size from 4–14 mm and may be accompanied by neurosensory retinal detachment and macular star formation (Fig 7-56). Choroidal tubercles may be one of the earliest signs of disseminated disease and are more commonly observed among immunocompromised hosts. On FA, active choroidal lesions display early hyperfluorescence with late leakage, and cicatricial lesions show early blocked fluorescence with late staining. ICG angiography reveals early- and late-stage hypofluorescence corresponding to the choroidal lesions, which are frequently more numerous than those seen on FA or even on clinical examination. Other manifestations of tuberculous infection of the choroid include multifocal choroiditis and a serpiginous-like choroiditis (Fig 7-57). In the setting of HIV/AIDS, tuberculous choroiditis may progress despite effective antituberculous therapy.

Retinal involvement in TB is usually secondary to extension of the choroidal disease or an immunologic response to mycobacteria. Eales disease is a peripheral retinal perivasculitis that presents in otherwise healthy young men aged 20–40 years with recurrent, unilateral retinal and vitreous hemorrhage and subsequent involvement of the fellow eye. A periphlebitis is most commonly observed, which may be accompanied by venous occlusion, peripheral nonperfusion, neovascularization, and the eventual development of tractional retinal detachment (Fig 7-58). The association between TB and retinal vasculitis is supported by the identification by PCR-based assays of *M tuberculosis* DNA from the aqueous, vitreous, and epiretinal membranes of patients with Eales disease. Other posterior segment findings of TB include subretinal abscess, CNV, optic neuritis, and acute panophthalmitis.

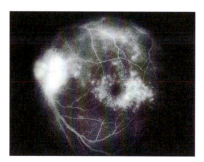

Figure 7-53 Chronic tuberculous uveitis with disc edema, vasculitis, periphlebitis, and cystoid macular edema (CME). *(Courtesy of John D. Sheppard, Jr, MD.)*

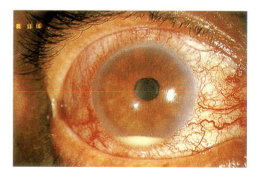

Figure 7-54 Acute tuberculous uveitis with hypopyon, posterior synechiae, vitritis, retinal vasculitis, and CME. *(Courtesy of John D. Sheppard, Jr, MD.)*

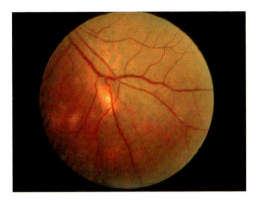

Figure 7-55 Multifocal, discrete, yellowish choroidal lesions in a patient with pulmonary tuberculosis. *(Reproduced with permission from Vitale AT, Foster CS. Uveitis affecting infants and children: infectious causes. In: Hartnett ME, Trese M, Capone A, Keats B, Steidl SM, eds.* Pediatric Retina. *Philadelphia, PA: Lippincott Williams & Wilkins; 2005:277; courtesy of Albert T. Vitale, MD.)*

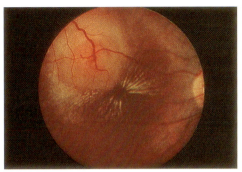

Figure 7-56 Choroidal tubercle with a macular star formation (miliary tuberculosis).

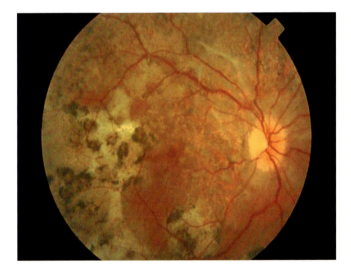

Figure 7-57 Tuberculous choroiditis masquerading as atypical serpiginous choroiditis. The patient showed progression and recurrence while on immunomodulatory agents; however, after antituberculous treatment, the patient showed improvement in vision and resolution of the vitritis without recurrences. *(Courtesy of Narsing A. Rao, MD.)*

Diagnosis

Definitive diagnosis of TB requires a finding of mycobacteria in bodily fluids or tissues. In many cases of ocular TB, this is not possible, and the diagnosis is instead presumptive, based on indirect evidence. A positive result on the PPD test or interferon gamma release assays such as the QuantiFERON-TB Gold test is indicative of prior exposure to TB but

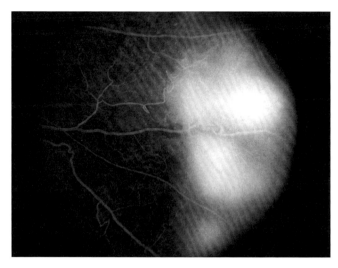

Figure 7-58 Eales disease. Fluorescein angiogram showing diffuse late leakage from peripheral retinal neovascularization. *(Courtesy of Albert T. Vitale, MD.)*

not necessarily of active systemic infection. In the United States, an induration of 5 mm or more, read 48–72 hours after intradermal injection of the standard 5-tuberculin-unit (5-TU), or intermediate-strength, test dose is considered to be a positive result in individuals with HIV infection, those exposed to active TB, or those whose radiographs are consistent with healed tuberculous lesions. An induration of 10 mm or more is considered indicative of a positive result for other high-risk groups, including patients with diabetes or renal failure, those on IMT, health care workers, and recent immigrants from high-prevalence countries. Patients with no known risks for tuberculosis are considered to exhibit a positive test result with an induration of 15 mm or more.

False-negative skin testing results occur at a rate of 25% because of patients with profound acute illness or immunocompromise, which can stem from corticosteroid use, advanced age, poor nutrition, and sarcoidosis. False-positive results may arise from patients infected with atypical mycobacteria, those immunized with bacille Calmette-Guérin (BCG), and treatment with intraluminal BCG injections for bladder carcinoma. Individuals recently immunized with BCG may present with an induration measuring around 10 mm, but the reaction is usually not sustained and tends to decrease with time compared to the reaction following the skin test after more recent systemic TB exposure. A Bayesian analysis predicts that routine screening of uveitis patients with PPD skin testing has a low probability of detecting disease in settings where the prevalence of TB is low. It is recommended, therefore, that skin testing be selectively used for patients in whom the index of suspicion has been heightened by a careful history, review of systems, and clinical examination.

A history of recent exposure to TB or a positive PPD test result warrants a concerted search for systemic infection, using chest radiography, PET scan, and/or microbiologic analysis of sputum, urine, or gastric aspirates, or a cervical lymph node biopsy for acid-fast bacilli. Failure to demonstrate systemic disease does not, however, exclude the possibility of intraocular infection. For cases of suspected ocular TB in which the results of the above-mentioned testing for systemic infection is negative, the patient is asymptomatic, or the infection is thought to be extrapulmonary, definitive diagnosis may require intraocular fluid analysis or tissue biopsy. Nucleic acid amplification techniques, with either transcription-mediated amplification of 16S ribosomal RNA or PCR amplification of unique DNA sequences of *M tuberculosis,* have been successfully used to diagnose intraocular TB. Chorioretinal biopsy used in conjunction with nucleic acid amplification techniques and routine histologic examination may be necessary in atypical cases where the differential diagnosis and therapeutic options are widely divergent. Recently, antibodies against purified cord factor, the most antigenic and abundant cell wall component of tubercle bacilli, have been detected by ELISA and may be useful for rapid serodiagnosis of pulmonary TB, in addition to providing supportive data for the diagnosis of ocular infection.

Treatment

Systemic antibiotic therapy is clearly indicated for patients with uveitis whose TB test results have recently converted to positive, those with an abnormal-appearing chest radiograph, or those with positive bacterial culture or PCR results. Multiple-agent therapy is recommended because of the increasing incidence of resistance to isoniazid (INH), as well as adherence problems associated with long-term therapy. These problems, together with the extremely slow growth rate of TB, contribute to the acquisition of multidrug-resistant tuberculosis (MDRTB). Patients at risk for MDRTB include nonadherent patients on single-agent therapy; migrant or indigent populations; immunocompromised patients, including those with HIV infection; and recent immigrants from countries where INH and rifampin are available over the counter. In brief, treatment entails an initial 2-month induction course of INH, rifampin, and pyrazinamide administered daily, followed by a continuation phase of 4–7 months. In the event of drug resistance, another agent, such as ethambutol or streptomycin, is added to the initial triple-drug regimen, followed by a 4-month continuation of INH and rifampin. More than 95% of immunocompetent patients may be successfully treated with a full course of therapy provided they remain adherent to this regimen. Directly observed therapy (DOT) plays a critical role in ensuring this success and is now the standard of care in the treatment of tuberculosis. Treatment protocols have been standardized and are available from the CDC.

More difficult is the treatment approach to patients with uveitis consistent with TB, normal chest radiograph appearance, and a positive TB test result. In this situation, a diagnosis of extrapulmonary TB may be entertained and treatment initiated, particularly in the setting of medically unresponsive uveitis or other findings supportive of the diagnosis, such as recent exposure to or inadequate treatment of the disease, a large area of induration, or skin test result recently converted to positive. Topical and systemic corticosteroids are frequently used in conjunction with antimicrobial therapy to treat the inflammatory component of the disease. Because intensive corticosteroid treatment administered without appropriate antituberculous cover may lead to progressive worsening of ocular disease, any patient suspected of harboring TB should undergo appropriate testing prior to beginning such therapy (Fig 7-59). Patients with a positive TB test result or abnormal chest film appearance in whom systemic corticosteroid treatment is being considered, or those who have received corticosteroids for longer than 2 weeks at doses greater than

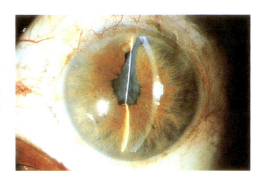

Figure 7-59 Long-standing, undiagnosed tuberculous uveitis with aphakia, dense pupillary membrane, posterior synechiae, CME, and chronic vitritis despite intensive corticosteroid therapy. *(Courtesy of John D. Sheppard, Jr, MD.)*

15 mg/day, may benefit from prophylactic treatment with INH for 6 months to a year. Likewise, patients with latent TB in whom anti–tumor necrosis factor therapy is being considered should be treated with INH prophylaxis beginning at least 3 weeks prior to the first infusion.

Diel R, Loddenkemper R, Nienhaus A. Evidence-based comparison of commercial interferon-γ release assays for detecting active TB: a metaanalysis. *Chest.* 2010;137(4):952–968.

Gupta A, Gupta V. Tubercular posterior uveitis. *Int Ophthalmol Clin.* 2005;45(2):71–88.

Mehta S, Gilada IS. Ocular tuberculosis in acquired immune deficiency syndrome (AIDS). *Ocul Immunol Inflamm.* 2005;13(1):87–89.

Morimura Y, Okada AA, Kawahara S, et al. Tuberculin skin testing in uveitis patients and treatment of presumed intraocular tuberculosis in Japan. *Ophthalmology.* 2002;109(5):851–857.

Sheu SJ, Shyu JS, Chen LM, Chen YY, Chirn SC, Wang JS. Ocular manifestations of tuberculosis. *Ophthalmology.* 2000;108(9):1580–1585.

Syed Ahamed Kabeer B, Raman B, Thomas A, Perumal V, Raja A. Role of QuantiFERON-TB gold, interferon gamma inducible protein-10 and tuberculin skin test in active tuberculosis diagnosis. *PLoS One.* 2010;5(2):e9051. doi: 10.1371/journal.pone.0009051

Thompson NJ, Albert DM. Ocular tuberculosis. *Arch Ophthalmol.* 2005;123(6):844–849.

Varma D, Anand S, Reddy AR, et al. Tuberculosis: an under-diagnosed aetiological agent in uveitis with an effective treatment. *Eye (Lond).* 2005;20(9):1068–1073.

Ocular Bartonellosis

Bartonella henselae (formerly *Rochalimaea henselae*), a small, fastidious, gram-negative rod, initially isolated from the tissue of patients with bacillary angiomatosis of AIDS, is now known to be the principal etiologic agent of cat-scratch disease (CSD) and is associated with an expanding spectrum of ocular manifestations. CSD is a feline-associated zoonotic disease found worldwide, with an estimated annual incidence rate in the United States of 9.3 cases per 100,000 persons; the highest age-specific incidence is among children younger than 10 years of age. Cats are the primary mammalian reservoir of *B henselae* and *Bartonella quintana,* and the cat flea is an important vector for the transmission of the organism among cats. The disease follows a seasonal pattern, occurring predominantly in the fall and winter, and is most prevalent in the southern states, California, and Hawaii. The disease is transmitted to humans by the scratches, licks, and bites of domestic cats, particularly kittens.

Systemic manifestations of CSD include a mild to moderate flulike illness associated with regional adenopathy that usually precedes the ocular manifestations of the disease. An erythematous papule, vesicle, or pustule usually forms at the primary site of cutaneous injury 3–10 days after primary inoculation and 1–2 weeks before the onset of lymphadenopathy and constitutional symptoms. Less commonly, more severe and disseminated disease may develop that is associated with encephalopathy, aseptic meningitis, osteomyelitis, hepatosplenic disease, pneumonia, and pleural and pericardial effusions.

Ocular involvement, which occurs in 5%–10% of patients with CSD, includes Parinaud oculoglandular syndrome (unilateral granulomatous conjunctivitis and regional lymphadenopathy) in approximately 5% of patients and a wide array of posterior segment and neuro-ophthalmic findings. Entities to be considered in the differential diagnosis of Parinaud oculoglandular syndrome include tularemia, tuberculosis, syphilis, sporotrichosis, and acute *Chlamydia trachomatis* infection.

The most well-known posterior segment manifestation of *B henselae* infection is neuroretinitis, a constellation of findings that includes abrupt visual loss, unilateral optic disc swelling, and macular star formation, which occurs in 1%–2% of patients with CSD (focal retinochoroiditis, however, is the most common uveitic manifestation of CSD). This syndrome, formerly known as *idiopathic stellate maculopathy* and later renamed *Leber idiopathic stellate neuroretinitis,* is now known to be caused by *B henselae* infection in approximately two-thirds of cases. See Table 7-5 for a list of other entities that may cause neuroretinitis. Visual acuity loss varies to between 20/25 and 20/200 or worse and follows

---

Table 7-5 Neuroretinitis: Other Associated Causes

Infectious
  Bartonellosis *(Bartonella henselae)*
  Syphilis
  Lyme disease
  Tuberculosis
  Diffuse unilateral subacute neuroretinitis (DUSN) *(Ancylostoma caninum, Baylisascaris procyonis)*
  Toxoplasmosis
  Toxocariasis
  Leptospirosis
  Salmonella
  Chickenpox (varicella)
  Herpes simplex
  Ehrlichiosis
  Rocky Mountain spotted fever

Noninfectious
  Sarcoidosis
  Acute systemic hypertension
  Diabetes mellitus
  Idiopathic increased intracranial hypertension
  Anterior ischemic optic neuropathy
  Leukemic infiltration of the optic nerve

Idiopathic
  Recurrent idiopathic neuroretintis

the onset of constitutional symptoms by approximately 2–3 weeks. Although the presentation is most often unilateral, bilateral cases of neuroretinitis have been reported and are frequently asymmetric in this setting. Optic disc edema, associated with peripapillary serous retinal detachment, has been observed 2–4 weeks before the appearance of the macular star and may be a sign of systemic *B henselae* infection. The development of the macular star is variable and may be partial or incomplete, usually resolving in approximately 8–12 weeks. When incomplete, a partial macular star is usually seen nasal to the macula (Fig 7-60).

Most patients with *Bartonella*-associated neuroretinitis exhibit some degree of anterior chamber inflammation and vitritis. Discrete, focal, or multifocal retinal and/or choroidal lesions measuring 50–300 μm are common posterior segment findings that may occur in the presence or absence of disc edema or exudates; when present, they provide strong support for the diagnosis of *B henselae* infection. Both arterial and venous occlusive disease, as well as localized neurosensory macular detachments, have been described in association with focal retinitis. Other posterior segment ocular complications include epiretinal membranes, inflammatory mass of the optic nerve head, peripapillary angiomatosis, intermediate uveitis, retinal white dot syndromes, orbital abscess, isolated optic disc swelling, and panuveitis.

The diagnosis of CSD is based on the characteristic clinical features together with confirmatory serologic testing. The indirect fluorescent antibody assay for the detection of serum anti–*B henselae* antibodies is 88% sensitive and 94% specific, with titers of greater than 1:64 being considered positive. Enzyme immunoassays with a sensitivity for IgG of 86%–95% and a specificity of 96%, together with Western blot analysis, have also been developed. A single positive indirect fluorescent antibody or enzyme immunoassay titer for IgG or IgM is sufficient to confirm the diagnosis of CSD. Other diagnostic approaches include bacterial cultures, which may require several weeks for colonies to become apparent; skin testing, with a sensitivity of up to 100% and a specificity of up to 98%; and PCR-based techniques that target the bacterial 16S ribosomal RNA gene or *B henselae* DNA.

Definitive treatment guidelines have not emerged for CSD because in most cases it is a self-limiting illness with an overall excellent systemic and visual prognosis. A variety of antibiotics, including doxycycline, erythromycin, rifampin, trimethoprim-sulfamethoxazole, ciprofloxacin, and gentamycin, have been used in the treatment of more severe systemic or

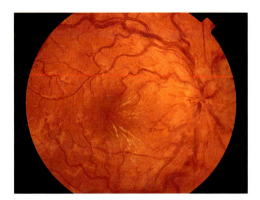

Figure 7-60 Partial macular star, optic disc swelling, and moderate vascular engorgement in a patient with cat-scratch disease. *(Reproduced with permission from Vitale AT, Foster CS. Uveitis affecting infants and children: infectious causes. In: Hartnett ME, Trese M, Capone A, Keats B, Steidl SM, eds.* Pediatric Retina. *Philadelphia, PA: Lippincott Williams & Wilkins; 2005:278; courtesy of Albert T. Vitale, MD.)*

ocular manifestations, despite the fact that their efficacy has not been conclusively demonstrated. A typical regimen for immunocompetent patients older than age 8 consists of doxycycline, 100 mg orally twice daily for 2–4 weeks. For more severe infections, doxycycline may be given intravenously or used in combination with rifampin, 300 mg orally twice daily; among immunocompromised individuals, this treatment is extended for 4 months. Children with CSD may be treated with azithromycin, but the safety of ciprofloxacin in individuals younger than age 18 has not been established. The efficacy of oral corticosteroids on the course of systemic and ocular disease is unknown. Finally, in the subset of patients with recurrent idiopathic neuroretinitis, long-term IMT may be of benefit.

Cunningham ET Jr, Koehler JE. Ocular bartonellosis. *Am J Ophthalmol.* 2000;130(3):340–349.

Purvin V, Ranson M, Kawasaki A. Idiopathic recurrent neuroretinitis: effects of long-term immunosuppression. *Arch Ophthalmol.* 2003;121(1):65–67.

Reed JB, Scales DK, Wong MT, Lattuada CP Jr, Dolan MJ, Schwab IR. *Bartonella henselae* neuroretinitis in cat-scratch disease. Diagnosis, management, and sequelae. *Ophthalmology.* 1998;105(3):459–466.

Suhler ED, Lauer AK, Rosenbaum JT. Prevalence of serologic evidence of cat scratch disease in patients with neuroretinitis. *Ophthalmology.* 2000;107(5):871–876.

Wade NK, Levi L, Jones MR, Bhisitkul R, Fine L, Cunningham ET Jr. Optic disc edema associated with peripapillary serous retinal detachment: an early sign of systemic *Bartonella henselae* infection. *Am J Ophthalmol.* 2000;130(3):327–334.

Whipple Disease

Whipple disease is a rare multisystem disease caused by the *Tropheryma whipplei* bacterium. It is most common in middle-aged white men. Migratory arthritis occurs in 80% of cases. Gastrointestinal symptoms, including diarrhea, steatorrhea, and malabsorption, occur in 75%. Intestinal loss of protein results in pitting edema and weight loss. Cardiomyopathy and valvular disease can also occur. Central nervous system involvement occurs in 10% of cases and results in seizures, dementia, and coma. Neuro-ophthalmic signs can include cranial nerve palsies, nystagmus, and ophthalmoplegia. Some patients develop a progressive supranuclear palsy–like condition.

Intraocular involvement is rare and occurs in less than 5% of cases. Patients can present with bilateral panuveitis and retinal vasculitis. Both anterior uveitis and moderate vitritis are present. Diffuse chorioretinal inflammation and diffuse retinal vasculitis in the perifoveal and midperipheral regions may occur. Retinal vascular occlusions and retinal hemorrhages may result from the vasculitis. Optic disc edema and, later, optic atrophy may occur. Unusual granular, crystalline deposits on the iris, capsular bag, and IOL have also been reported.

The gold standard for diagnosis of Whipple disease is a duodenal biopsy that demonstrates a periodic acid–Schiff–positive bacillus in macrophages within intestinal villi. PCR analysis of peripheral blood and vitreous may show *T whipplei* DNA and confirm the diagnosis. Culturing of *T whipplei* is difficult but possible. The differential diagnosis of uveitis associated with Whipple disease includes diseases that can cause retinal vasculitis with multisystem involvement, including SLE, polyarteritis nodosa, and Behçet disease.

Untreated Whipple disease can be fatal. Systemic trimethoprim-sulfamethoxazole is the preferred treatment. Patients allergic to sulfonamides may be treated with ceftriaxone, tetracycline, or chloramphenicol. Treatment duration may vary from 1 to 3 months, but relapses occur in 30% of cases, necessitating prolonged (up to 1 year) treatment. Retinal vasculitis can resolve with treatment, but neurologic deficits become permanent.

Chan RY, Yannuzzi LA, Foster CS. Ocular Whipple's disease: earlier definitive diagnosis. *Ophthalmology.* 2001;108(12):2225–2231.

Razonable RR, Pulido JS, Deziel PJ, Dev S, Salomão DR, Walker RC. Chorioretinitis and vitreitis due to *Tropheryma whipplei* after transplantation: case report and review. *Transpl Infect Dis.* 2008;10(6):413–418.

Williams JG, Edward DP, Tessler HH, Persing DH, Mitchell PS, Goldstein DA. Ocular manifestations of Whipple disease: an atypical presentation. *Arch Ophthalmol.* 1998;116(9):1232–1234.

Infectious Scleritis

Scleritis may occur in the setting of previous surgery or trauma, in which case an infectious etiology must be considered. Differentiation from noninfectious scleritis is important, as treatment regimens differ. See Chapter 6 in this volume and BCSC Section 8, *External Disease and Cornea,* for discussions of noninfectious scleritis.

Etiology

A wide variety of agents can infect the sclera, including *Pseudomonas* organisms (most common after pterygium excision), *Actinomyces* and *Nocardia* species, mycobacteria, fungi such as *Fusarium* and *Aspergillus* species, and gram-positive cocci (*Staphylococcus pneumococcus* and *Streptococcus* species). In addition, HSV and VZV can cause chronic infectious scleritis. Men and women appear to be equally affected. Infectious scleritis can occur after any previous ocular surgery, including pterygium surgery (especially when beta irradiation or mitomycin C is utilized), scleral buckling, cataract surgery, and pars plana vitrectomy. Trauma with a penetrating injury contaminated by soil or vegetable matter may also result in infectious scleritis.

Clinical Features

Infectious scleritis may present in a manner similar to noninfectious scleritis, with pain, redness, and decreased vision. The precipitating surgery may be recent or remote (in rare cases, many years). The sclera appears necrotic, thin, and avascular, with inflammation at edges (Fig 7-61), usually at the site of a surgical or traumatic wound. A mucopurulent discharge may be present depending on the microbiological agent responsible.

Diagnostic Workup

Cultures of the area of involvement, including the base and edges of the lesion, should be obtained. A lamellar scleral biopsy should be considered if the condition worsens on anti-inflammatory therapy alone. A diagnostic evaluation for noninfectious necrotizing scleritis should be performed, as detailed in Section 8, *External Disease and Cornea.*

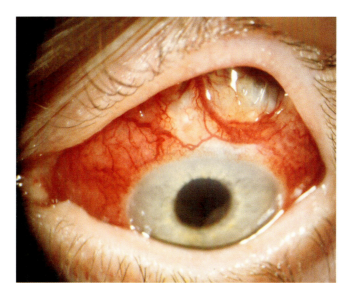

Figure 7-61 Necrotizing *Nocardia* scleritis occurring following cataract surgery. Note the violaceous hue to the sclera and localized avascular, necrotic sclera superiorly in the bed of the original corneoscleral contact wound. *(Courtesy of Ramana S. Moorthy, MD.)*

Treatment

The best outcome may be obtained when medical and surgical treatments are combined. Debridement of infected tissues may be needed. Antibiotics can be delivered topically, subconjunctivally, or systemically, and should be based on the suspected agent and culture results; microorganisms may be difficult to eradicate from the sclera and long-term treatment may be necessary. Corticosteroids should be avoided initially. Analgesics for pain control should be considered. Scleral patch grafting may be needed in patients who exhibit severe thinning in order to stabilize the eyewall.

Prognosis

Infectious scleritis is difficult to treat and multiple complications are common. If surgery is required, globe perforation may occur because of the thin necrotic sclera. Inadequate excision of infected tissues can result in disease recurrence, and an extension of the infection to the cornea may occur with inadequate or unsuccessful treatment. Endophthalmitis from intraocular extension can develop. Serous retinal detachment from concurrent inflammation of the eyewall is possible.

Lin CP, Su CY. Infectious scleritis and surgical induced necrotizing scleritis [letter]. *Eye (Lond)*. 2010;24(4):740.

Raiji VR, Palestine AG, Parver DL. Scleritis and systemic disease association in a community-based referral practice. *Am J Ophthalmol*. 2009;148(6):946–950.

CHAPTER 8

Endophthalmitis

Endophthalmitis is a clinical diagnosis made when intraocular inflammation involving both the posterior and anterior chambers is attributable to bacterial or fungal infection. The retina or the choroid may be involved; occasionally there is concomitant infective scleritis or keratitis. Acute postoperative and posttraumatic endophthalmitis are covered in BCSC Section 12, *Retina and Vitreous,* and will not be covered here. Chronic postoperative (infectious) endophthalmitis occurs weeks or months after surgery (usually cataract extraction) and is caused by a myriad of bacteria and fungi. Endogenous endophthalmitis occurs when bacteria or fungi are hematogenously disseminated into the ocular circulation. Sterile endophthalmitis describes cases in which infection is suspected but that return negative culture results.

Chronic Postoperative Endophthalmitis

Chronic postoperative endophthalmitis has a distinctive clinical course, with multiple recurrences of chronic indolent inflammation in an eye that had previously undergone surgery, typically cataract extraction. This recurrent indolent inflammation may occur at any point during the postoperative course, as early as 1 to 2 weeks after surgery, but it is often delayed by many weeks to months and sometimes years. This is quite different from the explosive onset of acute postoperative endophthalmitis. The incidence of acute postoperative endophthalmitis varies between 0.07% and 0.1%. The incidence of chronic endophthalmitis, however, has not been well established, as the condition may often go undiagnosed. Chronic postoperative endophthalmitis can be divided into bacterial and fungal varieties. Chronic postoperative fungal endophthalmitis should be distinguished from endogenous fungal endophthalmitis, which is typically caused by *Candida* and *Aspergillus* species.

Chronic postoperative bacterial endophthalmitis is most commonly caused by *Propionibacterium acnes.* Other bacteria with limited virulence, such as *Staphylococcus epidermidis* and *Corynebacterium* species, may also cause similar chronic infection. *P acnes,* a commensal, anaerobic, gram-positive, pleomorphic rod, is found on the eyelid skin or on the conjunctiva of normal patients. It is thought that *P acnes* may sequester itself between the intraocular lens (IOL) implant and the posterior capsule. In this relatively anaerobic environment, the organism grows and forms colonies, which manifest themselves as whitish plaques between the posterior capsule and the IOL implant (Fig 8-1). The patient may present with slight blurring of vision and a persistent granulomatous inflammation

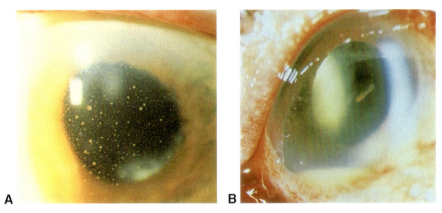

A B

Figure 8-1 **A** and **B,** Chronic postoperative endophthalmitis caused by *Propionibacterium acnes*. Note granulomatous keratic precipitates and white plaque in the capsular bag. *(Courtesy of David Meisler, MD.)*

that begins on average 3–4 months after surgery; this infection may respond initially to topical or regional corticosteroids, but often worsens or recurs when the corticosteroids are tapered. There may vitreous inflammation, corneal decompensation, and even iris neovascularization in the most severe untreated cases. Nd:YAG capsulotomy can trigger chronic endophthalmitis by liberating the organism into the vitreous cavity, resulting in a more severe vitreous inflammation and an exacerbation of underlying infection.

Chronic postoperative fungal endophthalmitis may present in a very similar fashion to that caused by *P acnes*. Multiple fungal organisms have been implicated in this chronic inflammatory process, including *Candida parapsilosis, Aspergillus flavus, Torulopsis candida, Paecilomyces lilacinus,* as well as *Verticillium* species. Most of these cases have occurred after cataract surgery, although other kinds of surgery may predispose to the development of fungal endophthalmitis. Patients may present with a delayed-onset, indolent, progressive inflammation that is not responsive to corticosteroids. Certain clinical signs may be helpful in differentiating a fungal from a bacterial etiology, including the presence of corneal infiltrate or edema, mass in the iris or ciliary body, or development of necrotizing scleritis. Presence of vitreous snowballs with a "string-of-pearls" appearance in the vitreous may also be indicative of a fungal infection. The intraocular inflammation may worsen after topical, periocular, or intraocular steroid therapy, which should automatically raise the suspicion of a possible infectious masquerade syndrome.

The diagnosis of chronic postoperative endophthalmitis is confirmed by obtaining aerobic, anaerobic, and fungal cultures of the aqueous, capsular plaques (if present), and undiluted vitreous at the time of therapeutic pars plana vitrectomy. Gram and Giemsa stains of undiluted specimens, capsular plaques, and vitreous snowballs should also be obtained along with polymerase chain reaction (PCR) studies of vitreous for *P acnes* or suspected fungi. The value of Gram and Giemsa stains cannot be underestimated, especially in cases of fungal endophthalmitis. The bacterial and fungal stains may yield immediate information enabling the clinician to tailor therapy and improve clinical prognosis long before the results of the cultures turn positive. Because of the slow-growing and fastidious nature of the organisms that cause chronic endophthalmitis, cultures must be retained by the microbiology laboratory for 2 or more weeks. PCR evaluation of aqueous, vitreous, and capsular plaques using pan-fungal and pan-bacterial primers is also of significant diagnostic value in these cases.

The differential diagnosis of chronic postoperative endophthalmitis includes noninfectious causes, such as lens-induced uveitis from retained cortical material or retained intravitreal lens fragments, intraocular inflammation from iris chafing resulting from IOL malposition, uveitis-glaucoma-hyphema syndrome, and intraocular lymphoma masquerade syndrome.

Pars plana vitrectomy and injection of intravitreal and endocapsular vancomycin is therapeutic in many cases of chronic postoperative bacterial endophthalmitis; however, this may not be completely successful in eradicating the infection, especially if equatorial lens capsule sequestrae of bacteria are present. In such cases IOL explantation, complete capsulectomy, and intravitreal vancomycin injection is curative. The decision to explant the IOL must be based in part on the clinical course, the severity of the intraocular inflammation, and the level of vision loss; it is made on a case-by-case basis. There is no preferred method for treating this condition, but it is clear from the existing literature that more than 1 surgery may be necessary in some cases to completely eradicate this chronic infection. The treatment of chronic fungal endophthalmitis is more difficult and requires the use of intravitreal antifungal agents (amphotericin and voriconazole) and, possibly, systemic antifungal agents in the most severe cases. Multiple surgeries may be necessary. The role of systemic therapy in this chronic form of fungal endophthalmitis is not well established or proven.

Lai J-Y, Chen K-H, Lin Y-C, Hsu W-M, Lee S-M. *Propionibacterium acnes* DNA from an explanted intraocular lens detected by polymerase chain reaction in a case of chronic pseudophakic endophthalmitis. *J Cataract Refract Surg.* 2006;32(3):522–535.

Meisler D, Mandelbaum S. *Propionibacterium*-associated endophthalmitis after extracapsular cataract extraction. Review of the reported cases. *Ophthalmology.* 1989;96(1):54–61.

Samson CM, Foster CS. Chronic postoperative endophthalmitis. *Int Ophthalmol Clin.* 2000; 40(1):57–67.

Endogenous Endophthalmitis

Endogenous Bacterial Endophthalmitis

Endogenous endophthalmitis is caused by hematogenous dissemination of bacterial organisms resulting in intraocular infection. This is an uncommon entity and accounts for less than 10% of all forms of endophthalmitis. Patients who have compromised immune systems are most at risk for developing endogenous endophthalmitis. Predisposing conditions include diabetes mellitus, systemic malignancy, sickle cell anemia, systemic lupus erythematosus, and human immunodeficiency virus (HIV) infection. Extensive gastrointestinal surgery, endoscopy, and dental procedures may all increase risk of endogenous endophthalmitis. Systemic immunomodulatory therapy and chemotherapy may also put patients at risk. Although the eye may be the only location where the infection can be found, there is an extraocular focus in 90% of cases. One must consider the possibility of pneumonia, urinary tract infection, bacterial meningitis, or a liver abscess as possible sources of infection. A wide variety of bacteria can cause endogenous endophthalmitis. The most common gram-positive organisms are *Streptococcus* species (endocarditis), *Staphylococcus aureus* (cutaneous infections), and *Bacillus* species (from intravenous drug use). The most common gram-negative organisms are *Neisseria meningitidis* (Fig 8-2), *Haemophilus influenzae,* and enteric organisms such as *Escherichia coli* and *Klebsiella* species. In Asia, infection from *Klebsiella* species in liver abscesses is the most common cause of endogenous endophthalmitis. It is important to also consider endogenous endophthalmitis in newborns and infants, especially those younger than 6 months.

The clinical features of endogenous bacterial endophthalmitis are suggestive of an ongoing systemic infection, and this may be associated with fever greater than 101.5°F, elevated peripheral leukocyte count, and positive bacterial cultures from extraocular sites (blood, urine, sputum). Patients are often ill and being treated for a primary underlying disease when they present with endogenous endophthalmitis. This disease may include cancer treated with prolonged intravenous chemotherapy or other chronic infections, which may subsequently sequester in the eye. A nonocular infection serving as a nidus for bacterial dissemination to the eye may be very difficult to diagnose, especially in cases of osteomyelitis, sinusitis, or pneumonia that is misdiagnosed as a simple upper respiratory tract infection. In these situations, laboratory tests are no substitute for a detailed history and review of systems; these continue to provide the most critical information for making the clinical diagnosis in any uveitic condition.

Clinical symptoms include acute onset of pain, photophobia, and blurred vision. Examination usually reveals severely reduced visual acuity, periorbital and eyelid edema, and fibrin in the anterior chamber; hypopyon may be present. There may be significant vitreous inflammation and vitreous cells. Sometimes, both eyes are affected simultaneously. Small microabscesses in the retina or subretinal space and white, centered retinal hemorrhages (Roth spots) may also be seen.

Diagnosis is based on anterior chamber paracentesis and vitrectomy with vitreous and aqueous cultures and Gram and Giemsa stains if fungal organisms are suspected. As with cases of chronic postoperative endophthalmitis, PCR evaluation of ocular fluids with pan-bacterial or pan-fungal primers is extremely useful. Blood and other body fluid cultures should be used together with ocular culture results to confirm the diagnosis and establish therapy. Intravitreal antibiotics are administered at the time of vitrectomy; if it is not clear whether or not fungal organisms may be involved, treatment of both fungal and

Figure 8-2 Endogenous endophthalmitis (meningococcal meningitis).

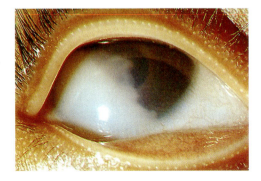

bacterial etiologies is indicated at the time of vitrectomy. In addition, intravenous antibiotic treatment is sometimes required for several weeks, depending on the organism that is isolated. Similarly, in patients who have endogenous fungal endophthalmitis, systemic antifungal therapy may be warranted for 6 weeks or more. Initial antimicrobial choices may be empiric and may be tailored to culture results.

The complications of endogenous endophthalmitis can be serious. If the diagnosis of systemic infection is missed, the patient may develop sepsis and even die. In severe cases, recurrent or persistent intraocular infection may require multiple surgeries and multiple injections of intravitreal antibiotics. In addition, complications such as cataract development, retinal detachment, suprachoroidal hemorrhage, vitreous hemorrhage, hypotony, and phthisis bulbi can occur in the most severe cases. The prognosis is directly related to the offending organism and the systemic status of the patient.

Chen YJ, Kuo HK, Wu PC, et al. A 10-year comparison of endogenous endophthalmitis outcomes: an east Asian experience with *Klebsiella pneumoniae* infection. *Retina.* 2004;24(3): 383–390.

Okada AA, Johnson RP, Liles WC, D'Amico DJ, Baker AS. Endogenous bacterial endophthalmitis. Report of a ten-year retrospective study. *Ophthalmology.* 1994;101(5):832–838.

Rodriguez-Adrian LJ, King RT, Tamayo-Derat LG, Miller JW, Garcia CA, Rex JH. Retinal lesions as clues to disseminated bacterial and candidal infections: frequency, natural history, and etiology. *Medicine (Baltimore).* 2003;82(3):187–202.

Endogenous Fungal Endophthalmitis

Endogenous fungal endophthalmitis develops slowly as focal or multifocal areas of chorioretinitis. Granulomatous or nongranulomatous inflammation is observed with keratic precipitates, hypopyon, and vitritis with cellular aggregates. The infection usually begins in the choroid, appearing as yellow-white lesions with indistinct borders that range in size from small cotton-wool spots to several disc diameters (Fig 8-3). It can subsequently break through into the vitreous, producing localized cellular and fungal aggregates overlying the original site(s). Iris nodules and rubeosis may also be seen in cases of severe fungal endophthalmitis.

Endogenous fungal endophthalmitis due to *Candida* (the most common cause), *Aspergillus*, and *Coccidioides* species can be considered a nonneoplastic masquerade syndrome because, in many patients, the condition is mistaken for noninfectious uveitis and

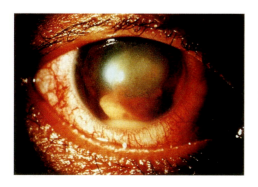

Figure 8-3 Fungal endophthalmitis.

treated with corticosteroids alone. This usually worsens the clinical course of the disease, necessitating further investigation to establish the correct diagnosis. The condition often requires aggressive systemic and local antifungal therapy as well as surgical intervention.

Endogenous fungal endophthalmitis caused by *Histoplasma capsulatum*, *Cryptococcus neoformans*, *Sporothrix schenkii*, and *Blastomyces dermatitidis* is less common than that caused by *Candida* and *Aspergillus* species.

Gonzales CA, Scott IU, Chaudhry NA, et al. Endogenous endophthalmitis caused by *Histoplasma capsulatum* var. capsulatum: a case report and literature review. *Ophthalmology.* 2000;107(2):725–729.

Candida *endophthalmitis*

Candida species are an important cause of nosocomial infections and are the most common fungal organisms, causing endogenous endophthalmitis in both the pediatric and adult populations. Although *Candida albicans* remains the most common pathogen, non-*albicans* species (eg, *Candida glabrata*) have also been identified in patients developing ocular disease. In patients with candidemia, the reported prevalence rates of intraocular candidiasis vary widely, ranging between 9% and 78%. However, when strict criteria are applied for the classification of chorioretinitis and endophthalmitis, these numbers drop precipitously; in 1 series, when patients were examined within 72 hours of a positive blood culture result, only 9% had chorioretinitis and none had endophthalmitis. Endogenous *Candida* endophthalmitis occurs in up to 37% of patients with candidemia if they are not receiving antifungal therapy. Ocular involvement drops to 3% in patients who are receiving treatment. Predisposing conditions associated with candidemia and the development of intraocular infection include hospitalization with a history of recent major gastrointestinal surgery, bacterial sepsis, systemic antibiotic use, indwelling catheters, hyperalimentation, debilitating diseases (eg, diabetes mellitus), immunomodulatory therapy, prolonged neutropenia, organ transplantation, or a combination of these. Hospitalized neonates and intravenous drug abusers are also at risk. Immunodeficiency per se does not appear to be a prominent predisposing factor, attested to by the paucity of reported cases of *Candida* chorioretinitis or endophthalmitis among patients with HIV infection or AIDS.

Patients may present with blurred or decreased vision resulting from macular chorioretinal involvement or pain arising from anterior uveitis, which may be severe. Typically, *Candida* chorioretinitis is characterized by multiple, bilateral, white, well-circumscribed lesions less than 1 mm in diameter, distributed throughout the postequatorial fundus and associated with overlying vitreous cellular inflammation (Fig 8-4). The chorioretinal lesions may be associated with vascular sheathing and intraretinal hemorrhages; the vitreous exudates may assume a "string-of-pearls" appearance.

Histologically, *Candida* species are recognized as budding yeast with a characteristic pseudohyphate appearance (Fig 8-5). The organisms reach the eye hematogenously through metastasis to the choroid. Fungi may then break through the Bruch membrane, form subretinal abscesses, and secondarily involve the retina and vitreous.

The diagnosis of ocular candidiasis is suggested by the presence of chorioretinitis or endophthalmitis in the appropriate clinical context and confirmed by positive results on either blood or vitreous cultures. Because earlier treatment of candidal endophthalmitis has been shown to be associated with better visual outcomes, and patients with ocular

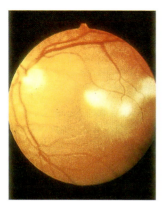

Figure 8-4 *Candida* retinitis.

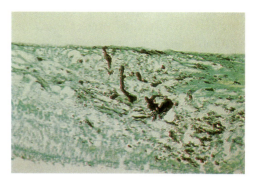

Figure 8-5 Pathology of *Candida* retinitis. Note fungi *(black)* in Gomori methenamine silver stain of retina.

lesions are likely to have infection involving a greater number of organ systems than those without eye lesions, it has been suggested that all patients with candidemia have baseline dilated funduscopic examinations and that these patients be followed up for the development of metastatic ocular candidiasis for at least 2 weeks after an initial eye examination. Presence of vitreous snowballs and endophthalmitis requires diagnostic and therapeutic vitrectomy. Giemsa stains, PCR for *Candida* species, and fungal cultures should be obtained on undiluted vitreous fluid samples.

The differential diagnosis of *Candida* endophthalmitis includes toxoplasmic retinochoroiditis, which exhibits posterior pole lesions that can appear yellow-white with fluffy borders and range in size from small cotton-wool spots to several disc diameters wide. *Candida* vitreous snowball lesions may also resemble pars planitis.

Treatment of intraocular candidiasis includes intravenous and intravitreal administration of antifungal agents. Consultation with an infectious disease specialist is essential. Chorioretinal lesions not yet involving the vitreous body may be effectively treated with the oral triazole antifungal agents fluconazole and voriconazole (200 mg bid for 2–4 weeks), with vigilant monitoring for evidence of progression. Voriconazole has good oral bioavailability, achieving therapeutic intravitreal levels with a broad spectrum of antifungal activity. Intravitreal injection of antifungal agents (amphotericin B, 5–10 μg/0.1 mL, or voriconazole, 100 μg/0.1 mL, with or without dexamethasone, 0.4 mg/0.1 mL) should be considered when the vitreous body is involved, usually in conjunction with pars plana vitrectomy. Vitrectomy may be useful diagnostically, allowing for the analysis of intraocular fluid by both microbiologic and molecular techniques, and therapeutically, by debulking the pathogen load. More severe infections may require intravenous amphotericin B with or without flucytosine. Significant dose-limiting toxicities (renal, cardiac, and neurologic) associated with conventional amphotericin B therapy have been greatly reduced with the development of liposomal lipid complex formulations. Finally, intravenously administered caspofungin, a novel antifungal of the echinocandin class (agents that inhibit synthesis of glucan in the cell wall) with activity against both *Candida* and *Aspergillus,* has been successfully employed in a small number of patients with *Candida* endophthalmitis;

however, some treatment failures have also been reported with this agent. Another echinocandin, intravenous micafungin, has also been approved for treatment of candidiasis. Oral voriconazole, flucytosine, fluconazole, or rifampin may be administered in addition to intravenous amphotericin B or caspofungin. Prompt treatment of both peripherally located lesions and those not involving the macular center may salvage useful vision.

Breit SM, Hariprasad SM, Mieler WF, Shah GK, Mills MD, Grand MG. Management of endogenous fungal endophthalmitis with voriconazole and caspofungin. *Am J Ophthalmol.* 2005;139(1):135–140.

Donahue SP, Greven CM, Zuravleff JJ, et al. Intraocular candidiasis in patients with candidemia. Clinical implications derived from a prospective multicenter study. *Ophthalmology.* 1994;101(7):1302–1309.

Hidalgo JA, Alangaden GJ, Eliott D, et al. Fungal endophthalmitis diagnosis by detection of *Candida albicans* DNA in intraocular fluid by use of species-specific polymerase chain reaction assay. *J Infect Dis.* 2000;181(3):1198–1201.

Krishna R, Amuh D, Lowder CY, Gordon SM, Adal KA, Hall G. Should all patients with candidemia have an ophthalmic examination to rule out ocular candidiasis? *Eye (Lond).* 2000; 14(Pt 1):30–34.

Menezes AV, Sigesmund DA, Demajo WA, Devenyi RG. Mortality of hospitalized patients with *Candida* endophthalmitis. *Arch Intern Med.* 1994;154(18):2093–2097.

Rao NA, Hidayat AA. Endogenous mycotic endophthalmitis: variations in clinical and histopathologic changes in candidiasis compared with aspergillosis. *Am J Ophthalmol.* 2001; 132(2):244–251.

Scherer WJ, Lee K. Implications of early systemic therapy on the incidence of endogenous fungal endophthalmitis. *Ophthalmology.* 1997;104(10):1593–1598.

Shah CP, McKey J, Spirn MJ, Maguire J. Ocular candidiasis: a review. *Br J Ophthalmol.* 2008; 92(4):466–468.

Aspergillus *endophthalmitis*

Endogenous *Aspergillus* endophthalmitis is a rare disorder associated with disseminated aspergillosis among patients with severe chronic pulmonary diseases, cancer, endocarditis, severe immunocompromise, or intravenous drug abuse. It is particularly common among patients following orthotopic liver transplantation. In rare instances, *Aspergillus* endophthalmitis may occur in immunocompetent patients with no apparent predisposing factors. Disseminated infection most commonly involves the lung, with the eye being the second most common site of infection. *Aspergillus fumigatus* and *A flavus* are the species most frequently isolated from patients with intraocular infection.

Aspergillus species are found in soils and decaying vegetation. The spores of these ubiquitous saprophytic molds become airborne and seed the lungs and paranasal sinuses of humans. Human exposure is very common, but infection is rare and depends on the virulence of the fungal pathogen and immunocompetence of the host. Ocular disease occurs via hematogenous dissemination of *Aspergillus* organisms to the choroid.

Endogenous *Aspergillus* endophthalmitis results in rapid onset of pain and visual loss. A confluent yellowish infiltrate is often seen in the macula, beginning in the choroid and subretinal space. A hypopyon can develop in the subretinal or subhyaloidal space (Fig 8-6A). Retinal hemorrhages, retinal vascular occlusions, and full-thickness retinal necrosis may occur. The infection can spread to produce a dense vitritis and variable degrees of cells, flare, and hypopyon in the anterior chamber. The macular lesions form a central atrophic scar when healed. In contrast to the lesions associated with *Candida* chorioretinitis and endophthalmitis, those produced by *Aspergillus* species are larger and more likely to be hemorrhagic, and they commonly invade the retinal and choroidal vessels, which may result in broad areas of ischemic infarction.

The diagnosis of endogenous *Aspergillus* endophthalmitis is based on clinical findings combined with positive results from pars plana vitreous biopsy and cultures and Gram and Giemsa stains. Coexisting systemic aspergillosis can be a strong clue, especially among high-risk patients. The diagnosis requires a high degree of suspicion within the correct clinical context and is confirmed by the demonstration of septate, dichotomously branching hyphae on analysis of vitreous fluid specimens. *Aspergillus* organisms may be difficult to culture from the blood.

The differential diagnosis of endogenous *Aspergillus* endophthalmitis includes *Candida* endophthalmitis, cytomegalovirus retinitis, *Toxoplasma* retinochoroiditis, coccidioidomycotic choroiditis or endophthalmitis, and bacterial endophthalmitis.

Aspergillus endophthalmitis lesions are histologically angiocentric. Mixed acute (polymorphonuclear leukocytes) and chronic (lymphocytes and plasma cells) inflammatory cells infiltrate the infected areas of the choroid and retina. Hemorrhage is present in all retinal layers. Granulomas contain rare giant cells. Branching fungal hyphae may be seen spreading on the surface of the Bruch membrane without penetrating it. Polymorphonuclear leukocytes are present in the vitreous. Fungal hyphae are often surrounded by macrophages and lymphocytes, which form small vitreous abscesses (Fig 8-6B). In *Candida* endophthalmitis, the vitreous is the prominent focus of infection, but in *Aspergillus* endophthalmitis, the principal foci are retinal and choroidal vessels and the subretinal or subretinal pigment epithelial space.

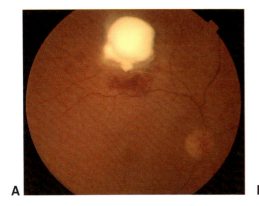 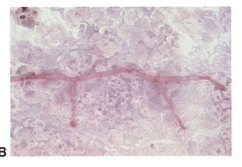

A   B

Figure 8-6   **A,** Biopsy-proven, culture-positive choroidal aspergilloma caused by endogenous *Aspergillus flavus* endophthalmitis in an immunocompetent patient with disseminated pulmonary aspergillosis. **B,** Light micrograph shows branching hyphae of *Aspergillus fumigatus* (periodic acid–Schiff × 220). *(Part A courtesy of Ramana S. Moorthy, MD. Part B reproduced with permission from Valluri S, Moorthy RS, Liggett PE, et al. Endogenous* Aspergillus *endophthalmitis in an immunocompetent individual.* Int Ophthalmol. *1993;17(3):133.)*

Endogenous *Aspergillus* endophthalmitis usually requires aggressive treatment with diagnostic and therapeutic pars plana vitrectomy combined with intravitreal injection of amphotericin B or voriconazole; intravitreal corticosteroids may be used in conjunction with these. Because most patients with this condition have disseminated aspergillosis, systemic treatment with oral voriconazole, intravenous amphotericin B, or caspofungin is often required. Other systemic antifungal agents, such as itraconazole, miconazole, fluconazole, and ketoconazole, may also be used. Systemic aspergillosis is best managed by an infectious disease specialist.

Despite aggressive treatment, the visual prognosis is poor because of frequent macular involvement. Final visual acuity is usually less than 20/200.

Hariprasad SM, Mieler WF, Holtz ER, et al. Determination of vitreous, aqueous, and plasmic concentration of orally administered voriconazole in humans. *Arch Ophthalmol.* 2004;122(1): 42–47.

Hunt KE, Glasgow BJ. *Aspergillus* endophthalmitis: an unrecognized endemic disease in orthotopic liver transplantation. *Ophthalmology.* 1996;103(5):757–767.

Rao NA, Hidayat AA. Endogenous mycotic endophthalmitis: variations in clinical and histopathologic changes in candidiasis compared with aspergillosis. *Am J Ophthalmol.* 2001; 132(2):244–251.

Weishaar PD, Flynn HW Jr, Murray TG, et al. Endogenous *Aspergillus* endophthalmitis: clinical features and treatment outcomes. *Ophthalmology.* 1998;105(1):57–65.

Cryptococcosis

Cryptococcus neoformans is a yeast that is found in high concentrations worldwide, in contaminated soil and in pigeon feces. Infection is acquired through inhalation of the aerosolized fungus. It has a predilection for the central nervous system and may produce severe disseminated disease among immunocompromised or debilitated patients. Although overall it remains an uncommon disease, cryptococcosis is the most common cause of fungal meningitis, as well as the most frequent fungal eye infection in patients with HIV infection or AIDS. The fungus probably reaches the eye hematogenously; however, the frequent association of ocular cryptococcosis with meningitis suggests that ocular infection may result from a direct extension from the optic nerve. Ocular infections may occur months after the onset of meningitis or, in rare instances, before the onset of clinically apparent central nervous system disease.

The most frequent presentation of ocular cryptococcosis is multifocal chorioretinitis, which appears as solitary or multiple discrete yellow-white lesions varying markedly in size in the postequatorial fundus. Associated findings include variable degrees of vitritis, vascular sheathing, exudative retinal detachment, papilledema, and granulomatous anterior cellular inflammation. It has been hypothesized that the infection begins as a focus in the choroid, with subsequent extension and secondary involvement of overlying tissues. Severe intraocular infection progressing to endophthalmitis may be observed in the absence of meningitis or clinically apparent systemic disease.

The clinical diagnosis requires a high degree of suspicion and is supported by demonstration of the organism with India ink stains or by culture of the fungus from cerebrospinal fluid. Intravenous amphotericin B and oral flucytosine are required to halt disease progression. With optic nerve or macular involvement, the prognosis is poor for visual recovery.

Sheu SJ, Chen YC, Kuo NW, Wang JH, Chen CJ. Endogenous cryptococcal endophthalmitis. *Ophthalmology.* 1998;105(2):377–381.

Shields JA, Wright DM, Augsburger JJ, Wolkowicz MI. Cryptococcal chorioretinitis. *Am J Ophthalmol.* 1990;89(2):210–217.

Coccidioidomycosis

Coccidioidomycosis is a disease produced by the dimorphic soil fungus *Coccidioides immitis,* which is endemic to the San Joaquin Valley of central California, certain parts of the southwestern United States, and parts of Central and South America. Infection follows inhalation of dust-borne arthrospores, most commonly resulting in pulmonary infection and secondary dissemination to the central nervous system, skin, skeleton, and eyes. Approximately 40% of infected patients are symptomatic; the vast majority presents with a mild upper respiratory tract infection or pneumonitis approximately 3 weeks after exposure to the organism. Erythema nodosum or multiforme may appear from 3 days to 3 weeks following the onset of symptoms; disseminated infection is rare, occurring in less than 1% of patients with pulmonary coccidioidomycosis.

Ocular coccidioidomycosis is likewise uncommon, even with disseminated disease. Disseminated disease usually causes blepharitis, keratoconjunctivitis, phlyctenular and granulomatous conjunctivitis, episcleritis and scleritis, and extraocular nerve palsies and orbital infection. Uveal involvement is still rarer: fewer than 20 pathologically verified cases have been reported. The anterior and posterior segments are equally involved. Intraocular manifestations include unilateral or bilateral granulomatous iridocyclitis, iris granulomas (Fig 8-7), and a multifocal chorioretinitis characterized by multiple, discrete, yellow-white lesions usually less than 1 disc diameter in size located in the postequatorial fundus. These choroidal granulomas may resolve, leaving punched-out chorioretinal scars. Vitreous cellular infiltration, vascular sheathing, retinal hemorrhage, serous retinal detachment, and involvement of the optic nerve have also been reported.

Serologic testing for anticoccidioidal antibodies in the serum, cerebrospinal fluid, vitreous, and aqueous, as well as skin testing for exposure to coccidioidin, establishes the diagnosis in the correct clinical context. One-half of patients with ocular involvement have

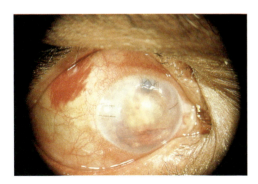

Figure 8-7 Coccidioidal iris granuloma in the pupil. This granuloma was biopsied and a peripheral iridectomy had just been performed because it was causing pupillary block and angle-closure glaucoma. *(Courtesy of Ramana S. Moorthy, MD.)*

systemic disease, and complement-fixation titers are often elevated (>1:32). With isolated anterior segment involvement, an anterior chamber tap may be useful. Culturing for the organism may delay diagnosis. The material from the anterior chamber tap may also be directly examined for coccidioidal organisms using the Papanicolaou stain.

Histologically, *C immitis* evokes pyogenic, granulomatous, and mixed reactions. Intraocular lesions from the anterior segment usually demonstrate zonal granulomatous inflammation that involves the uvea and angle structure, and *Coccidioides* organisms are usually seen.

The differential diagnosis of coccidioidal uveitis includes *Candida, Aspergillus,* and *Histoplasma* endophthalmitis and tuberculous uveitis. Coccidioidal uveitis should be considered in the differential diagnosis of any patient with apparent idiopathic granulomatous iritis who has lived in or traveled through the southwestern United States, southern California and the San Joaquin Valley, northern Mexico, or Argentina, where the organism is endemic.

The Infectious Diseases Society of America recommends initiating treatment with an oral azole antifungal such as fluconazole or itraconazole. Amphotericin B is usually reserved for patients with lesions that are worsening rapidly or that are located in vital sites like the spine. The visual prognosis is variable and determined in large part by the location of the chorioretinal lesions with respect to the optic nerve and foveal center. Surgical debulking of anterior chamber granulomas, pars plana vitrectomy, and intraocular injections of amphotericin and voriconazole may be required. With systemic disease, much higher doses and a longer duration of intravenous amphotericin therapy or oral voriconazole therapy may be needed. An infectious disease specialist is essential in the management of coccidioidomycosis.

Despite aggressive treatment, ocular coccidioidomycosis carries a poor visual prognosis, with most eyes requiring enucleation because of pain and blindness.

Glasgow BJ, Brown HH, Foos RY. Miliary retinitis in coccidioidomycosis. *Am J Ophthalmol.* 1987;104(1):24–27.

Moorthy RS, Rao NA, Sidikaro Y, Foos RY. Coccidioidomycosis iridocyclitis. *Ophthalmology.* 1994;101(12):1923–1928.

Vasconcelos-Santos DV, Lim JI, Rao NA. Chronic coccidioidomycosis endophthalmitis without concomitant systemic involvement: a clinicopathological case report. *Ophthalmology.* 2010;117(9):1839–1847.

CHAPTER 9

Masquerade Syndromes

Masquerade syndromes are those conditions that include the presence of intraocular cells but are not due to immune-mediated uveitic entities. These may be divided into neoplastic and nonneoplastic conditions. Masquerade syndromes account for nearly 5% of all patients with uveitis at tertiary referral.

Neoplastic Masquerade Syndromes

Neoplastic masquerade syndromes may account for 2%–3% of all patients seen in tertiary uveitis referral clinics. The vast majority of these are patients with intraocular involvement from primary CNS lymphoma.

Primary Central Nervous System Lymphoma

Nearly all (98%) primary central nervous system lymphomas (PCNSLs) are non-Hodgkin B-lymphocyte lymphomas. Approximately 2% are T-lymphocyte lymphomas. Although PCNSL mainly affects patients in their fifth to seventh decade of life, it also occurs, in rare instances, in children and adolescents. The incidence of PCNSL appears to be increasing and is projected to occur in 1 out of every 100,000 immunocompetent patients.

Clinical features and findings

Approximately 25% of patients with PCNSL have ocular involvement; approximately 15% may have ocular involvement alone. Sites of ocular involvement can include the vitreous, retina, subretinal pigment epithelium (sub-RPE), and any combination thereof. The most common complaints of presenting patients are decreased vision and floaters.

Examination reveals a variable degree of vitritis with the variable presence of anterior chamber cells. Retinal examination classically reveals creamy yellow subretinal infiltrates with overlying RPE detachments (Fig 9-1). They can look like discrete white lesions from acute retinal necrosis, toxoplasmosis, frosted branch angiitis, or retinal arteriolar obstruction with coexisting multifocal chorioretinal scars and retinal vasculitis. The lesions vary in thickness from about 1 mm to 2 mm.

Many of these patients are mistakenly diagnosed with an autoimmune uveitis and treated with anti-inflammatory medication. This can improve the vitreous cellular infiltration, but the effect is not long lasting and the uveitis often becomes resistant to therapy. Diagnosis is easier when retinal lesions are present (see Fig 9-1).

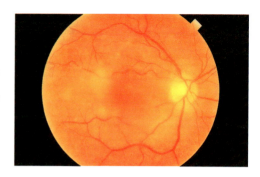

Figure 9-1 Primary central nervous system lymphoma. Fundus photograph of multifocal, subretinal pigment epithelial lesions. *(Courtesy of E. Mitchel Opremcak, MD.)*

CNS signs may be present and vary in nature. Behavioral changes appear to be the single most frequent sign, because of the periventricular location of many of the CNS lesions. Other neurologic signs include hemiparesis, cerebellar signs, epileptic seizures, and cranial nerve palsies. Cerebrospinal fluid seeding of lymphoma cells occurs in 42% of patients with PCNSL. Glaucoma, uveitis, and neurologic signs occurring together have been reported, and this is termed the *GUN syndrome.*

Diagnostic testing

Ultrasonography shows choroidal thickening, vitreous debris, elevated chorioretinal lesions, and serous retinal detachment. Fluorescein angiography shows hypofluorescent areas due to blockage from a sub-RPE tumor mass or from RPE clumping. Hyperfluorescent window defects may also be present caused by RPE atrophy from spontaneously resolved RPE infiltration. An unusual leopard-spot pattern of alternating hyperfluoresence and hypofluorescence may also be noted.

Magnetic resonance imaging (MRI) studies of the brain show isointense lesions on T1 and isointense to hyperintense lesions on T2. Computed tomography shows multiple diffuse periventricular lesions when no contrast is present. If intravenous contrast is used, these periventricular lesions may enhance. Cerebrospinal fluid analysis reveals lymphoma cells in one-third of patients.

Tissue diagnosis is the definitive method for establishing the presence of PCNSL. Lymphoma cells clearly identified from the cerebrospinal fluid may establish the diagnosis, obviating the need for pars plana vitreous biopsy. However, the presence of vitreous cells of unidentifiable source or cases of suspected uveitis not responding to therapy as expected (especially in a patient older than 65 years) necessitate a vitreous biopsy. Usually this is performed via a pars plana vitrectomy. Ideally, at least 1 mL of undiluted vitreous sample should be obtained. In addition, a retinal biopsy, an aspirate of sub-RPE material, or both may also be obtained during vitrectomy. This approach may improve diagnostic yield and is especially important when previous vitreous biopsy results have been negative. Communication with an experienced ophthalmic pathologist prior to surgery to determine his or her preferred method of fixation and delivery is mandatory. Portions of the specimen are typically prepared for both cytologic examination and cell surface marker determination by flow cytometry. Despite these measures, diagnostic yield from vitrectomy specimens is rarely more than 65% positive. A second biopsy of the vitreous may be performed if the clinical picture warrants.

Cytokine analysis in vitreous samples can be helpful in supporting the diagnosis of intraocular lymphoma. Interleukin-10 (IL-10) levels are elevated in the vitreous of patients with lymphoma because it is preferentially produced by malignant B lymphocytes. In contrast, high levels of IL-6 are found in the vitreous of patients with inflammatory uveitis. Thus, the relative ratio of IL-10 to IL-6 is often elevated in intraocular lymphoma and supports the diagnosis.

Histology

Cytologic specimens obtained from the vitreous or subretinal space often show pleomorphic cells with scanty cytoplasm, hyperchromatic nuclei with multiple irregular nucleoli, and an elevated nuclear/cytoplasmic ratio (Fig 9-2). Necrotic cellular debris is present in the background. Immunophenotyping by immunohistochemistry or flow cytometry is used to establish clonality of B lymphocytes by demonstrating the presence of abnormal immunoglobulin κ or λ light chain predominance and specific B-lymphocyte markers (CD19, CD20, and CD22). Monoclonal populations of cells are likely to be present in cases of PCNSL. Gene or oncogene translocations or gene rearrangements are often repeated in all cells in a given PCNSL.

Abnormal lymphocytes may be isolated manually or by laser capture, and polymerase chain reaction (PCR)-based assays performed to detect IgH, bcl-2 (a protein family that regulates apoptosis), or T-lymphocyte receptor gamma gene rearrangements. This improves the diagnostic yield of paucicellular samples.

If diagnosis by vitreous aspiration or subretinal aspiration cannot be performed, either internal or external chorioretinal biopsy techniques may be used to aid in the diagnosis of PCNSL.

Treatment

Treatment regimens vary by center. High-dose methotrexate delivered intravenously, along with intrathecal administration via an Ommaya reservoir in combination with radiation therapy and intravenous cytarabine, is 1 option. Others use intra-arterial therapy with blood–brain barrier disruption to facilitate access of the drug to the CNS. Approximately 56% of patients with ocular involvement eventually develop CNS involvement, prompting prophylactic treatment of the CNS even in cases of seemingly isolated ocular disease.

Local ocular treatment with repeated intravitreal injections of methotrexate (400 µg) can also be used in conjunction with systemic treatment. The role of this treatment alone

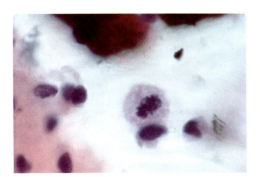

Figure 9-2 Vitreous aspirate showing mitotic figure and cellular atypia in large cell lymphoma. *(Courtesy of E. Mitchel Opremcak, MD.)*

in isolated ocular disease has been studied; it may be effective in controlling local disease, but its effect on median survival compared to that of systemic treatment is not known. Since these are predominately B-cell lymphomas, intraocular use of a monoclonal antibody against the CD20 antigen on B cells (rituximab) has been suggested and several reports of its use have been published; however, no long-term data are available.

Based on available information, chemotherapy alone is indicated for patients 60 years and older because of the potential CNS toxicity from radiation; for patients younger than 60 years, combination radiation therapy and chemotherapy is preferred. The negative effect of whole-brain radiation on quality of life is important when considering therapeutic options.

Itty S, Pulido JS. Rituximab for intraocular lymphoma. *Retina.* 2009;29(2):129–132.

Prognosis

Despite the availability of multiple treatment modalities and regimens, the long-term prognosis for patients with PCNSL remains poor; the median survival with supportive care alone is 2–3 months, and with surgery alone, median survival is in the range of 1–5 months. The longest median survival in various reports approaches 40 months with treatment. Factors that influence outcome include advancing age; worse neurologic functional classification level; single versus multiple lesions in the CNS (the latter indicating worse disease); and superficial cerebral and cerebellar hemispheric lesions versus deep nuclei/periventricular lesions (the latter indicating worse disease).

Chan CC, Fisson S, Bodaghi B. The future of primary intraocular lymphoma (retinal lymphoma). *Ocul Immunol Inflamm.* 2009;17(6):375–379.

Chan CC, Whitcup SM, Solomon D, Nussenblatt RB. Interleukin-10 in the vitreous of patients with primary intraocular lymphoma. *Am J Ophthalmol.* 1995;120(5):671–673.

Jahnke K, Thiel E. Treatment options for central nervous system lymphomas in immunocompetent patients. *Expert Rev Neurother.* 2009;9(10):1497–1509.

Raparia K, Chang CC, Chévez-Barrios P. Intraocular lymphoma: diagnostic approach and immunophenotypic findings in vitrectomy specimens. *Arch Pathol Lab Med.* 2009;133(6): 1233–1237.

Read RW, Zamir E, Rao NA. Neoplastic masquerade syndromes. *Surv Ophthalmol.* 2002; 47(2):81–124.

Rothova A, Ooijman F, Kerkhoff F, Van der Lelij A, Lokhorst HM. Uveitis masquerade syndromes. *Ophthalmology.* 2001;108(2):386–399.

Sen HN, Bodaghi B, Hoang PL, Nussenblatt R. Primary intraocular lymphoma: diagnosis and differential diagnosis. *Ocul Immunol Inflamm.* 2009;17(3):133–141.

Valluri S, Moorthy RS, Khan A, Rao NA. Combination treatment of intraocular lymphoma. *Retina.* 1995;15(2):125–129.

Zaldivar RA, Martin DF, Holden JT, Grossniklaus HE. Primary intraocular lymphoma: clinical, cytologic, and flow cytometric analysis. *Ophthalmology.* 2004;111(9):1762–1767.

Neoplastic Masquerade Syndromes Secondary to Systemic Lymphoma

Systemic lymphomas hematogenously spread to the choroid, to the subretinal space, into the vitreous, and occasionally into the anterior chamber. These entities often present with vitritis and creamy subretinal infiltrates of variable size, number, and extent. Retinal vasculitis, necrotizing retinitis, and diffuse choroiditis or uveal masses may also be present. All T-lymphocyte lymphomas (including mycosis fungoides, human T-cell lymphotropic virus type 1 [HTLV-1] lymphoma, systemic B-lymphocyte lymphoma, and anaplastic large cell lymphoma), Hodgkin disease, and primary intravascular lymphoma can present in this fashion. Reports of these entities are rare and scattered throughout the literature.

Neoplastic Masquerade Syndromes Secondary to Leukemia

Patients with leukemia may have retinal findings, including intraretinal hemorrhages, cotton-wool spots, white-centered hemorrhages, microaneurysms, and peripheral neovascularization. In rare instances, leukemic cells may invade the vitreous cavity. If the choroid is involved, exudative retinal detachment may be present and is angiographically similar to Vogt-Koyanagi-Harada (VKH) syndrome. Leukemia may also present with a hypopyon or hyphema, iris heterochromia, or a pseudohypopyon, which can be gray-yellow.

> Kincaid MC, Green WR. Ocular and orbital involvement in leukemia. *Surv Ophthalmol.* 1983;27(4):211–232.

Neoplastic Masquerade Syndromes Secondary to Uveal Lymphoid Proliferations

The uveal tract may be a site for lymphoid proliferations that can mimic chronic uveitis; these can range from benign reactive uveal lymphoid hyperplasia to frank lymphomas, associated or not with systemic lymphomas. Presenting symptoms may include gradual painless unilateral or bilateral vision loss. Early-stage disease shows multifocal creamy choroidal lesions that may mimic sarcoid uveitis or birdshot retinochoroidopathy, among others. Cystoid macular edema (CME) may be present. Anterior uveitis with acute symptoms of pain, redness, and photophobia may also be present. Glaucoma and elevated intraocular pressure (IOP) are common. Angle structures may be infiltrated by lymphocytes, resulting in elevation of IOP.

Fleshy episcleral or conjunctival masses that may be salmon pink in color may be present. Unlike subconjunctival lymphomas, these masses are not mobile and are attached firmly to the sclera. Differentiation from posterior scleritis and uveal effusion syndrome is important. Biopsy specimens demonstrate mature lymphocytes and plasma cells, quite different from the specimens seen with PCNSL. Therapy with corticosteroids, radiation, or both has been used with variable results. Systemic and periocular corticosteroid therapy can result in rapid regression of the lesions, as can external-beam radiation.

> Jakobiec FA, Sacks E, Kronish JW, Weiss T, Smith M. Multifocal static creamy choroidal infiltrates. An early sign of lymphoid neoplasia. *Ophthalmology.* 1987;94(4):397–406.

Nonlymphoid Malignancies

Uveal melanoma

Approximately 5% of patients with uveal melanoma present with ocular inflammation, including episcleritis, anterior or posterior uveitis, endophthalmitis, or panophthalmitis. Most tumors that present in this fashion are epithelioid cell or mixed cell choroidal melanomas. Ultrasonography is useful in diagnosing atypical cases because of the characteristic low internal reflectivity of these lesions. Management of uveal melanomas is discussed in BCSC Section 4, *Ophthalmic Pathology and Intraocular Tumors.*

Fraser DJ Jr, Font RL. Ocular inflammation and hemorrhage as initial manifestations of uveal malignant melanoma. Incidence and prognosis. *Arch Ophthalmol.* 1979;97(7):1311–1314.

Retinoblastoma

Approximately 1%–3% of retinoblastomas may present with the appearance of inflammation, most due to the relatively rare variant of diffuse infiltrating retinoblastoma. Patients are usually between age 4 and 6 years at presentation. These cases can be diagnostically confusing because of the limited visibility of the fundus and the lack of calcification on radiography or ultrasonography. Patients may have conjunctival chemosis, pseudohypopyon, and vitritis. The pseudohypopyon typically shifts with changes in head position and is usually white as opposed to the yellowish color of inflammatory hypopyon. Diagnostic aspiration of the aqueous humor may be required, but there is a significant risk of tumor spread through the needle tract. Histologic examination shows round cells with hyperchromatic nuclei and scanty cytoplasm.

Bhatnagar R, Vine AK. Diffuse infiltrating retinoblastoma. *Ophthalmology.* 1991;98(11): 1657–1661.

Juvenile xanthogranuloma

Juvenile xanthogranuloma is a histiocytic process affecting mainly the skin and eyes, and, in rare instances, viscera. Patients usually present before age 1 with characteristic skin lesions that are reddish yellow. Histologic investigation shows large histiocytes with foamy cytoplasm and Touton giant cells. Ocular lesions can involve the iris, from which spontaneous hyphema may occur. Iris biopsy shows fewer foamy histiocytes and fewer Touton giant cells than a skin biopsy. Other ocular structures may be involved, but this is rare. If the skin of the eyelids is involved, the globe is usually spared. Intraocular lesions may respond to topical, periocular, or systemic corticosteroid therapy. Resistant cases may require local resection, radiation, or immunomodulatory therapy.

Zamir E, Wang RC, Krishnakumar S, Aiello Leverant A, Dugel PU, Rao NA. Juvenile xanthogranuloma masquerading as pediatric chronic uveitis: a clinicopathologic study. *Surv Ophthalmol.* 2001;46(2):164–171.

Metastatic Tumors

Most intraocular malignancies in adults are metastatic tumors. The most common primary cancers include lung and breast. Choroidal metastasis may be marked by vitritis (which may be mild), serous retinal detachment, and, occasionally, CME. These lesions are often bilateral and multifocal.

Anterior uveal metastasis may present with cells in the aqueous humor, iris nodules, rubeosis iridis, and elevated IOP. Anterior chamber paracentesis may help confirm the diagnosis.

Retinal metastases are extremely rare. Primary cancers metastatic to the retina include cutaneous melanoma (the most common), followed by lung, gastrointestinal, and breast cancer. Metastatic melanoma often produces brown spherules in the retina, whereas other metastatic cancers are white to yellow and result in perivascular sheathing, simulating a retinal vasculitis or necrotizing retinitis.

Bilateral Diffuse Uveal Melanocytic Proliferation

Bilateral diffuse uveal melanocytic tumors have been associated with systemic malignancy. Such tumors can be accompanied by rapid vision loss; cataracts; multiple pigmented and nonpigmented, placoid iris and choroidal nodules; and serous retinal detachments. This condition can mimic VKH syndrome. Histologic investigation shows diffuse infiltration of the uveal tract by benign nevoid or spindle-shaped cells. Necrosis within the tumors may be present, and scleral involvement is common. The cause of this entity is unknown. Treatment should be directed at finding and treating the underlying primary lesion.

Barr CC, Zimmerman LE, Curtin VT, Font RL. Bilateral diffuse melanocytic uveal tumors associated with systemic malignant neoplasms: a recently recognized syndrome. *Arch Ophthalmol.* 1982;100(2):249–255.

Nonneoplastic Masquerade Syndromes

Retinitis Pigmentosa

Patients with retinitis pigmentosa (RP) often have variable numbers of vitreous cells and can develop CME. Distinguishing features of RP that differentiate it from uveitis include nyctalopia, positive family history, and on fundus examination, waxy disc pallor, attenuation of arterioles, and a bone-spicule pattern of pigmentary changes in the midperiphery (careful consideration of the entire clinical picture must be given, as these features can be seen in uveitis, especially retinal vasculitis, as well). Electroretinographic responses of patients with RP often appear severely depressed or extinguished, even early in the disease. See BCSC Section 12, *Retina and Vitreous,* for additional information.

Ocular Ischemic Syndrome

Ocular ischemic syndrome results from hypoperfusion of the entire eye and sometimes the orbit, usually due to carotid artery obstruction. Patients with ocular ischemic syndrome are typically males 65 or older. Patients present with decreased vision and mild ocular pain. Examination findings may include corneal edema, anterior chamber cells, and moderate flare, the latter often greater than and out of proportion to the number of cells. Neovascularization may be present on the iris and in the angle. IOP may be low from decreased aqueous production due to ischemia or high due to neovascular glaucoma. A cataract may be more prominent on the involved side. The vitreous is usually clear. Dilated fundus examination may show mild disc edema associated with dilated tortuous retinal venules, narrowed arterioles, and medium to large intraretinal scattered blot hemorrhages in the midperiphery and far periphery of the retina. Neovascularization may be present on the disc or elsewhere in the retina.

Fluorescein angiography shows delayed arteriolar filling, diffuse leakage in the posterior pole as well as from the optic disc, and signs of capillary nonperfusion. Retinal vascular staining may be present in the absence of any physical vascular sheathing on examination.

Diagnostic studies include carotid Doppler ultrasonography; ipsilateral carotid stenosis greater than 90% supports the diagnosis of ocular ischemic syndrome.

Definitive treatment involves carotid endarterectomy. Local treatment consists of both topical corticosteroids and cycloplegics, as well as panretinal photocoagulation treatment, especially if rubeosis or retinal neovascularization is present. Intraocular injection of vascular endothelial growth factors (VEGF) inhibitors may also be considered. The 5-year mortality rate of patients with ocular ischemic syndrome is 40%, usually due to cardiovascular disease and myocardial infarction. The visual prognosis is guarded, and many patients will transiently improve with treatment but eventually worsen.

Mendrinos E, Machinis TG, Pournaras CJ. Ocular ischemic syndrome. *Surv Ophthalmol.* 2010; 55(1):2–34.

Chronic Peripheral Rhegmatogenous Retinal Detachment

Chronic peripheral rhegmatogenous retinal detachment can be associated with anterior segment cell and flare and vitreous inflammatory and pigment cells. Patients often have good vision that can sometimes deteriorate because of CME. Careful dilated fundus examination with scleral depression is of paramount importance in establishing the diagnosis. Peripheral pigment demarcation lines, subretinal fluid, retinal breaks, subretinal fibrosis, and peripheral retinal cysts may be present. Photoreceptor outer segments liberated from the subretinal space may be present in the anterior chamber, simulating inflammatory cells. In such situations, IOP may be elevated as these photoreceptor outer segments are phagocytosed by the endothelial cells in the trabecular meshwork, resulting in secondary open-angle glaucoma. This condition is called *Schwartz syndrome.*

Matsuo N, Takabatake M, Ueno H, Nakayama T, Matsuo T. Photoreceptor outer segments in the aqueous humor in rhegmatogenous retinal detachment. *Am J Ophthalmol.* 1986;101(6): 673–679.

Schwartz A. Chronic open-angle glaucoma secondary to rhegmatogenous retinal detachment. *Am J Ophthalmol.* 1973;75(2):205–211.

Intraocular Foreign Bodies

Retained intraocular foreign bodies may produce chronic intraocular inflammation caused by mechanical, chemical, toxic, or inflammatory irritation of uveal tissues (particularly the ciliary body). A high index of suspicion followed by careful history; clinical examination; and ancillary testing, including gonioscopy, ultrasonography, and computed tomography of the eye and orbits, are essential. If this condition is suspected and recognized quickly, identification and removal of the foreign body often results in a cure. If the diagnosis is delayed, ocular complications such as proliferative vitreoretinopathy and endophthalmitis result in a poorer visual prognosis.

Pigment Dispersion Syndrome

Pigment dispersion syndrome is characterized by pigment granules that have been released from the iris and/or ciliary body floating in the anterior chamber; these granules may be confused with the cells of anterior uveitis. Refer to BCSC Section 10, *Glaucoma* for a complete discussion.

Other Syndromes

Certain infectious uveitic entities may also be mistaken for immunologic uveitis. Thus, nonneoplastic masquerade syndromes can also include bacterial uveitis due to *Nocardia* species and *Tropheryma whipplei* (Whipple disease), as well as fungal endophthalmitis due to *Candida* species, *Aspergillus* species, or *Coccidioides immitis*. These entities are discussed in Chapter 7 and Chapter 8.

CHAPTER 10

Complications of Uveitis

Calcific Band-Shaped Keratopathy

Patients with chronic uveitis lasting many years, especially those with childhood-onset uveitis, may develop calcium deposits in the epithelial basement membrane and the Bowman layer. Calcium deposits are usually found in the interpalpebral zone, often extending into the visual axis. This calcific band-shaped keratopathy may become visually significant in some cases and require removal. Subepithelial calcium is removed after epithelial debridement by chelation with 0.35% sodium ethylenediaminetetraacetic acid (EDTA). Visual improvement can be significant. Late recurrences may require repeat EDTA scrubs.

Cataracts

Any eye with chronic or recurrent uveitis may develop cataract as a result of both the inflammation itself and the corticosteroids used to treat it. Cataract surgery should be considered whenever functional benefit is likely. Cataract surgery in uveitic eyes is generally more complex and more likely to lead to postoperative complications. The key to a successful visual outcome in these cases is meticulous long-term control of preoperative and postoperative inflammation using corticosteroids and, more importantly, immunomodulatory therapy (IMT). The absence of inflammation for 3 or more months before surgery is a prerequisite for any elective intraocular surgery in uveitic eyes. The control of perioperative inflammation is as important as the technical feat of performing successful complex cataract extraction in uveitic eyes. See also BCSC Section 11, *Lens and Cataract,* for more information on many of the issues covered in this discussion.

Careful preoperative evaluation is necessary to ascertain how much the cataract is actually contributing to visual dysfunction, because visual loss in uveitis may stem from a variety of other ocular problems, such as macular edema or vitritis. Sometimes a cataract precludes an adequate view of the posterior segment of the eye, and surgery can be justified to permit examination, diagnosis, and treatment of posterior segment abnormalities.

Studies have shown that phacoemulsification with posterior chamber (in-the-bag) intraocular lens (IOL) implantation effectively improves vision and is well tolerated in many eyes with uveitis, even over long periods. For example, excellent surgical and visual results have been reported for eyes with Fuchs heterochromic iridocyclitis. Cataract surgery in other types of uveitis—including idiopathic uveitis; pars planitis; and uveitis associated with sarcoidosis, herpes simplex virus, herpes zoster, syphilis, toxoplasmosis, and spondyloarthropathies—can be more problematic, although such surgery may also yield very good results.

Management

Eyes with uveitis and visually significant cataract may fall into three broad surgical groups. Group 1 includes patients with few posterior synechiae, a long history of good inflammatory control, and no detectable flare. Group 2 comprises those with chronic flare, a history of poorly controlled inflammation, extensive posterior synechiae (>270°), and pupillary membranes (especially vascular ones). Group 3 consists of patients with JIA-associated uveitic cataracts. In all these categories, it is imperative to eliminate anterior chamber cells and to have the eye quiet, without inflammatory flare-ups, for at least 3 months prior to cataract surgery. Approximately 1–2 weeks before surgery, oral corticosteroids (0.5–1.0 mg/kg/day) and hourly topical corticosteroids should be administered. These may be tapered over 3–5 months after surgery, depending on the postoperative inflammatory response.

Group 1

In the first group, phacoemulsification using a clear corneal approach is preferred. This is particularly true in cases of scleritis that may be prone to postoperative scleral necrosis. Posterior synechiae and pupillary miosis may require mechanical or viscoelastic pupil stretching, sphincterotomies, or the use of flexible iris retractors. Pupillary membranes should be removed if possible. Continuous curvilinear capsulorrhexis is preferred, as it appears to reduce posterior synechiae formation, reduces the risk of posterior capsular tear, and facilitates placing IOL haptics in the capsular bag. A fibrotic anterior capsule may be more difficult to open with a capsulorrhexis. The zonules may be inherently weak, which may make phacoemulsification and lens implantation challenging or impossible. In such cases there may be few alternatives. It may be preferable in these cases to perform pars plana lensectomy and vitrectomy and, because of the lack of capsular support or zonular dehiscence, avoid placing an IOL. This scenario is fortunately rare. Nucleus extraction is performed using phacoemulsification, the preferred technique. Cortical cleanup should be meticulous. A hydrophobic acrylic posterior chamber IOL is preferred. The IOL may be placed in the capsular bag using a "shooter" through the small, clear corneal incision; or the corneal incision is enlarged to admit a forceps containing a folded IOL to be inserted into the capsular bag. Foldable silicone lenses should be avoided in uveitic eyes, because they may be associated with greater postoperative inflammation and because future vitreoretinal surgery may be necessary. If posterior segment pathology is present, silicone IOLs should be avoided because silicone oil would need to be used as a vitreous substitute. Ciliary sulcus and anterior chamber placement of IOLs must be avoided at all costs. Removal of IOLs, even after strict adherence to inflammatory control guidelines, may be unavoidable in 5%–10% of patients with uveitis, because of lens intolerance or dislocation. After IOL insertion, the ophthalmic viscoelastic device (OVD) must be removed. Periocular or intravitreal corticosteroids may be administered after surgery. Preoperative immunomodulation is continued after surgery and supplemented with liberal use of topical corticosteroids, which are slowly tapered. Phacoemulsification with IOL implantation can also be done in conjunction with pars plana vitrectomy if clinical or ultrasonographic examination suggests the presence of substantial vision-limiting vitreous debris or macular pathology such as epiretinal membranes. This scenario may occur in certain intermediate uveitis, posterior uveitis, and panuveitic syndromes.

Group 2

In the second group of uveitic cataract patients with historically much greater structural damage from inflammation, there is little recourse but to perform pars plana lensectomy and vitrectomy and leave the eye aphakic and essentially unicameral. Anterior segment pupillary management with synechiolysis is the same as for the first group. Meticulous removal of all lens material and capsular remnants assures better postoperative inflammatory control.

Group 3: JIA-associated uveitic cataracts

The third group—children with juvenile idiopathic arthritis (JIA)–associated uveitic cataracts—is more difficult to manage. There is also greater controversy and difference of opinion among specialists regarding IOL placement in these children. Consideration has to be given not only to the structural changes associated with these complex cataracts but also the management of preoperative and postoperative amblyopia and refractive axial length changes as the children age. Avoiding aphakia in children is desirable but may not always be achievable or in the best interest of the patient. In addition, choosing proper IOL power, especially in children under the age of 10, is difficult because of normal ocular/orbital growth. Regardless, the most important step in the treatment of these patients is absolute control of preoperative and postoperative intraocular inflammation with corticosteroids and, more importantly, IMT. Most ophthalmologists favor use of acrylic IOLs, which have good long-term success in visual rehabilitation and inflammatory control in these cases. Patients with JIA may be subdivided into subgroups similar to the first 2 groups and treated as indicated above. If IOLs are used, in-the-bag implantation of acrylic IOLs and primary posterior capsulorrhexis is preferred in children. Some surgeons may also perform a core anterior vitrectomy through the posterior capsulorrhexis prior to IOL placement. Intraocular corticosteroids at the end of the procedure are extremely useful for controlling postoperative inflammation and cystoid macular edema (CME). Using these methods, 75% of patients will obtain visual acuity of better than 20/40.

Complications

Postoperative complications commonly occur in uveitic eyes after cataract surgery. Their rates of occurrence may be reduced with effective perioperative inflammatory control using immunomodulators and corticosteroids. Visual compromise following phacoemulsification with posterior chamber lens implantation in patients with uveitis is usually attributed to posterior segment abnormalities, most commonly CME. Postoperative CME rates may be reduced by use of perioperative corticosteroids and control of uveitis for more than 3 months prior to surgery. The postoperative course may also be complicated by the recurrence or exacerbation of uveitis. Despite aggressive use of IMT, inflammatory cocooning of the IOL–lens capsule complex and uncontrolled inflammation may necessitate IOL explantation in 5%–10% of patients. The incidence of posterior capsule opacification is higher in uveitic eyes, leading to earlier use of Nd: YAG laser capsulotomy. In some uveitic conditions, such as pars planitis, inflammatory debris may accumulate and membranes may form on the surface of the IOL, necessitating frequent Nd:YAG laser procedures. On occasion, posterior chamber IOLs have been removed from these eyes. Frequent follow-up, a high index of suspicion, and aggressive IMT can optimize short- and long-term visual results.

Adán A, Gris O, Pelegrin L, Torras J, Corretger X. Explantation of intraocular lenses in children with juvenile idiopathic arthritis-associated uveitis. *J Cataract Refract Surg.* 2009;35(3): 603–605.

Alío JJ, Chipont E, BenEzra D, Fakhry MA. Comparative performance of intraocular lenses in eyes with cataract and uveitis. *J Cataract Refract Surg.* 2002;28(12):2096–2108.

Belair ML, Kim SJ, Thorne JE, et al. Incidence of cystoid macular edema after cataract surgery in patients with and without chronic uveitis using optical coherence tomography. *Am J Ophthalmol.* 2009;148(1):128–135.

Jancevski M, Foster CS. Cataracts and uveitis. *Curr Opin Ophthalmol.* 2010;21(1):10–14.

Nemet AY, Raz J, Sachs D, et al. Primary intraocular lens implantation in pediatric uveitis: a comparison of 2 populations. *Arch Ophthalmol.* 2007;125(3):354–360.

Quiñones K, Cervantes-Castañeda RA, Hynes AY, Daoud YJ, Foster CS. Outcomes of cataract surgery in children with chronic uveitis. *J Cataract Refract Surg.* 2009;35(4):725–731.

Glaucoma

Uveitic ocular hypertension is common and must be differentiated from uveitic glaucoma, a well-recognized complication of uveitis. Uveitic ocular hypertension refers to intraocular pressure (IOP) 10 mm Hg or greater above baseline without evidence of glaucomatous optic nerve damage. Uveitic glaucoma is defined as elevated IOP resulting in progressive neuroretinal rim loss and/or development of typical, perimetric, glaucomatous field defects.

Elevated IOP in uveitic eyes may be acute, chronic, or recurrent. In eyes with long-term ciliary body inflammation, the IOP may fluctuate between abnormally high and low values. Numerous morphologic, cellular, and biochemical alterations occur in the uveitic eye that cause uveitic glaucoma (Table 10-1) and ocular hypertension. Successful management of uveitic glaucoma and ocular hypertension requires the identification and treatment of each of these contributing factors.

Elevation of IOP to levels above 24 mm Hg seems to substantially increase the risk of glaucoma. However, most practitioners tend to treat IOPs greater than 30 mm Hg even without evidence of glaucomatous optic nerve damage. Assessment of patients with uveitis and elevated IOP should include, in addition to slit-lamp and dilated fundus examination, gonioscopy, disc photos and optical coherence tomography (OCT) evaluation of the optic nerve head, and serial automated visual fields.

Table 10-1 Pathogenesis of Uveitic Glaucoma

    I. Cellular and biochemical alterations of aqueous in uveitis
       A. Inflammatory cells
       B. Protein
       C. Prostaglandins
       D. Inflammatory mediators (cytokines) and toxic agents (oxygen free radicals)
    II. Morphologic changes in anterior chamber angle
       A. Angle closure
          1. Primary angle-closure glaucoma
          2. Secondary angle-closure glaucoma
             a. Posterior synechiae and pupillary block
             b. Peripheral anterior synechiae (PAS)
                i. PAS secondary to inflammation
                ii. PAS secondary to iris neovascularization
                iii. PAS secondary to prolonged iris bombé
             c. Forward rotation of ciliary body (due to inflammation)
       B. Open angle
          1. Primary open-angle glaucoma
          2. Secondary open-angle glaucoma
             a. Aqueous misdirection
             b. Mechanical blockage of trabecular meshwork
                i. Serum components (proteins)
                ii. Precipitates (cells, cellular debris)
             c. Trabeculitis (trabecular dysfunction)
             d. Damage to trabeculum and endothelium from chronic inflammation
             e. Corticosteroid-induced glaucoma
       C. Combined-mechanism glaucoma

Uveitic Ocular Hypertension

Early in the course of uveitis, ocular hypertension is treated with intensive corticosteroids. Clinicians should resist the tendency to reduce corticosteroids because of the unsubstantiated fear of corticosteroid-induced ocular hypertension. Corticosteroid-induced ocular hypertension rarely occurs before 3 weeks after initiation of corticosteroid therapy. Early IOP elevations with active inflammation are almost always caused by inflammation that requires aggressive treatment. When the inflammation becomes quiet but IOP is still 30 mm Hg or higher, topical corticosteroids may be slowly tapered and aqueous suppressants may be added.

Uveitic Glaucoma

Because many cellular, biochemical, and morphologic variables contribute to the development of uveitic glaucoma, many classification methods are possible. However, glaucoma associated with uveitis is best classified by morphologic changes in angle structure; thus, uveitic glaucoma may be divided into secondary angle-closure and secondary open-angle glaucoma. These entities may be further subdivided into acute and chronic types. Most cases of chronic uveitic glaucoma, however, result from a combination of mechanisms. In addition, corticosteroid-induced ocular hypertension and glaucoma are other components that must be addressed in cases of chronic uveitic glaucoma. Gonioscopic evaluation of the peripheral angle, optic nerve evaluation with disc photographs and OCT, and automated visual fields are essential in the treatment of all patients with uveitic glaucoma, especially those with chronic inflammation. See also BCSC Section 10, *Glaucoma*.

Secondary angle-closure glaucoma

Acute Acute secondary angle-closure glaucoma may occur when choroidal inflammation results in forward rotation of the ciliary body and lens–iris diaphragm. This can be the presenting sign of Vogt-Koyanagi-Harada (VKH) syndrome or sympathetic ophthalmia. Patients present with pain, elevated IOP, no posterior synechiae, and severe inflammation. Ultrasound biomicroscopy (UBM) or ultrasound evaluation showing choroidal thickening and anterior rotation of the ciliary body is diagnostic. Treatment with aggressive corticosteroid therapy and aqueous suppressants is required. As the inflammation subsides, the chamber deepens and the IOP normalizes. Peripheral iridotomy or iridectomy is not useful in these acute cases because the underlying cause is severe choroidal inflammation.

Subacute Chronic anterior segment inflammation may result in the formation of circumferential posterior synechiae, pupillary block, and iris bombé, resulting in subacute secondary peripheral angle closure. This condition occasionally occurs in patients with chronic granulomatous iridocyclitis associated with sarcoidosis or VKH syndrome and in those with recurrent nongranulomatous iridocyclitis, as is seen with ankylosing spondylitis. In patients with light-colored (blue, green, hazel) irides, peripheral iridotomy with the Nd:YAG or argon laser results in resolution of the bombé and angle closure if performed before permanent peripheral synechiae form. Iridotomies should be multiple and as large as possible. Considerable inflammation can be anticipated following laser iridotomy procedures in these eyes, making the iridotomies prone to close, requiring re-treatment. Intensive topical corticosteroid and cycloplegic therapy is given following the procedure. In patients with brown irides, or if laser iridotomy is not successful in patients with blue, green, or hazel irides, surgical iridectomy is the procedure of choice. The procedure may be supplemented with goniosynechialysis if peripheral anterior synechiae have started to develop. It is important that the iridectomy specimen be submitted for histologic, immunohistochemical, and possibly microbiologic studies to help determine or confirm the etiology of the uveitis. This step is often overlooked in uveitic eyes.

Chronic Chronic intraocular inflammation may result in insidious peripheral anterior synechiae and chronic secondary angle-closure glaucoma. These eyes often have superimposed chronic secondary open-angle glaucoma and corticosteroid-induced glaucoma. Topical aqueous suppressants may be inadequate to prevent progression of optic nerve head damage. These eyes may require goniosynechialysis and trabeculectomy with mitomycin C or glaucoma tube shunt placement.

Secondary open-angle glaucoma

Acute Inflammatory open-angle glaucoma occurs when the trabecular meshwork is inflamed (trabeculitis) or blocked by inflammatory cells and debris, as commonly occurs with infectious causes of uveitis such as *Toxoplasma* retinochoroiditis, necrotizing herpetic retinitis, herpes simplex and varicella-zoster iridocyclitis, cytomegalovirus iridocyclitis (including the Posner-Schlossman type), sarcoid uveitis, and Fuchs heterochromic iridocyclitis (rubella-associated). This type of glaucoma usually responds to topical cycloplegics, corticosteroids, and specific treatment of the infectious agent.

Chronic Chronic outflow obstruction is caused by inflammatory debris clogging the angle or direct damage to the trabecular meshwork. The management of chronic secondary open-angle glaucoma is similar to primary open-angle glaucoma (see BCSC Section 10, *Glaucoma*) with the added complexity of maintaining strict control of intraocular inflammation with IMT.

Combined-mechanism uveitic glaucoma

Multiple mechanisms may be responsible for most cases of uveitic glaucoma. Treatment should be aimed at controlling the inflammation and IOP through a multimodal approach, including both medical and surgical therapy aimed at the responsible mechanisms.

Corticosteroid-Induced Ocular Hypertension and Glaucoma

Early in the course of all types of uveitis, first priority should be given to the control of intraocular inflammation, even if the IOP is high. As the inflammation subsides and is brought under control, IOP will spontaneously decrease, if elevated on presentation. Clinicians must resist the temptation to reduce corticosteroid dosing and frequency prematurely.

However, progressive elevation of IOP after the inflammation is brought under control over the first 3–4 weeks may represent corticosteroid-induced ocular hypertension. Topical, periocular, intraocular (injection and sustained-release), and oral corticosteroid therapy for uveitis may all induce an elevation in IOP at any time, which may be difficult to distinguish from other causes of glaucoma in uveitis. This IOP rise may be avoided with a less-potent topical corticosteroid preparation, a less-frequent administration schedule, or both. Fluorometholone, loteprednol, and rimexolone may be less likely to induce an IOP elevation but may also be less effective in controlling intraocular inflammation than other topical ocular corticosteroid preparations. If these measures do not reduce IOP and prevent further optic nerve head damage, medical and possibly surgical treatment of the glaucoma may be required. This corticosteroid complication may be prevented by earlier institution of corticosteroid-sparing IMT in the treatment of chronic, recurrent intraocular inflammation.

Management

Medical management of uveitic glaucoma requires aggressive control of both intraocular inflammation and IOP, and prevention of glaucomatous optic nerve damage and visual field loss (see BCSC Section 10, *Glaucoma*). The prostaglandin analogues latanoprost, travoprost, and bimatoprost may be used to treat uveitic glaucoma and generally do not exacerbate intraocular inflammation, especially when used concomitantly with IMT and corticosteroids.

When medical management fails, glaucoma filtering surgery is indicated. Standard trabeculectomy has a greater risk of failure in these eyes. Results may be improved by using mitomycin C with intensive topical corticosteroids. However, intense and recurrent postoperative inflammation can often lead to filtering surgery failure in uveitic eyes. Overall, up to 90% of patients 1 year after surgery and around 62% 5 years after surgery have IOP control with 1 or 0 medications. Surgical complications include cataract formation, bleb leakage (early and late) that could lead to endophthalmitis, and choroidal effusions. Because peripheral iridotomy is performed with trabeculectomy, the excised trabecular block and iris should be submitted for pathologic evaluation, as discussed earlier.

Alternatives to classic trabeculectomy are numerous and have been used with some short-term success in uveitic glaucoma. Nonpenetrating deep sclerectomy with or without a drainage implant has been effective in controlling IOP in up to 90% of uveitic eyes for 1 year after surgery. Among pediatric uveitis patients, goniotomy has up to a 75% chance of reducing IOP to 21 mm Hg or less after 2 surgeries. This procedure may be complicated by transient hyphema and worsening of the preexisting cataract. Trabeculodialysis and laser sclerostomy have a high rate of failure because of recurrent postoperative inflammation. Viscocanalostomy has shown higher success rates in a limited number of studies.

Most cases of uveitic glaucoma, especially if pseudophakic or aphakic, require aqueous drainage devices such as Molteno (Molteno Ophthalmic), Ahmed valve (New World Medical), or Baerveldt (Abbott Medical Optics) implants. These tube shunts may be tunneled into the anterior chamber or placed directly into the vitreous cavity in eyes that have undergone previous vitrectomy. In addition, unidirectional valve design, such as the Ahmed valve implant, can prevent postoperative hypotony. These implants are more likely than trabeculectomy to successfully control IOP in the long term, with up to a 75% reduction of IOP from preoperative levels and with nearly 75% of patients achieving target IOPs with 0 or 1 topical antiglaucoma medications after 4 years. Complications of tube shunt surgery (10%/patient-year) include shallow anterior chamber, hypotony, suprachoroidal hemorrhage, and blockage of the tube by blood, fibrin, or iris. Long-term complications include tube erosion through the conjunctiva, valve migration, corneal decompensation, tube–cornea touch, and retinal detachment. Unlike trabeculectomy, these tube shunts have proven to be robust and continue to function despite chronic, recurrent inflammation; they provide excellent long-term IOP control in eyes with uveitic glaucoma.

Cyclodestructive procedures may worsen ocular inflammation and lead to hypotony and phthisis bulbi and are best avoided in uveitic eyes. Also, laser trabeculoplasty should be avoided in eyes with uveitis.

As with all surgeries in uveitic patients, tight and meticulous control of perioperative inflammation using immunomodulators and corticosteroids not only improves the success of glaucoma surgery but also improves visual acuity outcomes by limiting sight-threatening complications such as CME and hypotony.

Ceballos EM, Parrish RK 2nd, Schiffman JC. Outcome of Baerveldt glaucoma drainage implants for the treatment of uveitic glaucoma. *Ophthalmology.* 2002;109(12):2256–2260.

Fortuna E, Cervantes-Castañeda RA, Bhat P, Doctor P, Foster CS. Flare-up rates with bimatoprost therapy in uveitic glaucoma. *Am J Ophthalmol.* 2008;146(6):876–882.

Heinz C, Koch JM, Heiligenhaus A. Transscleral diode laser cyclophotocoagulation as primary surgical treatment for secondary glaucoma in juvenile idiopathic arthritis: high failure rate after short term follow up. *Br J Ophthalmol.* 2006;90(6):737–740.

Ho CL, Wong EY, Walton DS. Goniosurgery for glaucoma complicating chronic childhood uveitis. *Arch Ophthalmol.* 2004;122(6):838–844.

Kafkala C, Hynes A, Choi J, Topalkara A, Foster CS. Ahmed valve implantation for uncontrolled pediatric uveitic glaucoma. *J AAPOS.* 2005;9(4):336–340.

Markomichelakis NN, Kostakou A, Halkiadakis I, Chalkidou S, Papakonstantinou D, Georgopoulos G. Efficacy and safety of latanoprost in eyes with uveitic glaucoma. *Graefes Arch Clin Exp Ophthalmol.* 2009;247(6):775–780.

Papadaki TG, Zacharopoulos IP, Pasquale LR, Christen WB, Netland PA, Foster CS. Long-term results of Ahmed glaucoma valve implantation for uveitic glaucoma. *Am J Ophthalmol.* 2007;144(1):62–69.

Miserocchi E, Carassa RG, Bettin P, Brancato R. Viscocanalostomy in patients with glaucoma secondary to uveitis: preliminary report. *J Cataract Refract Surg.* 2004;30(3):566–570.

Molteno AC, Sayawat N, Herbison P. Otago glaucoma surgery outcome study: long-term results of uveitis with secondary glaucoma drained by Molteno implants. *Ophthalmology.* 2001;108(3):605–613.

Moorthy RS, Mermoud A, Baerveldt G, Minckler DS, Lee PP, Rao NA. Glaucoma associated with uveitis. *Surv Ophthalmol.* 1997;41(5):361–394.

Noble J, Derzko-Dzulynsky L, Rabinovitch T, Birt C. Outcome of trabeculectomy with mitomycin C for uveitic glaucoma. *Can J Ophthalmol.* 2007;42(1):89–94.

Yalvac IS, Sungur G, Turhan E, Eksioglu U, Duman S. Trabeculectomy with mitomycin-C in uveitic glaucoma associated with Behçet disease. *J Glaucoma.* 2004;13(6):450–453.

Hypotony

Hypotony in uveitis is usually caused by decreased aqueous production from the ciliary body and may follow intraocular surgery in patients with uveitis. Acute inflammation of the ciliary body may cause temporary aqueous hyposecretion, whereas chronic ciliary body damage with atrophic or absent ciliary processes results in permanent hypotony. Serous choroidal detachment often accompanies hypotony and complicates management.

Hypotony early in the course of uveitis usually responds to intensive corticosteroid and cycloplegic therapy, although prolonged choroidal effusions may require surgical drainage. Chronic hypotony in long-standing uveitis, with preservation of the ciliary process seen on UBM and with ciliary body traction from a cyclitic membrane or atrophy, may respond to pars plana vitrectomy and membranectomy, which may restore normal intraocular pressure. If ciliary processes are present, vitrectomy and intraocular silicone oil may help maintain ocular anatomy and increase IOP. In some of these cases, visual improvement after surgery can be significant; these gains may, however, be transient. Hypotony recurs in nearly one-half of eyes, requiring reinjection of silicone oil between 1 and 3 times over 1 year.

de Smet MD, Gunning F, Feenstra R. The surgical management of chronic hypotony due to uveitis. *Eye (Lond).* 2005;19(1):60–64.

Kapur R, Birnbaum AD, Goldstein DA, et al. Treating uveitis-associated hypotony with pars plana vitrectomy and silicone oil injection. *Retina.* 2010;30(1):140–145.

Ugahary LC, Ganteris E, Veckeneer M, et al. Topical ibopamine in the treatment of chronic ocular hypotony attributable to vitreoretinal surgery, uveitis, or penetrating trauma. *Am J Ophthalmol.* 2006;141(3):571–573.

Cystoid Macular Edema

Cystoid macular edema is a common cause of visual loss in eyes with uveitis. It most commonly occurs in pars planitis, birdshot retinochoroidopathy, and retinal vasculitis but can occur in any chronic uveitis. CME is usually caused by active intraocular inflammation and appears to be mediated by proinflammatory cytokines, namely vascular endothelial growth factor (VEGF) and interleukin-6, that cause retinal vascular leakage and retinal pigment epithelium dysfunction. CME may less commonly be caused by mechanical vitreomacular traction; the 2 causes can easily be differentiated by OCT. CME can also be quantitatively evaluated and followed by serial spectral-domain OCT and fluorescein angiography. A recent OCT study of uveitic macular edema divided the edema morphologically into diffuse macular edema (40%), CME (50%), and serous retinal detachment alone (10%). High correlation existed between CME thickness as measured by OCT and fluorescein angiographic leakage. Correlation between visual acuity and central thickness was significant only in the cystoid group. Serous retinal detachment did not significantly impact visual recovery. The severity of CME does not necessarily correspond to the level of inflammatory disease activity, but CME is often slow to respond and clear and often remains even after visible, active inflammation has resolved. Smoking appears to be associated with greater prevalence of CME, especially in intermediate uveitis and panuveitis.

Treatment of CME must first be directed toward meticulous control of intraocular inflammation with corticosteroids and IMT. Therapy that reduces intraocular inflammation in general often reduces CME. If CME persists despite adequate control of inflammation, more aggressive regional therapy may be required. When periocular therapy is used specifically to treat CME, a superotemporal posterior sub-Tenon injection of 20–40 mg of triamcinolone acetonide is preferred (see Chapter 5). Theoretically, this technique delivers juxtascleral corticosteroid closest to the macula. The injections may be repeated monthly. If CME still persists, then 2–4 mg of intravitreal preservative-free triamcinolone may be considered (see Chapter 5). Intravitreal triamcinolone can be highly effective in reducing CME, particularly in nonvitrectomized eyes, but its effect is time-limited; the drug is eliminated more quickly from the vitreous cavity of vitrectomized eyes. Maximum visual improvement and reduction of CME after intravitreal triamcinolone injection occurs within 4 weeks. Eyes with a longer duration of uveitic CME and worse vision on presentation tend to show the least amount of visual improvement after treatment with intravitreal triamcinolone. Corticosteroid-induced IOP elevation may occur in up to 40% of patients, especially in those younger than age 40. The fluocinolone acetonide implant dramatically reduced uveitic CME in 110 patients, with 25% demonstrating 3 or more lines of visual improvement but with high rate of cataract formation and glaucoma (see Chapter 5). An intravitreal sustained-release dexamethasone drug delivery system (700 µg) also shows promise for control of uveitic CME, with less risk of glaucoma (see Chapter 5). Intravitreal bevacizumab (Avastin, Genentech) also reduces inflammatory CME, but its action is of short duration and repeat injections are required. Intravitreal methotrexate (400 µg/0.1 mL) was recently shown to be effective in reducing uveitic CME in a limited number of patients and is under active investigation.

Other agents have been used to treat uveitic CME but with limited success. Topical ketorolac and nepafenac can be beneficial in treating pseudophakic CME. Their effectiveness in the treatment of uveitic CME has not been established. Oral acetazolamide, 500 mg once or twice daily, has also been effective in reducing uveitic CME, particularly in patients whose inflammation is well controlled.

Surgical therapy for uveitic CME is still controversial. Pars plana vitrectomy for uveitic CME in the presence of hyaloidal traction on the macula (as seen on OCT imaging) may be visually and anatomically beneficial. In the absence of vitreomacular traction, however, the efficacy of pars plana vitrectomy in treating CME is not well understood. There is some suggestion in recent literature reviews that vitrectomy may be beneficial in managing recalcitrant uveitic CME, but this requires further investigation. See BCSC Section 12, *Retina and Vitreous*.

Androudi S, Letko E, Meniconi M, Papadaki T, Ahmed M, Foster CS. Safety and efficacy of intravitreal triamcinolone acetonide for uveitic macular edema. *Ocul Immunol Inflamm.* 2005;13(2–3):205–212.

Angunawela RI, Heatley CJ, Williamson TH, et al. Intravitreal triamcinalone acetonide for refractory uveitic cystoid macular oedema: longterm management and outcome. *Acta Ophthalmol Scand.* 2005;83(5):595–599.

Becker M, Davis J. Vitrectomy in the treatment of uveitis. *Am J Ophthalmol.* 2005;140(6): 1096–1105.

Farber MD, Lam S, Tessler HH, Jennings TJ, Cross A, Rusin MM. Reduction of macular oedema by acetazolamide in patients with chronic iridocyclitis: a randomised prospective crossover study. *Br J Ophthalmol.* 1994;78(1):4–7.

Jennings T, Rusin MM, Tessler HH, Cunha-Vaz JG. Posterior sub-Tenon's injections of corticosteroids in uveitis patients with cystoid macular edema. *Jpn J Ophthalmol.* 1988;32(4): 385–391.

Kok H, Lau C, Maycock N, McCluskey P, Lightman S. Outcome of intravitreal triamcinolone in uveitis. *Ophthalmology.* 2005;112(11):1916–1921.

Lin P, Loh AR, Margolis TP, Acharya NR. Cigarette smoking as a risk factor for uveitis. *Ophthalmology.* 2010;117(3):585–590.

Rothova A. Inflammatory cystoid macular edema. *Curr Opin Ophthalmol.* 2007;18(6):487–492.

Schilling H, Heiligenhaus A, Laube T, Bornfeld N, Jurklies B. Long-term effect of acetazolamide treatment of patients with uveitic chronic cystoid macular edema is limited by persisting inflammation. *Retina.* 2005;25(2):182–188.

Taylor SR, Habot-Winer Z, Pacheco P, Lightman SL. Intraocular methotrexate in the treatment of uveitis and uveitic cystoid macular edema. *Ophthalmology.* 2009;116(4):797–801.

Tran TH, de Smet MD, Bodaghi B, Fardeau C, Cassoux N, Lehoang P. Uveitic macular oedema: correlation between optical coherence tomography patterns with visual acuity and fluorescein angiography. *Br J Ophthalmol.* 2008;92(7):922–927.

Vitreous Opacification and Vitritis

Permanent vitreous opacification affecting vision occasionally occurs in uveitis, particularly in eyes with *Toxoplasma* retinitis and pars planitis. In fact, in a review of 39 recent studies of eyes with chronic uveitis that had undergone pars plana vitrectomy, visual acuity improved in 68%. In other cases of vitritis, the diagnosis is uncertain. Pars plana vitrectomy may be therapeutic or diagnostic in eyes with vitritis.

A standard small (25- or 23-gauge) 3-port pars plana vitrectomy is the preferred technique, with a few minor variations. See BCSC Section 12, *Retina and Vitreous*.

Becker M, Davis J. Vitrectomy in the treatment of uveitis. *Am J Ophthalmol.* 2005;140(6): 1096–1105.

Davis JL, Miller DM, Ruiz P. Diagnostic testing of vitrectomy specimens. *Am J Ophthalmol.* 2005;140(5):822–829.

Manku H, McCluskey P. Diagnostic vitreous biopsy in patients with uveitis: a useful investigation? *Clin Experiment Ophthalmol.* 2005;33(6):604–610.

Rhegmatogenous Retinal Detachment

Rhegmatogenous retinal detachment (RRD) occurs in 3% of patients with uveitis. The high prevalence of RRD means that uveitis itself may be an independent risk factor for the condition. Panuveitis and infectious uveitis are the entities most frequently associated with RRD. Pars planitis and posterior uveitis can also be associated with rhegmatogenous or tractional retinal detachments. Uveitis is often still active in eyes that present with RRD. Up to 30% of patients with uveitis and RRD may have proliferative vitreoretinopathy (PVR) at presentation; this percentage is significantly higher than in primary RRD in patients without uveitis. Repair is often complicated by preexisting PVR, vitreous organization, and poor visualization. Scleral buckling with cryoretinopexy is still useful in cases of retinal detachment associated with pars planitis. Acute retinal necrosis and cytomegalovirus retinitis frequently lead to retinal detachments that are difficult to repair because of multiple large posterior retinal breaks. Pars plana vitrectomy and endolaser treatment with internal silicone oil tamponade are required to repair the detachment. When PVR is present, combined scleral buckling and pars plana vitrectomy is often required to reattach the retina. The retinal reattachment rate after 1 surgery in uveitic eyes with RRD is 60%. Final vision was less than 20/200 in 70% of eyes in 1 study, and 10% of these had no light perception. Thus, the prognosis in eyes with uveitis and RRD is particularly poor compared to that in nonuveitic eyes with RRD.

Kerkhoff FT, Lamberts QJ, van den Biesen PR, Rothova A. Rhegmatogenous retinal detachment and uveitis. *Ophthalmology.* 2003(2);110:427–431.

Nussenblatt RB, Whitcup SM. *Uveitis: Fundamentals and Clinical Practice.* 3rd ed. Philadelphia, PA: Mosby; 2004.

Retinal and Choroidal Neovascularization

Retinal neovascularization may develop in any chronic uveitic condition but is particularly common in pars planitis, sarcoid panuveitis, and retinal vasculitis of various causes, including Eales disease. Retinal neovascularization occurs from chronic inflammation or capillary nonperfusion. Treatment is directed toward the underlying etiology. The presence of uveitic retinal neovascularization does not always require panretinal photocoagulation. Some cases of sarcoid panuveitis, for example, may present with neovascularization of the disc that resolves completely with immunomodulatory and corticosteroid therapy alone. Thus, treatment must first be directed against reduction of inflammation. If ischemia is angiographically extensive, as in retinal vasculitis or Eales disease, scatter laser photocoagulation in the ischemic areas is therapeutic. Recent studies have shown dramatic regression of neovascularization of the disc and elsewhere in various inflammatory disorders after 1 or 2 injections of intravitreal bevacizumab, a VEGF inhibitor. This treatment may be used as an adjunct to IMT and scatter laser photocoagulation.

Choroidal neovascularization (CNV) can develop in posterior uveitis and panuveitis. It can commonly occur in ocular histoplasmosis syndrome, punctate inner choroidopathy, idiopathic multifocal choroiditis, and serpiginous choroiditis. CNV can also occur in VKH syndrome and other panuveitic entities. In such cases, CNV results from a disruption of the Bruch membrane from choroidal inflammation and the presence of inflammatory cytokines that promote angiogenesis. The prevalence of CNV varies among different entities. It can occur in up to 10% of patients with VKH syndrome. Patients present with metamorphopsia and scotoma. Diagnosis is based on clinical and angiographic findings. Treatment should be directed toward reducing inflammation as well as on anatomical ablation of the CNV. Focal laser photocoagulation of peripapillary, extrafoveal, and juxtafoveal CNV may be performed. The treatment of subfoveal CNV is more difficult. Corticosteroids (systemic, periocular, and intraocular) and immunomodulators alone may be used in an attempt to promote involution of CNV by controlling underlying intraocular inflammation. Recent studies have suggested significant long-term benefit from intravitreal pharmacotherapy with bevacizumab; 2–3 intravitreal injections improved vision in nearly all patients, significantly reduced central subfield thickness on OCT for 24 months, and reduced the size of subfoveal CNV in nearly all patients. If these approaches do not work, pars plana vitrectomy and subfoveal CNV extraction may be considered in selected cases (see Chapter 7).

Doctor PP, Bhat P, Sayed R, Foster CS. Intravitreal bevacizumab for uveitic choroidal neovascularization. *Ocul Immunol Inflamm.* 2009;17(2):118–126.

Kuo IC, Cunningham ET. Ocular neovascularization in patients with uveitis. *Int Ophthalmol Clin.* 2000(2);40:111–126.

Lott MN, Schiffman JC, Davis JL. Bevacizumab in inflammatory eye disease. *Am J Ophthalmol.* 2009;148(5):711–717.

Mansour AM, Arevalo JF, Ziemssen F, et al. Long-term visual outcomes of intravitreal bevacizumab in inflammatory ocular neovascularization. *Am J Ophthalmol.* 2009;148(2):310–316.

O'Toole LL, Tufail A, Pavesio C. Management of choroidal neovascularization in uveitis. *Int Ophthalmol Clin.* 2005;45(2):157–177.

Sanislo SR, Lowder CY, Kaiser PK, et al. Corticosteroid therapy for optic disc neovascularization secondary to chronic uveitis. *Am J Ophthalmol.* 2000;130(6):724–731.

Vision Rehabilitation

Despite optimal treatment, inflammatory disorders of the eye can lead to decreased vision. Worldwide, inflammatory disease is a significant cause of blindness and low vision, and even in the United States, 10% of all blindness is attributed to inadequately treated uveitis. Clinicians can assist their patients by enquiring if vision loss secondary to inflammation is affecting day-to-day function, such as reading or enjoying leisure activities, and by advising patients about vision rehabilitation resources. Referral to vision rehabilitation is recommended for patients with acuity less than 20/40, reduced contrast sensitivity, or central or peripheral field loss (American Academy of Ophthalmology; Vision Rehabilitation for Adults: Preferred Practice Pattern). The SmartSight patient handout on the American Academy of Ophthalmology website outlines how patients can identify vision rehabilitation resources in their community.

CHAPTER 11

Ocular Involvement in AIDS

Acquired immunodeficiency syndrome (AIDS) is caused by the human immunodeficiency virus (HIV), which infects and results in the depletion of CD4$^+$ helper T lymphocytes. This loss of CD4$^+$ T lymphocytes causes profound immune deficiency with subsequent opportunistic infections. Refer to BCSC Section 1, *Update on General Medicine,* for a full discussion of AIDS and HIV.

Ophthalmic Manifestations

Ocular manifestations may be the first sign of disseminated systemic HIV infection and have been reported in up to 70% of infected people. These ocular manifestations include

- HIV-related microangiopathy of the retina
- opportunistic viral, bacterial, and fungal infections
- Kaposi sarcoma
- lymphomas involving the retina (primary intraocular lymphoma), adnexal structures, and orbit
- squamous cell carcinoma of the conjunctiva

Reports also suggest that HIV itself may cause anterior or intermediate uveitis that is not responsive to corticosteroids but improves with antiretroviral therapy.

HIV retinopathy is the most common ocular finding in patients with AIDS, occurring in up to 70% of cases. It is characterized by retinal hemorrhages, microaneurysms, and cotton-wool spots (Fig 11-1). HIV has been isolated from the human retina, and its antigen has been detected in retinal endothelial cells by immunohistochemistry. It is thought that such HIV endothelial infection and/or rheologic abnormalities such as increased leukocyte activation and rigidity may play a role in the development of cotton-wool spots and other vascular alterations.

Other infectious agents that can affect the eye in patients with AIDS include cytomegalovirus (CMV), herpes zoster virus, *Toxoplasma gondii, Mycobacterium tuberculosis, Mycobacterium avium-intracellulare, Cryptococcus neoformans, Pneumocystis jiroveci* (formerly known as *Pneumocystis carinii*), *Histoplasma capsulatum, Candida* species, molluscum contagiosum virus, microsporida, and others. These pathogens can infect the ocular adnexa, anterior segment, or posterior segment. Visual morbidity, however, occurs primarily with posterior segment involvement, particularly retinitis caused by CMV, herpes zoster virus, or *T gondii.*

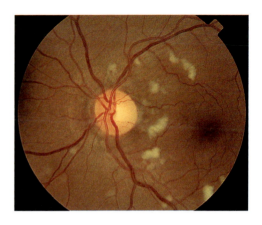

Figure 11-1 HIV retinopathy with numerous cotton-wool spots. *(Reprinted with permission from Cunningham ET Jr, Belfort R Jr. HIV/AIDS and the Eye: A Global Perspective. Ophthalmology Monograph 15. San Francisco, CA: American Academy of Ophthalmology; 2002:55.)*

Cunningham ET Jr. Uveitis in HIV positive patients. *Br J Ophthalmol.* 2000;84(3):233–235.

Goldenberg DT, Holland GN, Cumberland WG, et al. An assessment of polymorphonuclear leukocyte rigidity in HIV-infected individuals after immune recovery. *Invest Ophthalmol Vis Sci.* 2002;43(6):1857–1861.

Cytomegalovirus Retinitis

Disseminated CMV infection was the most common opportunistic infection in AIDS before the advent of highly active antiretroviral therapy (HAART), and retinal infection was its most clinically important manifestation, occurring in up to 40% of patients with AIDS. CMV retinitis remains the most common opportunistic ocular infection in patients with AIDS and occasionally is the first AIDS-defining infection seen in an individual. See Chapter 7 for a full discussion of CMV retinitis.

Immune recovery uveitis

Immune recovery uveitis (IRU) may occur in patients with previous CMV retinitis whose immune status improves with HAART. IRU occurs only in eyes infected with CMV, manifests as anterior or intermediate uveitis, and appears to be proportional to the surface area of retina involved.

A large prospective cohort study recorded IRU in 10% of patients with previous CMV retinitis. Immune recovery was defined as an increase in the CD4+ T-lymphocyte count of at least 50 cells/μL to at least 100 cells/μL. IRU was associated with a CMV retinitis surface area of 25% or more. The likelihood of developing IRU was significantly greater (odds ratio, 10.6) in patients who had ever used cidofovir.

Eyes with IRU were much more likely to have macular edema or epiretinal membrane. The macular edema can be resistant to treatment with sub-Tenon injections of depot corticosteroids, although such injections do not seem to cause reactivation of CMV infection. Intravitreal injections of corticosteroids must be avoided. IRU has been associated with moderate vision loss in the eyes in which it occurs but has not been linked to active replication of CMV or with the continuation or discontinuation of anti-CMV medication.

Retinal detachment

Retinal detachment occurs in up to 50% of patients with CMV retinitis. It may occur during active disease or after successful treatment. In the HAART era, the rate of retinal detachment has been reduced to 0.06 per patient-year. Involvement of all 3 retinal zones, lower CD4+ T-lymphocyte count, and more extensive retinitis are risk factors for developing retinal detachment. The retinal detachments in patients with CMV retinitis may be difficult to repair because of extensive retinal necrosis and multiple, often posterior, hole formation. Most require pars plana vitrectomy with long-term silicone oil tamponade. Anatomical reattachment can be achieved in 90% of patients.

El-Bradey MH, Cheng L, Song MK, Torriani FJ, Freeman WR. Long-term results of treatment of macular complications in eyes with immune recovery uveitis using a graded treatment approach. *Retina.* 2004;24(3):376–382.

Holland GN, Vaudaux JD, Shiramizu KM, et al, and the Southern California HIV/Eye Consortium. Characteristics of untreated AIDS-related cytomegalovirus retinitis. II. Findings in the era of highly active antiretroviral therapy (1997 to 2000). *Am J Ophthalmol.* 2008;145(1): 12–22.

Jabs DA, Van Natta ML, Thorne JE, et al. Course of cytomegalovirus retinitis in the era of highly active antiretroviral therapy: 1. Retinitis progression. *Ophthalmology.* 2004;111(12): 2224–2231.

Jabs DA, Van Natta ML, Thorne JE, et al. Course of cytomegalovirus retinitis in the era of highly active antiretroviral therapy: 2. Second eye involvement and retinal detachment. *Ophthalmology.* 2004;111(12):2232–2239.

Kempen JH, Min YI, Freeman WR, et al. Risk of immune recovery uveitis in patients with AIDS and cytomegalovirus retinitis. *Ophthalmology.* 2006;113(4):684–694.

Schrier RD, Song MK, Smith IL, et al. Intraocular viral and immune pathogenesis of immune recovery uveitis in patients with healed cytomegalovirus retinitis. *Retina.* 2006;26(2):165–169.

Song MK, Azen SP, Buley A, et al. Effect of anti-cytomegalovirus therapy on the incidence of immune recovery uveitis in AIDS patients with healed cytomegalovirus retinitis. *Am J Ophthalmol.* 2003;136(4):696–702.

Necrotizing Herpetic Retinitis

Patients with AIDS may develop aggressive forms of necrotizing herpetic retinitis, which appear to manifest as a spectrum of disease; the severity of these forms is directly proportional to the level of immunologic compromise. Hence, patients with HIV infection with profound reductions in CD4+ T-lymphocyte counts may develop more severe forms of necrotizing herpetic retinitis.

A rare infection in HIV-positive patients—progressive outer retinal necrosis (PORN), a variant of necrotizing herpetic retinitis—may be caused by the varicella-zoster virus or herpes simplex virus (Fig 11-2). It may occur in the absence of, at the same time as, or subsequent to a cutaneous varicella-zoster infection. (See also Chapter 7.)

In its early stages, PORN may be difficult to differentiate from peripheral CMV retinitis. However, PORN's characteristic rapid progression and relative absence of vitreous inflammation usually allow this entity to be distinguished from CMV retinitis and acute

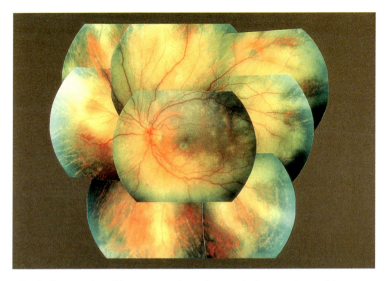

Figure 11-2 Retinal necrosis with preservation of vessels in a patient with progressive outer retinal necrosis (PORN). *(Courtesy of Narsing A. Rao, MD.)*

retinal necrosis (ARN). PORN is associated with a high incidence of retinal detachment, and bilateral involvement is common. Treatment with the ganciclovir implant, intravitreal foscarnet, intravenous acyclovir, and HAART has been reported to preserve vision.

Engstrom RE Jr, Holland GN, Margolis TP, et al. The progressive outer retinal necrosis syndrome. A variant of necrotizing herpetic retinopathy in patients with AIDS. *Ophthalmology.* 1994;101(12):1488–1502.

Kim SJ, Equi R, Belair ML, Fine HF, Dunn JP. Long-term preservation of vision in progressive outer retinal necrosis treated with combination antiviral drugs and highly active antiretroviral therapy. *Ocul Immunol Inflamm.* 2007;15(6):425–427.

Toxoplasma Retinochoroiditis

Toxoplasmosis in patients with AIDS differs from toxoplasmosis in immunocompetent patients in several ways. In general, the lesions are larger in patients with AIDS, with up to one-third of lesions greater in size than 5 disc diameters. Bilateral disease is seen in up to 40% of cases. Solitary, multifocal, and miliary patterns of retinitis have been observed (Fig 11-3). A vitreous inflammatory reaction usually appears overlying the area of active retinochoroiditis, but the degree of vitreous reaction may be less than that observed in immunocompetent patients. (See also Chapter 7.)

The diagnosis of ocular toxoplasmosis may also be more difficult in patients with AIDS. In immunocompetent patients, this diagnosis is frequently helped by the presence of old retinochoroidal scars; in patients with AIDS, however, such preexisting scars are rarely seen (present in 6% of patients at most). Because the clinical manifestations in this latter population are so varied and may be more severe than those seen in immunocompetent patients, ocular toxoplasmosis in patients with AIDS may be difficult to distinguish from ARN, necrotizing herpetic retinitis, or syphilitic retinitis.

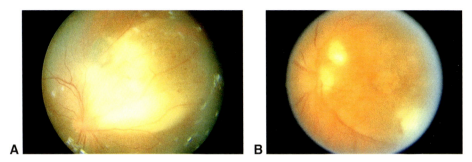

Figure 11-3   A, A large area of macular toxoplasmic retinochoroiditis in a patient infected with HIV. **B,** Multifocal toxoplasmic retinochoroiditis in another patient infected with HIV. *(Courtesy of Emmett T. Cunningham, Jr, MD.)*

The histologic features of ocular specimens from patients with AIDS reflect the immunologic abnormalities of the host. In general, the inflammatory reaction in the choroid, retina, and vitreous is less prominent than in patients with an intact immune system. Trophozoites and cysts can be observed in greater numbers within areas of retinitis, and *T gondii* organisms can occasionally be seen invading the choroid, which is not the case in immunocompetent patients.

Ocular toxoplasmosis in immunocompetent patients is usually the result of reactivation of a congenital infection. In contrast, newly acquired infections or dissemination from nonocular sites are the most likely causes among patients with AIDS.

The prompt diagnosis of ocular toxoplasmosis is especially important in patients who are immunocompromised, because the condition inevitably progresses if left untreated, in contrast to the self-limiting disease in immunocompetent patients. In addition, ocular toxoplasmosis in immunocompromised patients may be associated with cerebral or disseminated toxoplasmosis, an important cause of morbidity and mortality in patients with AIDS. HIV-infected patients with active ocular toxoplasmosis should therefore undergo magnetic resonance imaging (MRI) of the brain to rule out central nervous system (CNS) involvement.

Antitoxoplasmic therapy with various combinations of pyrimethamine, sulfadiazine, and clindamycin is required. Corticosteroids should be used with caution and only in the presence of appropriate antimicrobial cover because of the risk of further immunosuppression in this population. In selecting the therapeutic regimen, the physician should consider the possibility of coexisting cerebral or disseminated toxoplasmosis as well as the toxic effects of pyrimethamine and sulfadiazine on bone marrow. Continued maintenance therapy may be necessary for patients with poor immune status that is not improving.

Moshfeghi DM, Dodds EM, Couto CA, et al. Diagnostic approaches to severe, atypical toxoplasmosis mimicking acute retinal necrosis. *Ophthalmology.* 2004;111(4):716–725.

Syphilitic Chorioretinitis

The clinical presentations of ocular syphilitic chorioretinitis include uveitis, optic neuritis, and nonnecrotizing retinitis. Patients may also experience dermatologic and CNS symptoms. A classic manifestation of syphilis in patients with AIDS is unilateral or bilateral pale yellow placoid retinal lesions that preferentially involve the macula (syphilitic posterior placoid chorioretinitis). Exudative retinal detachment can also be seen. Some HIV-positive patients with syphilis may present with dense vitritis without clinical evidence of chorioretinitis. In these patients, vitritis can be the first manifestation of syphilis. (See also Chapter 7.)

The course of syphilis may be more aggressive in patients with AIDS. These patients require treatment with 18–24 million units of intravenous penicillin G administered daily for 10–14 days, followed by 2.4 million units of intramuscular benzathine penicillin G administered weekly for 3 weeks. Monitoring of the quantitative rapid plasma reagin (RPR) test is recommended, as symptomatic disease can recur.

Browning DJ. Posterior segment manifestations of active ocular syphilis, their response to a neurosyphilis regimen of penicillin therapy, and the influence of human immunodeficiency virus status on response. *Ophthalmology.* 2000;107(11):2015–2023.

Pneumocystis jiroveci Choroiditis

Patients with AIDS are at much greater risk for *P jiroveci* pneumonia. In rare instances, this infection can disseminate, and patients with such disseminated infection may present with choroidal infiltrates containing the responsible microorganisms.

Fundus changes characteristic of *P jiroveci* choroiditis consist of slightly elevated, plaquelike, yellow-white lesions located in the choroid with minimal vitritis (Figs 11-4, 11-5). On fluorescein angiography, these lesions tend to be hypofluorescent in the early phase and hyperfluorescent in the later phases. If disseminated *P jiroveci* infection is suspected, an extensive examination is required, including chest radiography, arterial blood gas analysis, liver function testing, and abdominal computed tomography.

Treatment of *P jiroveci* choroiditis involves a 3-week regimen of intravenous trimethoprim (20 mg/kg/day) and sulfamethoxazole (100 mg/kg/day) or pentamidine (4 mg/kg/day). Within 3–12 weeks, most of the yellow-white lesions disappear, leaving mild overlying pigmentary changes. Vision is usually not affected.

Cryptococcus neoformans Choroiditis

The dissemination of *C neoformans* in patients with AIDS may result in a multifocal choroiditis similar to *P jiroveci* choroiditis. Some patients with *C neoformans* choroiditis show choroidal lesions before they develop clinical evidence of dissemination. More typically,

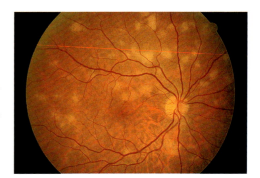

Figure 11-4 *Pneumocystis jiroveci* choroiditis. The fellow eye revealed similar findings. *(Reprinted with permission from Cunningham ET Jr, Belfort R Jr. HIV/AIDS and the Eye: A Global Perspective. Ophthalmology Monograph 15. San Francisco, CA: American Academy of Ophthalmology; 2002:67.)*

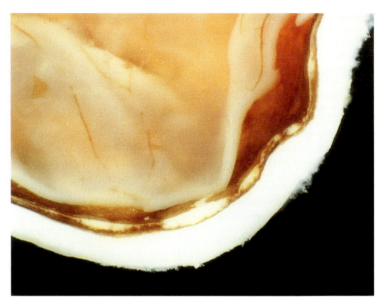

Figure 11-5 Gross appearance of multifocal infiltrates of *Pneumocystis jiroveci* in the choroid.

C neoformans infection involves the cerebrospinal fluid and there is secondary optic nerve edema from increased intracranial pressure that can slowly lead to optic atrophy. Direct invasion of the optic nerve by organisms is also possible and can lead to more rapid vision loss.

Kestelyn P, Taelman H, Bogaerts J, et al. Ophthalmic manifestations of infections with *Cryptococcus neoformans* in patients with the acquired immunodeficiency syndrome. *Am J Ophthalmol.* 1993;116(6):721–727.

Multifocal Choroiditis and Systemic Dissemination

Multifocal choroidal lesions from a variety of infectious agents, including those just discussed, are seen in up to 10% of patients with AIDS. Most of these lesions are caused by *C neoformans, P jiroveci, M tuberculosis,* or atypical mycobacteria. Due to the profound immunosuppression, multiple infectious agents may cause simultaneous infectious multifocal choroiditis.

The choroid is often a site of opportunistic disseminated infections and thus needs to be carefully examined in patients with AIDS. Although nonspecific, multifocal choroiditis should prompt an exhaustive workup because it frequently is a sign of disseminated infection.

External Eye Manifestations

Other ophthalmic manifestations of AIDS include Kaposi sarcoma; molluscum contagiosum; herpes zoster ophthalmicus; and keratitis caused by various viruses, protozoa, conjunctival infections, and microvascular abnormalities. All of these conditions affect mainly the anterior segment of the globe and the ocular adnexa. These conditions are also discussed in BCSC Section 8, *External Disease and Cornea.*

Ocular Adnexal Kaposi Sarcoma

Human herpesvirus 8 is associated with Kaposi sarcoma.Two aggressive variants of this tumor have been described: an endemic variety especially prevalent in Kenya and Nigeria and a second variant, *epidemic Kaposi sarcoma,* which was first noted in renal transplant recipients and currently occurs in 30% of patients with AIDS. AIDS-associated Kaposi sarcoma may disseminate to visceral organs (the gastrointestinal tract, lung, and liver) in up to 50% of patients. In the era before HAART, ocular adnexal involvement occurred in approximately 20% of patients with AIDS-associated systemic Kaposi sarcoma (Fig 11-6). Histologic investigation shows spindle cells mixed with vascular structures (Fig 11-7).

Treatment of Kaposi sarcoma consists of excision, cryotherapy, radiation, or a combination of these methods, based on the clinical stage of the tumor as well as its location and the presence or absence of disseminated lesions.

Molluscum Contagiosum

Molluscum contagiosum is caused by a DNA virus of the poxvirus family. The characteristic skin lesions show a small elevation with central umbilication. Molluscum contagiosum lesions in healthy individuals are few, unilateral, and involve the eyelids. In patients with AIDS, however, these lesions may be numerous and bilateral. If molluscum contagiosum

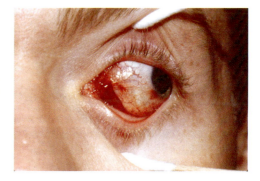

Figure 11-6 Conjunctival involvement in Kaposi sarcoma; hemorrhagic conjunctival tumor. *(Courtesy of Elaine Chuang, MD.)*

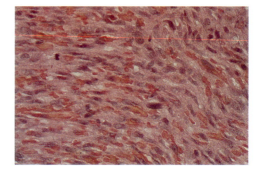

Figure 11-7 Histologically, Kaposi sarcoma is made up of large spindle cells forming slitlike spaces. These spaces contain erythrocytes.

lesions in patients with AIDS are symptomatic or cause conjunctivitis, surgical excision may be necessary.

Herpes Zoster

People younger than age 50 presenting with herpes zoster lesions of the face or eyelids should be tested for HIV. Corneal involvement can cause a persistent, chronic epithelial keratitis; treatment consists of intravenous and topical acyclovir. These patients should be followed up periodically with retinal examinations to ensure that posterior segment involvement does not occur.

Other Infections

HIV infection does not appear to predispose patients to bacterial keratitis. However, infections appear to be more severe and are more likely to cause corneal perforation in patients with AIDS than in immunocompetent patients. Bacterial and fungal keratitis can occur in patients with AIDS who have no obvious predisposing factors such as trauma or topical corticosteroid use. Although herpes simplex keratitis does not appear to have a higher incidence in patients with AIDS, it may have a prolonged course or multiple recurrences and involve the limbus (Fig 11-8). Microsporidia have been shown to cause a coarse, superficial punctate keratitis with a minimal conjunctival reaction in patients with AIDS (Fig 11-9). Electron microscopy of epithelial scrapings has revealed the organism, which is an obligate, intracellular, protozoal parasite.

Solitary granulomatous conjunctivitis from cryptococcal or mycotic infections or tuberculosis can occur in persons infected with HIV. As with all other infections in patients with AIDS, the possibility of dissemination must be considered, aggressively investigated,

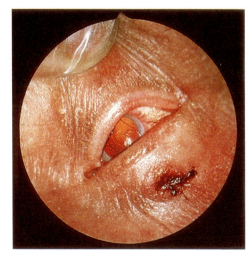

Figure 11-8 Lesions of the eyelid and cornea in a patient with AIDS and disseminated herpes simplex.

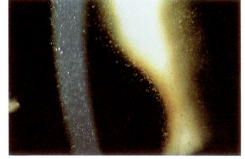

Figure 11-9 Superficial punctate keratitis caused by microsporidia.

and, if present, treated. Orbital lymphomas and intraocular lymphomas have been described in patients with AIDS. These neoplasms are mostly large B-cell lymphomas. Conjunctival squamous cell carcinomas have been reported, and in some patients these neoplasms show spindle cells with frequent abnormal mitotic figures.

Precautions in the Health Care Setting

Universal precautions as advocated in the United States by the Centers for Disease Control and Prevention (CDC) and other governmental agencies, including the Occupational Safety and Health Administration (OSHA), should always be followed.

Precautions in Ophthalmic Practice

There are no published reports of HIV transmission in ophthalmic health care settings. Regardless, the American Academy of Ophthalmology advocates that ophthalmic health care practitioners take precautionary measures against HIV infection. Hands should be washed or a hand sterilizer solution used between tests on an individual and between patients. Tonometers, diagnostic contact lenses, and contact lens trial sets should be appropriately disinfected according to the manufacturers' guidelines. BCSC Section 10, *Glaucoma,* gives more specific instructions for infection control in tonometry.

> Minimizing transmission of bloodborne pathogens and surface infectious agents in ophthalmic offices and operating rooms. Information Statement. San Francisco, CA: American Academy of Ophthalmology; 2002.

Diagnostic Survey for Uveitis

(to be filled in by patient)

FAMILY HISTORY

These questions refer to your grandparents, parents, aunts, uncles, brothers and sisters, children, or grandchildren

Has anyone in your family ever had any of the following?

Cancer	Yes	No
Diabetes	Yes	No
Allergies	Yes	No
Arthritis or rheumatism	Yes	No
Syphilis	Yes	No
Tuberculosis	Yes	No
Sickle cell disease or trait	Yes	No
Lyme disease	Yes	No
Gout	Yes	No

Has anyone in your family had medical problems in any of the following areas?

Eyes	Yes	No
Skin	Yes	No
Kidneys	Yes	No
Lungs	Yes	No
Stomach or bowel	Yes	No
Nervous system or brain	Yes	No

SOCIAL HISTORY

Age (years): Current job:		
Have you ever lived outside of the United States?	Yes	No
If yes, where?		
Have you ever owned a dog?	Yes	No
Have you ever owned a cat?	Yes	No
Have you ever eaten raw meat or uncooked sausage?	Yes	No
Have you ever had unpasteurized milk or cheese?	Yes	No
Have you ever been exposed to sick animals?	Yes	No
Do you drink untreated stream, well, or lake water?	Yes	No
Do you smoke cigarettes?	Yes	No
Have you ever used intravenous drugs?	Yes	No
Have you ever had bisexual or homosexual relationships?	Yes	No
Have you ever taken birth control pills?	Yes	No

PERSONAL MEDICAL HISTORY

Are you allergic to any medications?	Yes	No
If yes, which medications?		

Please list the medications that you are currently taking, including nonprescription drugs such as aspirin, ibuprofen, antihistamines, etc:

_____
_____

Please list all the eye operations you have had (including laser surgery) and the dates of the surgeries:

_____
_____
_____
_____

Please list all operations you have had and the dates of the surgeries:

_____
_____
_____
_____

Have you ever been told that you have the following conditions?

Anemia (low blood count)	Yes	No
Cancer	Yes	No
Diabetes	Yes	No
Hepatitis	Yes	No
High blood pressure	Yes	No
Pleurisy	Yes	No
Pneumonia	Yes	No
Ulcers	Yes	No
Herpes (cold sores)	Yes	No
Chickenpox	Yes	No
Shingles (zoster)	Yes	No
German measles (rubella)	Yes	No
Measles (rubeola)	Yes	No
Mumps	Yes	No
Chlamydia or trachoma	Yes	No
Syphilis	Yes	No
Gonorrhea	Yes	No
Any other sexually transmitted disease	Yes	No
Tuberculosis	Yes	No
Leprosy	Yes	No
Leptospirosis	Yes	No
Lyme disease	Yes	No
Histoplasmosis	Yes	No
Candida infection or moniliasis	Yes	No
Coccidioidomycosis	Yes	No
Sporotrichosis	Yes	No
Toxoplasmosis	Yes	No
Toxocariasis	Yes	No
Cysticercosis	Yes	No
Trichinosis	Yes	No

Whipple disease	Yes	No
AIDS	Yes	No
Hay fever	Yes	No
Allergies	Yes	No
Vasculitis	Yes	No
Arthritis	Yes	No
Rheumatoid arthritis	Yes	No
Lupus (systemic lupus erythematosus)	Yes	No
Scleroderma	Yes	No

Have you ever had any of the following illnesses?

Reactive arthritis	Yes	No
Colitis	Yes	No
Crohn disease	Yes	No
Ulcerative colitis	Yes	No
Behçet disease	Yes	No
Sarcoidosis	Yes	No
Ankylosing spondylitis	Yes	No
Erythema nodosa	Yes	No
Temporal arteritis	Yes	No
Multiple sclerosis	Yes	No
Serpiginous choroiditis	Yes	No
Fuchs heterochromic iridocyclitis	Yes	No
Vogt-Koyanagi-Harada syndrome	Yes	No

Have you ever had any of the following illnesses?

GENERAL HEALTH

Chills	Yes	No
Fever (persistent or recurrent)	Yes	No
Night sweats	Yes	No
Fatigue (tire easily)	Yes	No
Poor appetite	Yes	No
Unexplained weight loss	Yes	No
Do you feel sick?	Yes	No

HEAD

Frequent or severe headaches	Yes	No
Fainting	Yes	No
Numbness or tingling in your body	Yes	No
Paralysis in parts of your body	Yes	No
Siezures or convulsions	Yes	No

EARS

Hard of hearing or deafness	Yes	No
Ringing or noise in your ears	Yes	No
Frequent or severe ear infections	Yes	No
Painful or swollen ear lobes	Yes	No

NOSE AND THROAT

Sore in your nose or mouth	Yes	No
Severe or recurrent nosebleeds	Yes	No

Frequent sneezing	Yes	No
Sinus trouble	Yes	No
Persistent hoarseness	Yes	No
Tooth or gum infections	Yes	No

SKIN

Rashes	Yes	No
Skin sores	Yes	No
Sunburn easily (photosensitivity)	Yes	No
White patches of skin or hair	Yes	No
Loss of hair	Yes	No
Tick or insect bites	Yes	No
Painfully cold fingers	Yes	No
Severe itching	Yes	No

RESPIRATORY

Severe or frequent colds	Yes	No
Constant coughing	Yes	No
Coughing up blood	Yes	No
Recent flu or viral infection	Yes	No
Wheezing or asthma attacks	Yes	No
Difficulty breathing	Yes	No

Have you ever had any of the following symptoms?

CARDIOVASCULAR

Chest pain	Yes	No
Shortness of breath	Yes	No
Swelling of your legs	Yes	No

BLOOD

Frequent or easy bruising	Yes	No
Frequent or easy bleeding	Yes	No
Have you received blood transfusions?	Yes	No

GASTROINTESTINAL

Trouble swallowing	Yes	No
Diarrhea	Yes	No
Bloody stools	Yes	No
Stomach ulcers	Yes	No
Jaundice or yellow skin	Yes	No

BONES AND JOINTS

Stiff joints	Yes	No
Painful or swollen glands	Yes	No
Stiff lower back	Yes	No
Back pain while sleeping or awakening	Yes	No
Muscle aches	Yes	No

GENITOURINARY

Kidney problems	Yes	No
Bladder trouble	Yes	No
Blood in your urine	Yes	No

Urinary discharge	Yes	No
Genital sores or ulcers	Yes	No
Prostatitis	Yes	No
Testicular pain	Yes	No
Are you pregnant?	Yes	No
Do you plan to be pregnant in the future?	Yes	No

Adapted with permission from Foster CS, Vitale AT. *Diagnosis and Treatment of Uveitis.* Philadelphia, PA: WB Saunders; 2002.

Basic Texts

Intraocular Inflammation and Uveitis

Albert DM, Miller JW, Azar DT, Blodi BA, eds. *Albert & Jakobiec's Principles and Practice of Ophthalmology*. 3rd ed. Philadelphia, PA: Saunders; 2008.

Delves PJ, Martin S, Burton D, Roitt IM. *Roitt's Essential Immunology*. 11th ed. Malden, MA: Blackwell Publishing; 2006.

Dick A, Forrester J, Okada A. *Practical Manual of Intraocular Inflammation*. New York, NY: Informa Healthcare USA Inc; 2008.

Foster CS, Vitale AT, eds. *Diagnosis and Treatment of Uveitis*. Philadelphia, PA: WB Saunders; 2002.

Giles CL. Uveitis in childhood. In: Tasman W, Jaeger EA, eds. *Duane's Clinical Ophthalmology*. Philadelphia, PA: Lippincott Williams & Wilkins; 2005.

Kanski JJ. *Clinical Ophthalmology: A Systematic Approach*. 6th ed. London. Butterworth-Heinemann; 2007.

Michelson JB. *Color Atlas of Uveitis Diagnosis*. 2nd ed. St Louis, MO: Mosby; 1992.

Nussenblatt RB, Whitcup SM. *Uveitis: Fundamentals and Clinical Practice*. 4th ed. St Louis, MO: Mosby; 2010.

Pepose JS, Holland GN, Wilhelmus KR, eds. *Ocular Infection and Immunity*. St Louis, MO: Mosby; 1996.

Rao NA, section ed. Part 7: Uveitis and Other Intraocular Inflammations. In: Yanoff M, Duker JS, eds. *Ophthalmology*. 3rd ed. St Louis, MO: Mosby; 2009.

Related Academy Materials

Focal Points: Clinical Modules for Ophthalmologists

Ahmed M, Foster CS. Steroid therapy for ocular inflammatory disease (Module 7, 2006).

Arellanes-Garcia L. Infectious posterior uveitis (Module 3, 2005).

Buggage RR. White dot syndrome (Module 4, 2007).

Cunningham ET. Diagnosis and management of anterior uveitis (Module 1, 2002).

Dodds EM. Ocular toxoplasmosis: clinical presentations, diagnosis, and therapy (Module 10, 1999).

Doft BH. Managing infectious endophthalmitis: results of the Endophthalmitis Vitrectomy Study (Module 3, 1997).

Dunn JP. Uveitis in children (Module 4, 1995).

Jampol LM. Nonsteroidal anti-inflammatory drugs: 1997 update (Module 6, 1997).

Lightman S, McCluskey P. Cystoid macular edema in uveitis (Module 8, 2003).

Margo CE. Nonpigmented lesions of the ocular surface (Module 9, 1996).

Moshfeghi DM, Muccioli C, Belfort R Jr. Laboratory evaluation of patients with uveitis (Module 12, 2001).

Read RW. Sympathetic ophthalmia (Module 5, 2004).

Samples JR. Management of glaucoma secondary to uveitis (Module 5, 1995).

Smith JR, Rosenbaum JT. Immune-mediated systemic diseases associated with uveitis (Module 11, 2003).

Tessler HH, Goldstein DA. Update on systemic immunosuppressive agents (Module 11, 2000).

Print Publications

Arnold AC, ed. *Basic Principles of Ophthalmic Surgery* (2006).

Dunn JP, Langer PD, eds. *Basic Techniques of Ophthalmic Surgery* (2009).

Rockwood EJ, ed. *ProVision: Preferred Responses in Ophthalmology, Series 4.* Self-Assessment Program, 2-vol set (2007).

Wilson FM II, ed. *Practical Ophthalmology: A Manual for Beginning Residents.* 6th ed (2009).

Academy Maintenance of Certification (MOC)

MOC Exam Review Course (2011).

CDs/DVDs

Johns KJ, ed. *Eye Care Skills: Presentations for Physicians and Other Health Care Professionals* (CD-ROM; 2009).

Online Materials

Focal Points modules; http://one.aao.org/CE/EducationalProducts/FocalPoints.aspx

Hebson CB, Martin DF. Academy Grand Rounds: Blurry Vision Following Cat Scratch (January 2009). ONE Network interactive online case; http://one.aao.org/CE/EducationalContent/Cases.aspx

Practicing Ophthalmologists Learning System (2011); http://one.aao.org/CE/POLS/Default.aspx

Rockwood EJ, ed. *ProVision: Preferred Responses in Ophthalmology, Series 4.* Self-Assessment Program. 2-vol set (2007); http://one.aao.org/CE/EducationalProducts/Provision.aspx

---

To order any of these materials, please order online at www.aao.org/store or call the Academy's Customer Service toll-free number 866-561-8558 in the U.S. If outside the U.S., call 415-561-8540 between 8:00 AM and 5:00 PM PST.

Requesting Continuing Medical Education Credit

The American Academy of Ophthalmology is accredited by the Accreditation Council for Continuing Medical Education to provide continuing medical education for physicians.

The American Academy of Ophthalmology designates this enduring material for a maximum of 10 *AMA PRA Category 1 Credits™*. Physicians should claim only the credit commensurate with the extent of their participation in the activity.

The American Medical Association requires that all learners participating in activities involving enduring materials complete a formal assessment before claiming continuing medical education (CME) credit. To assess your achievement in this activity and ensure that a specified level of knowledge has been reached, a posttest for this Section of the Basic and Clinical Science Course is provided. A minimum score of 80% must be obtained to pass the test and claim CME credit.

To take the posttest and request CME credit online:

1. Go to www.aao.org/cme and log in.
2. Select the appropriate Academy activity. You will be directed to the posttest.
3. Once you have passed the test with a score of 80% or higher, you will be directed to your transcript. *If you are not an Academy member, you will be able to print out a certificate of participation once you have passed the test.*

To take the posttest and request CME credit using a paper form:

1. Complete the CME Posttest Request Form on the following page and return it to the address provided. *Please note that there is a $20.00 processing fee for all paper requests.* The posttest will be mailed to you.
2. Return the completed test as directed. Once you have passed the test with a score of 80% or higher, your transcript will be updated automatically. To receive verification of your CME credits, be sure to check the appropriate box on the posttest.

   Please note that test results will not be provided. If you do not achieve a minimum score of 80%, another test will be sent to you automatically, at no charge. If you do not reach the specified level of knowledge (80%) on your second attempt, you will need to pay an additional processing fee to receive the third test.

Note: Submission of the CME Posttest Request Form does not represent claiming CME credit.

• Credit must be claimed by June 1, 2014 •

For assistance, contact the Academy's Customer Service department at 866-561-8558 (US only) or 415-561-8540 between 8:00 AM and 5:00 PM (PST), Monday through Friday, or send an e-mail to customer_service@aao.org.

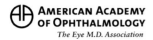
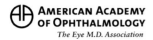AMERICAN ACADEMY
OF OPHTHALMOLOGY
The Eye M.D. Association

CME Posttest Request Form
Basic and Clinical Science Course, 2012–2013
Section 9

Please note that requesting CME credit with this form will incur a fee of $20.00. (Prepayment required.)

☐ Yes, please send me the posttest for BCSC Section 9. I choose not to report my CME credit online for free. I have enclosed a payment of **$20.00** for processing.

Academy Member ID Number (if known): _____

Name: _____
      First   Last

Address: _____

_____
      City   State/Province   ZIP/Postal Code   Country

Phone Number: _____ Fax Number: _____

E-mail Address: _____

Method of Payment: ☐ Check   ☐ Credit Card   Make checks payable to AAO.

Credit Card Type: ☐ Visa   ☐ MasterCard   ☐ American Express   ☐ Discover

Card Number: _____ Expiration Date: _____

Credit must be claimed by June 1, 2014. Please note that submission of this form does not represent claiming CME credits.

Test results will not be sent. If a participant does not achieve an 80% pass rate, one new posttest will be sent at no charge. Additional processing fees are incurred thereafter.

Please mail completed form to:
American Academy of Ophthalmology, CME Posttest
Dept. 34051
PO Box 39000
San Francisco, CA 94139

Please allow 3 weeks for delivery of the posttest.

Academy use only:

PN: _____ MC: _____

Study Questions

Please note that these questions are *not* part of your CME reporting process. They are provided here for self-assessment and identification of personal professional practice gaps. The required CME posttest is available online or by request (see "Requesting CME Credit").

Following the questions are a blank answer sheet and answers with discussions. Although a concerted effort has been made to avoid ambiguity and redundancy in these questions, the authors recognize that differences of opinion may occur regarding the "best" answer. The discussions are provided to demonstrate the rationale used to derive the answer. They may also be helpful in confirming that your approach to the problem was correct or, if necessary, in fixing the principle in your memory. The Section 9 faculty would like to thank the Self-Assessment Committee for working with them to provide these study questions and discussions.

1. Experimental immune uveitis (EIU) is an animal model in which a transient anterior uveitis is induced in rodents following foot-pad administration of lipopolysaccharide (LPS). What is the likely mechanism of the inflammation induced by LPS?
   a. LPS generates a T helper-1 (Th1) response against specific ocular antigens
   b. LPS induces increased B-cell and plasma cell activity with generation of autoantibodies
   c. recognition of lipid A, O polysaccharide, and core oligosaccharide by toll-like receptors triggers up-regulation of cytokines by innate effector cells
   d. LPS is directly chemotactic for dendritic cells and macrophages

2. What is the principal mechanism of phacolytic glaucoma?
   a. granulomatous inflammation occurring around retained cortical lens fragments
   b. lens-protein–laden macrophages populating the anterior chamber and blocking aqueous outflow in the trabecular meshwork
   c. anaphylactic response to previously sequestered lens proteins
   d. monocyte cytokine release leading to ciliary body edema with forward rotation, causing angle closure

3. What is the most likely immune mechanism of Vogt-Koyanagi-Harada (VKH) syndrome?
   a. Th1 and other T-cell–mediated pathways
   b. Th2 and other T-cell–mediated pathways
   c. antigen-antibody complexes
   d. a complement- and polymorphonuclear-cell–mediated process

4. What is the immune mechanism involved in *Toxocara canis*–induced uveitis?

   a. molecular mimicry inducing severe inflammation to epitopes shared by parasite and choroidal cells

   b. a Th1 delayed hypersensitivity response resulting in clonal T-cell proliferation in the choroid

   c. basophil and mast cell degranulation leading to increased retinal vascular permeability

   d. a Th2-mediated response resulting in local eosinophilia

5. What is the critical local (ocular) process in anterior chamber–associated immune deviation (ACAID)?

   a. removal of antigen from the anterior chamber

   b. use of an adjuvant along with specific antigenic peptide

   c. exposure of antigen-presenting cells in the anterior chamber to transforming growth factor β_2 (TGF-β_2) results in ultimate suppression of delayed-type hypersensitivity to specific antigens

   d. pharmacologic treatment of preexisting delayed-type hypersensitivity

6. All of the following are thought to increase risk of corneal allograft rejection *except*

   a. the presence of central corneal vascularization

   b. the presence of Fas ligand on corneal endothelium

   c. contamination of the graft with donor-derived antigen-presenting cells at the time of transplantation

   d. induction of major histocompatability complex (MHC) antigens by the corneal stroma

7. Which of these human leukocyte antigen (HLA) genes confers the highest relative risk (RR) for its associated disease?

   a. Behçet disease and HLA-B51

   b. reactive arthritis and HLA-B27

   c. tubulointerstitial nephritis and uveitis (TINU) syndrome and HLA-DRB1*0102

   d. birdshot retinochoroidopathy and HLA-A29

8. A major side effect of systemic cyclosporine is

   a. elevated intraocular pressure

   b. cataracts

   c. osteoporosis

   d. systemic hypertension

9. Which statement best applies regarding the use of nonsteroidal anti-inflammatory drugs (NSAIDs)?

   a. oral NSAIDs may adversely affect renal function and elevate systemic blood pressure

   b. selective cyclooxygenase-2 (COX-2) inhibitors have been demonstrated to be safer and more effective for treating scleritis than nonselective inhibitors

   c. topical NSAIDs have been demonstrated in controlled studies to be an effective treatment for uveitic cystoid macular edema (CME)

   d. topical NSAIDs are effective in treating scleritis

10. What age group had the highest incidence and prevalence of uveitis overall in a study population from northern California in the United States?

   a. patients in the first and second decades of life

   b. patients in the third and fourth decades of life

   c. patients older than age 65 years

   d. patients in the fifth decade of life

11. What is the mediator of the anti-inflammatory effects of methotrexate?

   a. inhibition of folate metabolism

   b. nucleotide cross-linking during DNA replication

   c. inhibition of calcineurin

   d. extracellular release of adenosine

12. A patient has uveitic glaucoma that is not controlled with maximally tolerated medical therapy. There are extensive posterior synechiae but 1 clock hour is open and there is no iris bombé. The uveitis is controlled on antimetabolite medication. What is the next step in the management of the glaucoma?

   a. laser trabeculoplasty

   b. laser iridotomy

   c. glaucoma implant (aqueous drainage device) or mitomycin trabeculectomy

   d. stop the antimetabolite

13. What is the initial surgical management of a patient with uveitis and iris bombé?

   a. laser iridotomy or surgical iridectomy

   b. laser trabeculoplasty

   c. trabeculectomy

   d. glaucoma implant

14. Florid bilateral CME in a patient with bilateral, chronic, granulomatous anterior uveitis with 2+ cells in the anterior chamber, posterior synechiae, and 2+ vitreous cells is most effectively managed by which of the following?

    a. oral acetazolamide

    b. topical ketorolac

    c. systemic corticosteroids and systemic immunomodulatory therapy

    d. pars plana vitrectomy

15. Which of following is the most appropriate instruction to a patient beginning daily oral cyclophosphamide therapy?

    a. The patient should use 1 mg per day of folic acid supplementation.

    b. The patient should undergo annual influenza immunization with an intranasal live vaccine.

    c. The patient should maintain adequate hydration.

    d. The patient should avoid taking the medication with a fatty meal.

16. The fluocinolone acetonide implant releases therapeutic levels of corticosteroids to the vitreous cavity for approximately how many days?

    a. 500

    b. 1000

    c. 5000

    d. 100

17. What is the specific concern about using a tumor necrosis factor (TNF) inhibitor in a 25-year-old woman with intermediate uveitis and no evidence of tuberculosis or other systemic disease or infection?

    a. congestive heart failure

    b. risk of neoplasia

    c. lupuslike syndrome

    d. demyelinating disease

18. Chronic postoperative endophthalmitis is most commonly caused by which organism?

    a. *Candida glabrata*

    b. *Nocardia* species

    c. *Klebsiella pneumoniae*

    d. *Propionibacterium acnes*

19. Which of the following findings is most likely to be seen in a patient with systemic lupus erythematosus?

    a. chronic anterior uveitis

    b. intraretinal hemorrhages and cotton-wool spots

    c. intermediate uveitis

    d. acute anterior uveitis

20. A 25-year-old Brazilian man presents with a history of decreased vision in his left eye for 1 week. Visual acuity is 20/70 and moderate vitritis is present. On dilated examination, a pigmented scar in the posterior pole with adjacent focal white chorioretinitis is present. What is the most appropriate treatment?
    a. oral corticosteroids
    b. pyrimethamine, sulfadiazine, and prednisone
    c. intravenous acyclovir
    d. amphotericin B

21. Which of the following statements most likely applies to a patient newly diagnosed with serpiginous choroiditis?
    a. vasculitis is a prominent feature
    b. old, scarred lesions may be present in the newly diagnosed eye
    c. intense vitritis is common
    d. multiple, isolated lesions occur, with recurrences

22. Which clinical finding is associated with acute retinal necrosis?
    a. extensive choroidal scarring
    b. natural history of rapid progression
    c. occlusive vasculopathy mostly involving retinal venules
    d. minimal vitritis

23. The white dot lesions of which disease are least apparent on fluorescein angiography?
    a. serpiginous choroiditis
    b. punctate inner choroidopathy (PIC)
    c. acute posterior multifocal placoid pigment epitheliopathy (APMPPE)
    d. birdshot retinochoroidopathy

24. In patients with VKH syndrome, the presence of diffuse choroiditis is most likely to be found during which stage of the disease?
    a. recurrent
    b. prodromal
    c. late (chronic)
    d. early (acute uveitic)

25. A patient with bilateral anterior and intermediate uveitis is suspected of having sarcoidosis. There are no conjunctival or eyelid granulomata. Chest x-ray shows no abnormalities and serum angiotensin-converting enzyme (ACE) level is normal. Which of the following is the most appropriate examination for confirming the diagnosis of sarcoidosis?
    a. biopsy of the conjunctiva
    b. evaluation of HLA-B27 status
    c. repeat serum ACE test to rule out laboratory error
    d. high-resolution computed tomographic scan of the chest

26. Which statement is correct regarding patients with West Nile virus infection?

    a. Ocular involvement is limited to anterior uveitis without chorioretinal lesions.

    b. In the United States, West Nile virus is most commonly acquired in the winter.

    c. West Nile virus is most often contracted via mosquito bites.

    d. Ocular involvement requires antiviral therapy.

27. What is the triad of reactive arthritis syndrome?

    a. urethritis, polyarthritis, and conjuctival inflammation

    b. ulcerative colitis, polyarthritis, and conjunctival inflammation

    c. genital ulcers, polyarthritis, and vasculitis

    d. palmar rashes, pauciarticular arthritis, and fevers

28. What class of microorganisms has been associated with glaucomatocyclitic crisis?

    a. viruses

    b. bacteria

    c. fungi

    d. parasites

29. What serologic test is most likely to suggest a specific cause of uveitis, may be curative, and must be considered for all patients with uveitis?

    a. a treponemal-specific serologic test

    b. antinuclear antibody (ANA)

    c. rheumatoid factor (RF)

    d. antineutrophil cytoplasmic antibody (ANCA)

30. What is the most common infectious condition or agent associated with neuroretinitis?

    a. tuberculosis

    b. syphilis

    c. *Bartonella henselae*

    d. toxoplasmosis

31. What is the most common ocular manifestation of stage 3 Lyme disease?

    a. keratitis

    b. anterior uveitis

    c. intermediate uveitis

    d. panuveitis

32. A patient with uveitis and strongly positive rapid plasma regain (RPR) and fluorescent treponemal antibody absorption (FTA-ABS) tests has a history of resolved penile chancre, and recently developed a rash on his palms. What is the most likely diagnosis?

   a. primary syphilis

   b. false-positive FTA-ABS result

   c. secondary syphilis

   d. tertiary syphilis

33. When submitting a vitreous biopsy specimen to rule out intraocular lymphoma, the most important factor that will ensure the highest chance of obtaining reliable information is

   a. preoperative magnetic resonance imaging (MRI) to determine if central nervous system (CNS) lesions exist

   b. preoperative consultation with the ophthalmic pathologist

   c. obtaining a large enough specimen to allow vitreous cytokine analyses

   d. performance of polymerase chain reaction (PCR) studies to determine heavy chain rearrangement

34. Which of the following is a common presentation of CNS/intraocular lymphoma?

   a. weight loss and fever

   b. decreased vision and floaters

   c. pain radiating to jaw or forehead

   d. enlarged blind spot

35. Which of the following patients is the most likely to have primary CNS/intraocular lymphoma?

   a. a 40-year-old man with cotton-wool spots and hard exudates

   b. a 59-year-old man with hemorrhagic retinitis and retinal vasculitis

   c. a 65-year-old woman with dense vitritis, subretinal infiltrates, and mental confusion

   d. a 29-year-old woman with pars plana exudates and retinal vasculitis

36. An individual infected with the human immunodeficiency virus (HIV) has a necrotizing retinitis. Which of the following tests would be most helpful in making the diagnosis?

   a. blood and urine cultures for herpes viruses, including CMV

   b. vitreous biopsy for polymerase chain reaction evaluation, cultures, and cytologic testing

   c. purified protein derivative testing for tuberculosis

   d. serologic testing for herpes viruses, including CMV

37. What is the most common intraocular infection in patients with AIDS?

   a. acute retinal necrosis

   b. toxoplasmosis

   c. candidiasis

   d. CMV retinitis

38. What test may suggest a specific surgical approach to persistent macular edema in an eye with a long-standing (several years' duration) intermediate uveitis that has no active inflammation under treatment with immunosuppressive agents?

    a. fluorescein angiography

    b. MRI of the head and orbit

    c. optical coherence tomography (OCT)

    d. Lyme titers

Answer Sheet for Section 9
Study Questions

Question	Answer		Question	Answer
1	a b c d		20	a b c d
2	a b c d		21	a b c d
3	a b c d		22	a b c d
4	a b c d		23	a b c d
5	a b c d		24	a b c d
6	a b c d		25	a b c d
7	a b c d		26	a b c d
8	a b c d		27	a b c d
9	a b c d		28	a b c d
10	a b c d		29	a b c d
11	a b c d		30	a b c d
12	a b c d		31	a b c d
13	a b c d		32	a b c d
14	a b c d		33	a b c d
15	a b c d		34	a b c d
16	a b c d		35	a b c d
17	a b c d		36	a b c d
18	a b c d		37	a b c d
19	a b c d		38	a b c d

Answers

1. **c.** Lipopolysaccharide, also known as endotoxin, is a component of the cell walls of gram-negative bacteria. It is composed of lipid A, O polysaccharide, and core oligosaccharide. Recognition of LPS by cells of the innate and adaptive immune system leads to up-regulation of immune effector genes including interleukin-1, interleukin-6, tumor necrosis factor, and chemokines. LPS can also directly affect vascular permeability and can cause degranulation of granuolcytes. LPS activity functions through the innate immune system, and does not induce antigen-specific effects per se.

2. **b.** In phacolytic glaucoma, soluble lens proteins leak through the intact capsule, and appear to serve as chemokines for monocytic cells. Macrophages engulfing this lens protein become swollen and may block normal aqueous outflow, leading to acute ocular hypertension and, potentially, glaucoma. This is in contrast to other forms of lens-induced uveitis, which typically feature zonal granulomatous inflammation.

3. **a.** Antigen-specific Th1 T cells have been implicated in VKH syndrome, and more recently Th17 cells were also shown to possibly play a role. Th2 T cells are found in parasitic infections, including toxocariasis. Mucous membrane pemphigoid is thought to result from antigen-antibody deposition and complement activation in the basement membrane of mucous membranes including the conjunctiva; some forms of vasculitis may have similar mechanisms. Polymorphonuclear cells may be found in acute anterior chamber inflammation, especially in infectious diseases such as endophthalmitis.

4. **d.** *Toxocara canis* is a parasite typically carried by dogs. Ocular involvement occurs following visceral larval migrans and lodging of the larvae in the choroid. Like many parasites, *T canis* induces a strong Th2-mediated response typified by eosinophil and macrophage infiltration, immunoglobulin E production, and granuloma formation.

5. **c.** ACAID is thought to be a major mechanism contributing to immune privilege in the anterior chamber of the eye. Injection of antigen into the anterior chamber results in normal B-cell and antibody-mediated responses but a specific loss of delayed-type hypersensitivity responses. ACAID is thought to result from aberrant activation of macrophages in the anterior chamber due to the presence of TGF-β_2. Antigen presented in the spleen then induces a tolerogenic T-cell response rather than inducing delayed-type sensitivity.

6. **b.** Corneal allografts enjoy a 90% or greater success rate and uniquely can be transplanted without histocompatability matching. The presence of Fas ligand on the donor graft is thought to lead to apoptosis of immune effector cells in the anterior chamber, protecting the graft from rejection. Corneal vascularization, the presence of donor-derived antigen-presenting cells, and increased expression of MHC genes by donor stroma all increase the likelihood of T-cell mediated graft rejection.

7. **c.** Each of these pairs represents a relatively strong association between a specific HLA allele and disease. HLA-B51 has the weakest risk conferral of this group, with an RR for Behçet disease of 4–6. HLA-B27 is strongly associated with reactive arthritis (RR = approximately 60). Both birdshot retinochoroidopathy and TINU syndrome have among the strongest HLA associations of any known disease: HLA-A29 confers an RR of approximately 150 for birdshot disease, and HLA-DRB1*0102 an RR of about 167 for TINU syndrome. It is important to remember, however, that the HLA association for TINU syndrome was based only on 1 small cohort and the RR is therefore just an estimate. Even

the risks for well-established entities such as birdshot retinochoroidopathy are estimates that vary in different cohorts. An important question is whether the HLA associations have sufficient negative or positive predictive value to be useful clinically. It does appear that HLA-A29 has sufficient negative predictive value to suggest that birdshot retinochoroidopathy is less likely than an alternative diagnosis if the patient is HLA-A29 negative, but in itself HLA-A29–negative status does not rule out birdshot disease. It is possible that the negative predictive value of the HLA subtype associated with TINU syndrome is sufficiently strong to suggest that if it is not present the diagnosis may be questioned, but there are not sufficient data to verify that in this rare disease.

8. **d.** The main potential toxicities of cyclosporine are systemic hypertension and nephrotoxicity. Additional side effects include paresthesia, gastrointestinal upset, fatigue, hypertrichosis, and gingival hyperplasia. Blood pressure measurement, assessment of serum creatinine levels, and complete blood counts are performed monthly to monitor patients on cyclosporine.

9. **a.** Several studies have shown that systemic NSAIDs may be efficacious in the treatment of chronic iridocyclitis (eg, juvenile idiopathic arthritis–associated iridocyclitis) and possibly CME; they may allow the practitioner to maintain the patient on a lower dose of topical corticosteroids. Systemic NSAIDs may be used to treat nonnecrotizing, noninfectious scleritis. Potential complications of prolonged systemic NSAID use include myocardial infarction, hypertension, and stroke (especially with selective COX-2 inhibitors); gastric ulceration; gastrointestinal bleeding; nephrotoxicity; and hepatotoxicity. COX-2 inhibitors should only be used with caution and after obtaining detailed informed consent, if no alternative agents are effective.

10. **c.** Anterior uveitis is the most common morphologic form of uveitis worldwide. Men and women appear to be equally affected. In the epidemiologic study from northern California by Gritz and Wong, the pediatric age group had the lowest incidence and prevalence and the group older than age 65 had the highest incidence and prevalence.

11. **d.** Methotrexate, a folic acid analogue and inhibitor of dihydrofolate reductase, inhibits DNA replication, but its anti-inflammatory effects result from extracellular release of adenosine.

12. **c.** Laser trabeculoplasty in any form (argon, diode, elective) is not indicated in patients with uveitis and glaucoma. It is ineffective, may exacerbate intraocular inflammation, and may cause severe intraocular pressure elevation. Trabeculectomy, use of a glaucoma implant (aqueous drainage device), and trabeculodialysis have all been successfully used in the surgical management of these patients.

13. **a.** The initial management of patients with uveitis and iris bombé should include laser iridotomy or surgical iridectomy if the laser procedure is difficult (eg, due to iris–corneal touch or corneal edema), glaucoma medications as needed, and intensive application of topical corticosteroids. Surgical iridectomy may also become necessary if a patent laser iridotomy cannot be successfully maintained. A trabeculectomy or glaucoma implant may later become necessary if there is a patent laser iridotomy and medically uncontrolled intraocular pressure. Laser trabeculoplasty is of no benefit in uveitic angle closure or iris bombé.

14. **c.** Meticulous control of intraocular inflammation with topical, regional, intraocular, and systemic corticosteroids and, if necessary, systemic immunomodulatory agents is best for long-term eradication of uveitic CME. Other ancillary agents may be used when CME

persists despite control of all visible active inflammation or for short-term management of CME. The severity of CME can but does not necessarily correspond to the level of inflammatory disease activity, but it is often slow to respond and clear and often remains even after visible active inflammation has resolved. Topical NSAIDs and acetazolamide provide marginal benefits in controlling CME in an eye that is actively inflamed. Intravitreal triamcinolone shows promise in eliminating CME, at least temporarily, and is under active investigation. The value of pars plana vitrectomy in the management of uveitic CME is controversial, although it may have some role in refractory cases.

15. **c.** Myelosuppression and hemorrhagic cystitis are the most common side effects of cyclophosphamide treatment; the latter is more common when the drug is administered orally. Complete blood count and urinalysis are performed weekly to monthly. Patients must be encouraged to drink more than 2 liters of fluid per day while on this regimen. Microscopic hematuria is a warning to increase hydration, while gross hematuria warrants discontinuation of therapy. If white cell counts fall below 2500 cells/μL, cyclophosphamide should be discontinued until the counts recover. Other toxicities include teratogenicity, sterility, and reversible alopecia. Opportunistic infections such as *Pneumocystis* pneumonia occur more commonly in patients who are receiving cyclophosphamide; trimethoprim-sulfamethoxazole prophylaxis is recommended.

16. **b.** The duration of the anti-inflammatory efficacy of the fluocinolone implant is about 3 years. The implant is effective for a mean of 38 months before first recurrence. At that point, implantation of another fluocinolone implant or reinstitution of systemic immunomodulatory therapy must be considered if durable remission has not been achieved.

17. **d.** While congestive heart failure, malignancy, and lupuslike syndrome are all concerns, the specific controversy in treating intermediate uveitis, especially in the patient described, is demyelinating disease. Because women in this age group have a greater likelihood of developing multiple sclerosis, and intermediate uveitis is associated with multiple sclerosis in up to 15% of cases, demyelinating disease is a specific concern in the choice of TNF inhibitor therapy in this instance. Multiple sclerosis may present years after the onset of the intermediate uveitis, so even if there was no evidence of demyelinating disease at onset, that could change while the patient is under therapy.

18. **d.** Chronic postoperative bacterial endophthalmitis is most commonly due to *Propionibacterium acnes.* Many other bacteria and fungi, such as *Staphylococcus epidermidis* and *Corynebacterium* species, also cause similar chronic endophthalmitis. *P acnes,* a commensal, anaerobic, gram-positive, pleomorphic rod, is found on the eyelid skin and conjunctiva of healthy patients.

19. **b.** Lupus retinopathy is considered an important marker of systemic disease activity, and consists of cotton-wool spots with or without intraretinal hemorrhages occurring independently of hypertension; it is thought to be due to the underlying microangiopathy of the disease. Severe retinal vascular occlusive disease (both arterial and venous thromboses) may result in retinal nonperfusion ischemia, secondary retinal neovascularization, and vitreous hemorrhage and appears to be associated with central nervous system lupus disease and the presence of antiphospholipid antibodies. Lupus choroidopathy, characterized by serous elevation of the neurosensory retina, pigment epithelium, or both; choroidal infarction; and choroidal neovascularization may be observed in patients with severe systemic vascular disease due to either hypertension from lupus nephritis or systemic vasculitis. Uveitis per se is distinctly uncommon in patients with lupus erythematosus.

20. **b.** This patient presents with the characteristic lesion of ocular toxoplasmosis: focal retinochoroiditis with overlying vitreous inflammation adjacent to a pigmented chorioretinal scar. Moreover, the patient is from Brazil, an area where toxoplasmosis is endemic. The presence of significantly reduced visual acuity and vitritis are indications for treatment. While numerous agents have been used to treat toxoplasmosis, there is no single drug or combination that should be applied categorically to every patient, nor is there consensus as to the most effective regimen. The classic regimen for the treatment of ocular toxoplasmosis consists of "triple therapy" with pyrimethamine, sulfadiazine, and prednisone; because sulfonamides and pyrimethamine inhibit folic acid metabolism, folinic acid is added to try to prevent the decreases in white blood cells and platelets that may result from treatment. Some clinicians advocate adding clindamycin to this regimen as "quadruple" therapy. Alternative regimens include the use of trimethoprim-sulfamethoxazole, azithromycin alone or in combination with pyrimethamine, and atovaquone. Intravitreal clindamycin has been used successfully in patients in whom systemic therapy is either undesirable or not tolerated. Oral corticosteroids are frequently added after 24–48 hours of antimicrobial therapy to treat the inflammatory component of the disease, but are never used as monotherapy. Similarly, periocular injections of steroids are contraindicated in patients with ocular toxoplasmosis. Intravenous acyclovir is the gold standard for the treatment of herpetic necrotizing retinitis, and amphotericin B is used in the treatment of fungal endophthalmitis, particularly that caused by *Aspergillus* organisms.

21. **b.** Old, scarred lesions may be present in the newly diagnosed eye. Funduscopic findings in patients with serpiginous choroidopathy include characteristic gray-white lesions at the level of the retinal pigment epithelium (RPE) projecting in a pseudopodial manner from the optic nerve in the posterior fundus. Less commonly, macular or peripheral lesions may present without peripapillary involvement. Typically, disease activity is confined to the leading edge of the advancing lesion; it may be associated with shallow subretinal fluid. Occasionally, vascular sheathing has been reported along with RPE detachment and disc neovascularization. Significant vitritis is distinctly uncommon. Late findings include atrophy of the choriocapillaris, RPE, and retina, with extensive RPE hyperpigmentation and subretinal fibrosis; choroidal neovascularization occurs in some patients at the border of the old scar.

22. **b.** Acute retinal necrosis presents with a classic triad of retinal arteriolitis, vitritis, and multifocal yellow-white peripheral retinitis. Early in the course of the disease, the peripheral retinal lesions are discontinuous and have a scalloped edge that appears to arise in the retina. Within days, they coalesce to form a confluent 360° area of peripheral retinitis that progresses rapidly towards the posterior pole, leaving full-thickness retinal necrosis in its wake.

23. **d.** Fluorescein angiography in birdshot retinochoroidopathy reveals inconsistent findings depending on the age of the lesions and the phase of the study. Early birdshot lesions may show initial hypofluorescence with subtle late staining. However, in general, fluorescein angiography does not typically highlight the birdshot lesions themselves, but rather is useful in identifying more subtle types of active inflammation such as retinal vasculitis, CME, and optic nerve head leakage. In contrast, in patients with APMPPE it shows characteristic early blockage with late staining of the lesions, and in those with PIC it reveals early hyperfluorescence with late staining of the lesions. In patients with serpiginous choroiditis, fluorescein angiography reveals blockage of the choroidal flush in the early stage of the study and staining of the active edge of the lesion in the later stage of the angiogram. Early

hyperfluorescence with late leakage is indicative of choroidal neovascular membranes, which are seen frequently in patients with PIC and less often in those with serpiginous choroiditis and birdshot retinochoroidopathy.

24. **d.** VKH syndrome has been divided into four stages: prodromal, acute uveitic, convalescent, and chronic recurrent; histologic findings vary depending upon the stage of the disease. During the acute uveitic stage, there is a diffuse, nonnecrotizing, granulomatous inflammation (virtually identical to that seen in sympathetic ophthalmia) consisting of lymphocytes and macrophages mixed with epithelioid and multinucleate giant cells with preservation of the choriocapillaris. The convalescent stage is characterized by nongranulomatous inflammation with uveal infiltration of lymphocytes and plasma cells and the absence of epithelioid histiocytes. The number of choroidal melanocytes decreases with the loss of melanin and pigment, corresponding to the "sunset glow" fundus seen clinically. In addition, one sees numerous atrophic depigmented lesions in the peripheral retina erroneously thought to be Dalen-Fuchs nodules. The chronic recurrent stage reveals granulomatous choroiditis with damage to the choriocapillaris.

25. **d.** The definitive diagnosis of sarcoidosis relies on histologic confirmation of noncaseating granulomata. A chest radiograph is probably the best single screening test for sarcoidosis, as it reveals abnormal results in approximately 90% of the patients with active disease. Thin-cut spiral computed tomographic (CT) imaging is a more sensitive imaging modality and may be particularly valuable in the patient with a normal-appearing chest radiograph in whom there remains a high clinical suspicion for disease. In such cases, parenchymal, mediastinal, and hilar structures with distinctive CT patterns highly suggestive for sarcoidosis may lead to the diagnosis. Although serum ACE and lysozyme levels may be abnormally elevated, neither is diagnostic or specific.

26. **c.** The most common ocular manifestation of West Nile virus infection is a characteristic multifocal chorioretinitis with nongranulomatous anterior uveitis and vitreous cellular inflammation. The chorioretinal lesions vary in size and number and are distributed throughout the midperiphery, frequently in linear arrays following the course of retinal nerve fibers. Active chorioretinal lesions appear whitish to yellow, are flat and deep, and evolve with varying degrees of pigmentation and atrophy, not infrequently becoming targetoid in appearance. West Nile virus is maintained in an enzootic cycle mainly involving the *Culex* genus of mosquitoes and birds. Although birds are the natural host of the virus, it is most often transmitted from them to humans and other vertebrates through the bite of an infected mosquito. Peak disease onset occurs in late summer, but the disease can happen anytime between July and December. There is currently no proven treatment for West Nile virus infection; in patients with severe disease therapy is supportive.

27. **a.** Reactive arthritis syndrome is defined as urethritis, polyarthritis, and conjunctival inflammation.

28. **a.** Glaucomatocyclitic crisis has been associated with cytomegalovirus (CMV) infection and the virus has been isolated from the eyes of patients with this disease. Topical corticosteroids and aqueous suppressants are utilized to treat the acute anterior uveitis and intraocular pressure elevation, respectively, with which these patients present. Presenting intraocular pressure may be very high (>40 mm Hg) and should be treated. The inflammation responds readily to topical corticosteroids.

29. **a.** Whereas false-positive and false-negative results may occur with treponemal-specific serologic tests, syphilis is the great imitator and screening syphilis serologies have an

unacceptably high false-negative rate in patients with uveitis. ANA and RF testing rarely contribute to uncovering the cause of uveitis in the absence of scleritis, keratitis, or vasculitis, and then rarely suggest specific therapy. ANCA testing is most important when Wegener granulomatosis is suspected (although patients with other vasculitides may test positive for ANCA), but again is rarely useful in a patient with isolated uveitis. Therapy is more directed in a patient with Wegener granulomatosis, but treatment for this entity is not curative in the sense that appropriate antibiotic treatment would be for an infectious disease such as syphilis.

30. **c.** While all of these conditions or agents may be associated with neuroretinitis, *Bartonella henselae* is the most common cause (of course, *B henselae* may not be the cause of neuroretinitis for an individual from an area in which a specific disease such as tuberculosis is endemic). *B henselae* is a gram-negative rod that causes the anthropozoonosis cat-scratch disease (CSD); another *Bartonella* species *(Bartonella quintana)* is the causative agent in trench fever. Systemic antibiotic treatment for CSD can be helpful in curtailing the course of systemic disease but may not be needed, as the illness can be self limiting. The most common uveitic manifestation of CSD is focal choroiditis, which can look exactly like *Toxoplasma* retinochoroiditis.

31. **a.** Although Lyme disease can be associated with neuro-ophthalmic abnormalities as well as any of the forms of uveitis (anterior, intermediate, and panuveitis) in the answers, and is most often thought of in the context of intermediate uveitis, keratitis that responds to topical corticosteroids is the most common form of ocular manifestation in stage 3 Lyme disease.

32. **c.** Uveitis may be seen in any stage of syphilis but most commonly occurs in the secondary and tertiary stages of the disease. Thus, laboratory evaluation for syphilis in patients with uveitis should use treponemal-specific tests such as FTA-ABS or the microhemagglutination assay for *Treponema pallidum* antibodies (MHA-TP) rather than nontreponemal screening tests such as the VDRL or RPR evaluations. A chancre is seen at the site of inoculation in primary syphilis. In secondary syphilis a rash may be seen on the palms. This rash may allow transfer of the spirochete and should not be touched. Tertiary or latent syphilis is manifested by gummatous inflammation of the viscera and neurosyphilis.

33. **b.** Vitrectomy specimens from suspected cases of intraocular lymphoma must be processed promptly by an experienced ophthalmic pathologist in order to preserve the cytology for examination. Prolonged time between obtaining a specimen and its processing by the pathologist increases the degeneration of the specimen and greatly reduces its value for obtaining a diagnosis. It is thus important that the surgeon clearly communicate to the pathologist the clinical suspicion of lymphoma and indicate that a specimen will be submitted so that arrangements can be made for timely evaluation. In addition, depending on the clinical scenario, the pathologist may want special fixatives to be used to allow special studies, such as flow cytometry, in addition to cytologic examination.

34. **b.** Nonspecific symptoms are most common in intraocular lymphoma and relate to the presence of vitreous cells and debris. Patients with lymphoma may have extraocular symptoms, but fever is uncommon. Pain radiating to the jaw or forehead is more consistent with giant cell arteritis. An enlarged blind spot is also not a typical finding in intraocular lymphoma.

35. **c.** Vitritis, subretinal (especially sub-RPE) infiltrates, and CNS manifestations such as confusion are hallmarks of primary CNS lymphoma. This disease typically occurs in older

individuals. A 40-year-old person with cotton-wool spots and exudates would more likely have diabetic retinopathy; a hemorrhagic retinitis and retinal vasculitis could be infectious or autoimmune, but is less likely to be malignant; and a 29-year-old patient with pars plana exudates likely has pars planitis.

36. **b.** A necrotizing retinitis in any immunocompromised person should be presumed infectious until proven otherwise. Viral or parasitic (eg, *Toxoplasma canis*) agents are most likely, but any infectious pathogen can be responsible. Blood and urine cultures may show the presence of virus but do not provide information about the intraocular process. These tests might be useful in the negative; ie, a negative result would argue against CMV as the cause, but a positive result does not prove that it is the cause. In addition, culturing samples is slow. Tuberculosis skin testing is unreliable in patients with AIDS due to anergy. Similar to the case with blood and urine cultures, serologic evidence of herpes is not proof of intraocular infection. A direct sample from intraocular fluid is the most specific way to determine the cause of an infectious necrotizing retinitis.

37. **d.** Cytomegalovirus retinitis remains the most common intraocular infection in patients with AIDS, despite a decline in the number of new AIDS cases.

38. **c.** OCT can show vitreoretinal traction, which may require vitreoretinal surgery. Fluorescein angiography may suggest the same (as of course may clinical examination), but this possibility is best evaluated by OCT. Fluorescein angiography or OCT may suggest a subretinal neovascular membrane, but that would be exceedingly rare in a patient with intermediate uveitis (as opposed to chorioretinopathy). MRI may be useful if demyelinating disease is suspected, but that would not result in macular edema in and of itself. Measurement of Lyme titers may be appropriate, but if the inflammation is currently controlled even a positive test result would not suggest a surgical treatment for the macular edema, and it is not clear that macular edema in late Lyme disease would respond to antibiotics (although they should be given to prevent possible systemic complications).

Index

(*f* = figure; *t* = table)

347

Cytomegalovirus, 204–208
congenital infection caused by, 204, 205, 206
Fuchs heterochromic iridocyclitis/uveitis associated with, 134
in HIV infection/AIDS, 204, 205, 206, 306–307
retinitis caused by, 204–207, 205f, 206f, 306–307
acute retinal necrosis, 202
congenital (cytomegalic inclusion disease), 204, 205, 206
foscarnet for, 207
ganciclovir for, 207
in HIV infection/AIDS, 204, 205, 206, 306–307
immune recovery uveitis and, 306
retinal detachment and, 302, 307
Cytotoxic hypersensitivity (type II) reaction, 44, 44t. See also Cytotoxic T lymphocytes
Cytotoxic T lymphocytes, 42f, 43, 51, 53f
in viral conjunctivitis, 60
Cytotoxicity, antibody-dependent, 51–55, 54f
Cytoxan. See Cyclophosphamide

Daclizumab, for uveitis, 108t, 115
Dalen-Fuchs nodules/spots
in sympathetic ophthalmia, 178, 179, 180
in Vogt-Koyanagi-Harada (VKH) syndrome, 184, 186f
Daraprim. See Pyrimethamine
DCs. See Dendritic cells
Delayed hypersensitivity (type IV) reaction, 42–43, 42f, 44, 44t, 48–51, 49f, 50t
response to poison ivy as, 35
in sympathetic ophthalmia, 52–53
in Toxocara granuloma, 52
tuberculin form of, 35
Delayed hypersensitivity (DH) T lymphocytes, 42–43, 42f, 48–51, 49f, 50t
Dendritic cells, 11–12
Dengue fever, 219–220
Depo-Medrol. See Methylprednisolone
Depot injections, corticosteroid
for pars planitis, 137
for uveitis, 102
Dexamethasone, for uveitis, 101t, 106
cystoid macular edema and, 301
Dexamethasone implant, for uveitis, 106
DH. See Delayed hypersensitivity (type IV) reaction
Diethylcarbamazine
uveitis caused by, 128
Diffuse unilateral subacute neuroretinitis (DUSN), 239–241, 240f, 241f
Diffuse uveitis. See Panuveitis
Difluprednate, for uveitis, 100, 101t
Discoid systemic lupus erythematosus, 140, 141t
Dog hookworm (Ancylostoma caninum), diffuse unilateral subacute neuroretinitis caused by, 239
Domains, immunoglobulin, 45f, 46
Donor cornea, rejection of, 63, 64, 64f, 65
Doppler imaging, in ocular ischemic syndrome, 288
Doxycycline
for leptospirosis, 256
for Lyme disease, 253t
for onchocerciasis, 242
Drug-induced uveitis, 128
Drug resistance, in tuberculosis, 261
Dry-eye syndrome, sarcoidosis and, 174
DUSN. See Diffuse unilateral subacute neuroretinitis

E-selectin, in neutrophil rolling, 18
Eales disease, 258, 260f

Early latent syphilis, 244, 248t
EAU. See Experimental uveitis, autoimmune
EBV. See Epstein-Barr virus
Effector blockade, 62
Effector cells, 42–43, 42f
basophils and mast cells as, 10
dendritic cells and Langerhans cells as, 11–12
eosinophils as, 10
locations of, 58t
lymphocytes as, 12, 42–43, 42f, 48–51, 49f, 50t, 52–53, 53f
monocytes and macrophages as, 11, 20
neutrophils as, 9, 17
Effector phase of immune response arc, 33–36, 36f, 42–43, 42f
adaptive immunity and, 42–43, 42f, 44–55, 44t
in anterior chamber–associated immune deviation, 62
antibody-mediated, 45–48, 45f, 47t, 48
cells in. See Effector cells
combined antibody and cellular, 51–55, 54f
innate immunity and, 14–23, 14t, 23t
lymphocyte-mediated, 42–43, 42f, 48–51, 49f, 50t, 52–53, 53f
mediator systems and, 23–31, 23t
response to poison ivy and, 34, 35
response to tuberculosis and, 35
in viral conjunctivitis, 60–61
Efferent lymphatic channels, 33, 34
Eicosanoids, 25, 25–27, 26f
EIU. See Experimental uveitis, immune
Electrophysiologic testing, in inflammatory chorioretinopathies, 150t
Electroretinogram
in birdshot retinochoroidopathy, 150t, 153
in multiple evanescent white dot syndrome, 168
in uveitis, 95
Elevated intraocular pressure
corticosteroids causing, uveitis and, 103, 105, 295, 297
in glaucoma
phacolytic glaucoma and, 126
uveitis and, 294, 295
in uveitis, 294, 295
corticosteroid-induced, 103, 105, 295, 297
herpetic infection and, 199
ELISA. See Enzyme-linked immunosorbent assay
Elschnig spots, in polyarteritis nodosa/microscopic polyangiitis, 143
Encephalitis, herpes, acute retinal necrosis and, 202
Endarterectomy, carotid, for ocular ischemic syndrome, 288
Endemic Kaposi sarcoma, 312
Endocrine action, of cytokines, 27
Endogenous endophthalmitis, 269, 271–280. See also Endophthalmitis
Endophthalmitis, 269–280
bacterial
endogenous, 271–273, 272f
postoperative, 269–270, 270f
toxins affecting severity of, 16
endogenous, 269, 271–280
Aspergillus causing, 273–274, 276–278, 277f
bacterial, 271–273, 272f
Candida causing, 273–274, 274–276, 275f
in coccidioidomycosis, 273–274, 279–280, 279f
in cryptococcosis, 278–279
fungal, 273–280, 273f, 275f, 277f, 279f
fungal
endogenous, 273–280, 273f, 275f, 277f, 279f
postoperative, 270